Practical Diagnosis

HEMATOLOGIC DISEASE

William C. Maslow, MD
Ernest Beutler, MD
Carol A. Bell, MD
Cecil Hougie, MD
Carl R. Kjeldsberg, MD

HM MD Houghton Mifflin Professional Publishers
Two Park Street, Boston, Massachusetts

Library of Congress Cataloging in Publication Data

Hematologic disease.
    (Practical diagnosis)
    Includes index.
    1. Blood—Diseases—Diagnosis.   I.   Maslow,
William C.   II.   Series.
RC633.H42   616.1'5   79-19373
ISBN 0-89289-203-X

ISBN 0-89289-203-X

LCCCN 79-19373

AUTHORS

William C. Maslow, MD
Chairman, Division of Clinical Pathology
Director of Clinical Laboratories
City of Hope National Medical Center
Duarte, California

Ernest Beutler, MD
Chairman, Department of Clinical Research
Scripts Clinic and Research Foundation
La Jolla, California

Carol A. Bell, MD
Clinical Professor of Pathology
University of California, Irvine
Director, Clinical Laboratories
Dr. David M. Brotman Memorial Hospital
Culver City, California

Cecil Hougie, MD
Professor of Pathology
University of California, San Diego
School of Medicine
La Jolla, California

Carl R. Kjeldsberg, MD
Associate Professor of Pathology
University of Utah, College of Medicine
Chief, Laboratory Service
Veterans Administration Hospital
Salt Lake City, Utah

CONTENTS

Preface

PREFACE

The diagnosis of hematologic disorders has become a complex (and often confusing) multidisciplinary endeavor. Blood counts and conventional morphologic studies have been augmented by diagnostic tools from the fields of biochemistry, immunology, immunohematology, and genetics and by the application of radioisotope tracers to laboratory testing. This situation presents the clinician with problems as well as solutions. When confronted with the patient who has a blood disorder, he or she now has the often difficult task of choosing the most useful and practical procedures from a growing array of laboratory tests. The related tasks of interpreting test results and integrating these results with the clinical findings are no less problematic. Nevertheless, we have not yet found a concise source of guidelines to the selection, use, and interpretation of laboratory tests that at the same time correlates the laboratory and clinical pictures. For this reason, Drs. Beutler, Bell, Hougie, Kjeldsberg, and I have sought to provide the clinician with such a source.

During the development of this handbook, we have continually struggled to make it a truly useful source of problem-solving information. We have, in fact, given considerable thought to our format in order to make this information as logical, succinct, and accessible as possible. Each chapter dealing with a disease or a category of disease begins with a discussion of the salient pathogenetic and clinical considerations. The chapter then outlines the laboratory approach to diagnosis, providing explicit guidelines to the primary and ancillary laboratory tests. These guidelines are clearly formatted under the subheadings *Purpose, Principle, Procedure, Specimen, Interpretation,* and *Notes and Precautions.* In addition, the morphologic features of the blood and bone marrow are discussed whenever appropriate, and we have provided references that guide the reader to more detailed discussions of procedures and their clinical utility.

Finally, as a corollary to our recommendations to clinicians, this handbook also offers laboratorians a perspective as to their role in the overall diagnostic effort and therapeutic decisions. It is our hope that both groups will find this handbook of value in solving the clinical and laboratory problems that confront them.

William C. Maslow, MD

PART A / DISORDERS OF THE ERYTHROCYTES

chapter 1

The Diagnosis of Anemia

The primary function of the erythrocyte is to provide a mode of transport for hemoglobin to deliver oxygen to the tissues. The physiologic consequences of anemia result from the associated total reduction of oxygen delivery capacity by the blood. Conceptually, therefore, anemia is correctly defined as a reduction in the total quantity of red cells or hemoglobin in the circulation; this can be measured most accurately as a reduction in red cell mass. Because this reduction (for whatever reason) generally results in a compensatory expansion of plasma volume, measurements of concentration of red cells or of hemoglobin very nearly reflect red cell mass. Exceptions include factitious anemia caused by increased plasma volume, as in pregnancy; masked anemia caused by decreased plasma volume, as in dehydration; and absence of anemia during the early period after hemorrhage before compensatory expansion in plasma volume.

CLINICAL FINDINGS

Anemia itself is not a diagnosis but merely a sign of disease. The two most common causes are iron deficiency resulting from excessive menstrual bleeding and chronic disease states. In the first instance, since women are often not aware of excessive bleeding, a detailed menstrual history may be required. In chronic disease, anemia is usually mild; however, when it is unexpectedly severe, complications such as bleeding or, in the case of malignancy,

3

marrow infiltration should be considered (see Chapter 2). In both iron deficiency and chronic disease, the etiologic diagnosis can usually be made by careful clinical evaluation using routine hematologic tests. In all obscure cases of anemia, an adequate history and physical examination are crucial for an intelligent and direct approach to diagnosis (Tables 1-1 and 1-2).

EXAMINATION OF THE BLOOD

The basic hematologic tests for evaluation of anemia include (a) red cell measurements, including hemoglobin concentration (Hb), hematocrit (HCT), red cell count with an electronic counter, and red cell indices; (b) leukocyte count; (c) reticulocyte count; (d) examination of stained blood smear, including leukocyte differential count and platelet count estimate; and (e) platelet count, particularly with abnormal platelet count estimate. Ancillary tests that are helpful in the initial laboratory evaluation of anemia are tests for serum bilirubin and serum creatinine.

Blood Cell Measurements

The routine use of automated counting equipment in the laboratory has greatly increased the precision and efficiency of counting blood cells (1, 2). The error ($\pm$ 2 coefficients of variations, 95% confidence limits) of counting is 3%–4% with electronic counters, while errors with manual counting frequently range from 16%–25%. This increased precision is especially important for the red cell count, which can now be used with confidence for calculating the mean corpuscular volume (MCV) and mean corpuscular hemoglobin (MCH). Hemoglobin concentration and hematocrit are also measured in multiple parameter, automated blood-counting machines. The reproducibility of these measurements by manual procedures is also excellent, however; the error of $\pm$ 2% is comparable to the precision obtained with automated methods. Reliable procedures for measuring hemoglobin concentration are based on the measurement of the derivative cyanmethemoglobin by its absorbance at

4

Table 1-1. **Patient History in Diagnosis of Anemia**

Considerations	Related Concerns
Age of onset	History of anemia, jaundice, gall bladder disease
Duration of illness	Results of last medical examination
	Last known normal blood count
	Last time accepted or rejected as blood donor
	Prior prescriptions of hematinics (iron, folate, B_{12}?)
Suddenness and severity of anemia; symptoms of respiratory and circulatory decompensation	Dyspnea on exertion
	Palpitation
	Dizziness
	Faintness on arising from sitting or lying position
	Marked fatigue; may be only symptom with insidious onset
Presence of chronic blood loss	Excessive menstrual bleeding, frequent pregnancy
	Black stools, bloody stools
	Gastrointestinal symptoms
Hemolytic episodes	Episodes of weakness with slight icterus and dark urine
Toxic exposure	Occupation, hobbies, drugs
Dietary history	Milk feeding without supplements for long period in infants—iron deficiency
	Chronic alcoholism, dietary idiosyncrasy; folate deficiency in the elderly
Family history	History of anemia, splenomegaly, splenectomy; early gall bladder disease in parents, siblings, or offspring

Table 1-2. **Physical Examination in Diagnosis of Anemia**

Anatomic Location	Finding	Disease
Skin and mucous membrane	Pallor	
	Scleral icterus	Hemolytic anemia
	Smooth tongue	Pernicious anemia, severe iron deficiency
	Petechiae	Associated thrombocytopenia, e.g., leukemia
Lymph nodes	Lymphadenopathy	Infectious mononucleosis, leukemia, lymphoma
Heart	Cardiac dilatation, tachycardia, loud murmur	Severe anemia
	Murmurs	Subacute bacterial endocarditis; anemia, usually mild
Abdomen	Spenomegaly	Infectious macronucleosis, leukemia, lymphoma, subacute bacterial endocarditis
	Massive splenomegaly	Chronic granulocytic leukemia, myelofibrosis with myeloid metaplasia
	Hepatosplenomegaly with ascites	Liver disease
Central nervous system	Subacute combined degeneration of the spinal cord	Pernicious anemia
	Delayed Achilles tendon reflexes	Hypothyroidism

540 nm in a photometer. Both macro and micro methods for determination of hematocrit are satisfactory. The micro procedure is generally preferred because it requires a smaller amount of blood, shorter centrifugation time, and smaller, less expensive equipment.

Many clinicians prefer the hematocrit over other red cell measurements for monitoring a patient's course because of the speed and precision of the manual HCT determination. The hematocrit is a derived or indirect measurement in most of the automated blood-counting systems. In the Coulter Counter Model S,* for example, hematocrit is derived from the MCV and hemoglobin. Although HCT obtained in this manner provides reliable results, automated hemoglobin and red cell counts offer comparable precision.

Automated blood-counting machines, particularly those offering multiple parameters, are complex and require careful calibration, quality control, and maintenance, together with an awareness of the special circumstances that can result in erroneous results. Thus, with the Coulter Counter Model S, high white cell counts in the range of 35,000–50,000 mm^3 result in significant errors in the MCV and the derived hematocrit as well as in the hemoglobin. In the presence of large, bizarre platelets, machine platelet counts are spuriously low.

Peripheral Blood Smear

Examination of the blood smear by a physician who knows the patient clinically is a central part of the laboratory evaluation of anemia. When a blood smear is inspected as part of a routine examination, even highly proficient laboratory personnel may overlook abnormalities that are apparent to an examiner who is familiar with the clinical background. Red cells are examined for size and shape and for hemoglobin concentration, distribution, and staining properties. Although red cell indices provide useful information regarding morphology, they are measurements of mean red cell size

---

*Manufactured by Coulter Diagnostics, a division of Coulter Electronics, Inc., Hialeah, FL.

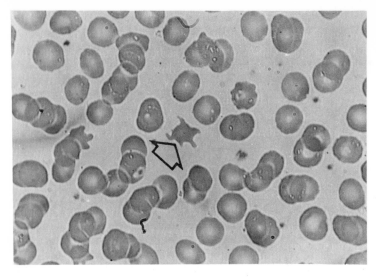

Figure 1-1. Acanthocyte (*arrow*).

and hemoglobin concentration. This information is inadequate when there is a mixed red cell population, as in the presence of prominent anisocytosis or poikilocytosis (i.e., abnormal variations in size or shape (Figures 1-1–1-8). The significance of various morphologic changes on routine smear with Wright's stain is shown in Table 1-3. Some red cell inclusions can be demonstrated only by supravital staining. These include reticulocytes, Heinz bodies, and hemoglobin H inclusions. Examination of a smear should always include a rough estimate of the number of platelets. On the average, the ratio of platelets to red cells is between 1:10–1:20.

Red Cell Indices

With the use of electronic counting of red cells, the application of standardized procedures for hemoglobin determination, and the use of the microhematocrit technique, red cell indices provide useful and reliable information for the morphologic classification of anemia. The indices are generally consistent with the findings on

Table 1-3. Changes in Red Cell Morphology

Red Cell	Description	Underlying Change	Disease States
Acanthocyte spur cell	Irregularly spiculated red cells with projections of varying length	Altered lipids in cell membrane	Abetalipoproteinemia, liver disease, postsplenectomy
Basophilic stippling	Punctate basophilic inclusions	Precipitated ribosomes	Course stippling—lead intoxication, thalassemia; diffuse stippling—a variety of anemia
Burr cell (echinocyte)	Red cells with short, evenly spaced spicules	May be associated with altered membrane lipids	Uremia, bleeding peptic ulcer, carcinoma, artifact in case of crenated red cells
Cabot's rings	Blue threadlike inclusion		Postsplenectomy, hemolytic anemia, megaloblastic anemia
Ovalocyte (elliptocyte)	Elliptically shaped cell		Hereditary elliptocytosis, minor degree may be seen in various anemias
Howell-Jolly bodies	Small, discrete dense inclusions, usually single	Nuclear remnant	Postsplenectomy, hemolytic anemia, megaloblastic anemia

9

Table 1-3. Changes in Red Cell Morphology (Continued)

Red Cell	Description	Underlying Change	Disease States
Hypochromic cell	Reduced central pallor	Diminished hemoglobin synthesis	Iron deficiency anemia, thalassemia, sideroblastic anemia
Leptocyte	Flat, waferlike, thin, hypochromic cell		Liver disease, thalassemia
Macrocyte	Red cells larger than normal (> 8.5 μm), well filled with hemoglobin	Young red cells; abnormal red cell maturation	Increased erythropoiesis, megaloblastic anemia
Microcyte	Red cells smaller than normal (< 7.0 μm)		See hypochromia
Pappenheimer bodies	Small, dense basophilic granules	Iron-containing body	Sideroblastic anemia
Polychromatophilia	Greyish or blue hue frequently seen with macrocytes	Ribosomal material	Reticulocytosis, reflects premature marrow release
Rouleaux	Red cell aggregates resembling stack of coins	Red cell clumping by circulating paraprotein	Paraproteinemia

Cell Type	Description	Mechanism	Associated Disorders
Schistocyte (helmet cell)	Distorted, fragmented cell	Mechanical distortion in microvasculature by fibrin strands, mechanical disruption by prosthetic heart valve	Microangiopathic hemolytic anemia (disseminated intravascular coagulation, thrombotic thrombocytopenic purpura) prosthetic heart valves, severe burns
Sickle cell	Bipolar, spiculated forms, shape of sickle	Molecular aggregation of HbS	Sickle cell disorders—SS, SC, S-thalassemia, SD disease, etc.
Spherocyte	Spherical cell, dense appearance, absent central pallor, usually decreased diameter	Decreased membrane redundancy	Hereditary spherocytosis, immunohemolytic anemia
Stomatocyte	Mouth-or cuplike deformity	Membrane defect with abnormal cation permeability	Hereditary stomatocytosis, liver disease
Target cell (codocyte)	Targetlike appearance, often hypochromic	Increased redundancy of cell membrane	Liver disease, postsplenectomy, thalassemia, HbC disease
Teardrop cell	Distorted, fragmented, drop-shaped cell		Myelofibrosis

11

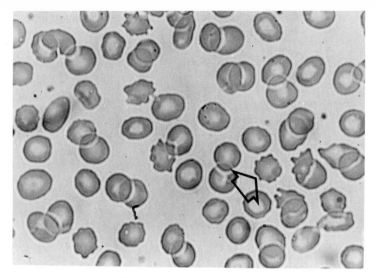

Figure 1-2. Burr cell (*arrow*).

examination of the blood smear. However, as was previously noted, they may be misleading in the presence of mixed red cell morphology since they represent mean values.

Calculations for red cell indices and their normal values are shown in Table 1-4. Mean corpuscular volume is a measure of red cell size and mean corpuscular hemoglobin concentration (MCHC) is a measure of hemoglobin concentration. Since MCH reflects both size and hemoglobin concentration, it is the least useful of the indices. A low MCV indicates microcytosis and a high MCV denotes macrocytosis. A low MCHC indicates hypochromia, and a low MCH means hypochromia, microcytosis, or both. A high MCH is always seen with a high MCV, reflecting the presence of macrocytosis. A high MCHC is seen only with prominent spherocytosis and reflects the decreased red cell volume associated with decreased redundancy of the cell membrane.

Table 1-4. Calculations of Red Cell Indices in the Adult and Normal Values

Index	Calculation	Normal Values
Mean corpuscular volume (MCV)	$MCV = \dfrac{HCT\ (\%)}{RBC\ (million/\mu l)} \times 10$	81–100 μm^3
Mean corpuscular hemoglobin concentration (MCHC)	$MCHC = \dfrac{Hb\ (g/dl)}{HCT\ (\%)} \times 100$	31%–36%
Mean corpuscular hemoglobin (MCH)	$MCH = \dfrac{Hb\ (g/dl)}{RBC\ (millions/\mu l)} \times 10$	26–34 pg

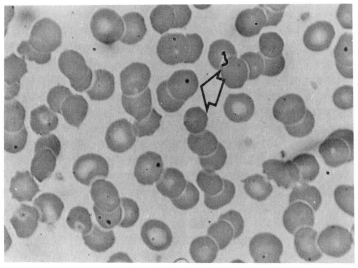

Figure 1-3. Howell-Jolly bodies (*arrow*).

13

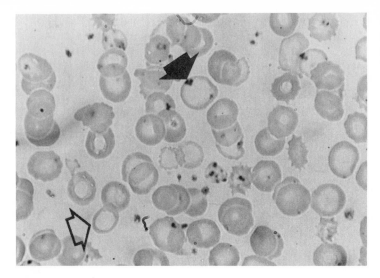

Figure 1-4. Hypochromic cell (*open arrow*) and Pappenheimer bodies (*solid arrow*).

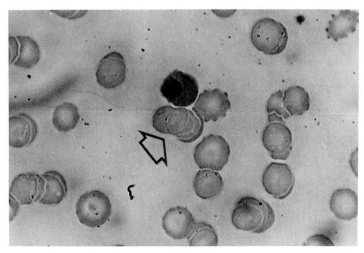

Figure 1-5. Rouleaux (*arrow*).

The Reticulocyte Count

Erythrocytes are released into the circulation by the marrow as cells with residual ribosomes, the reticulocytes. Ribosomes aggregate and stain with dyes such as new methylene blue (Figure 1-9).

Reticulocytes are counted by noting the number seen per 1000 red cells. Generally this number is reported as a percentage of the red cells counted; the normal percentage of reticulocytes is 1.0 ± 0.5. However, this percentage is not an adequate assessment of effective red cell production. Rather, production of red cells is reflected by the absolute number of reticulocytes released into the circulation daily, or the reticulocyte birth rate, independent of the red cell count. On the average, the normal daily reticulocyte birth rate, or the absolute reticulocyte count, is 1% of 5×10^6 red cells/mm^3, or 50,000 reticulocytes/mm^3. In practice, the corrected percentage reticulocyte count is used more often than the absolute count:

$$\text{Corrected reticulocyte count} = \% \text{ reticulocytes} \times \frac{\% \text{ patient's HCT}}{45}$$

Even the corrected reticulocyte count, however, can be a misleading index of effective erythropoiesis, because it assumes a one-day survival for red cells in the form of reticulocytes. In fact, in the presence of anemia, marrow reticulocytes may be released into the blood prematurely, appearing as large polychromatophilic cells on routine smear. They therefore spend a larger proportion of their life span than the normal one-day period in the circulation, resulting in a spurious elevation in the reticulocyte count.

A second correction factor corresponding to the assumed true circulating reticulocyte life span in days can be applied to the corrected reticulocyte count to obtain the *reticulocyte production index* (RPI) (Table 1-5):

$$\text{RPI} = \% \text{ reticulocytes} \times \frac{\% \text{ patient's HCT}}{45} \div \text{correction factor}$$

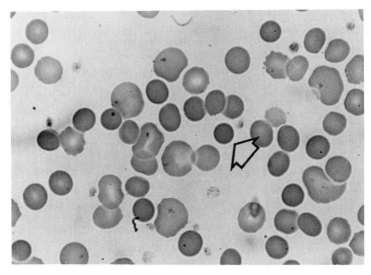

Figure 1-6. Spherocyte (*arrow*).

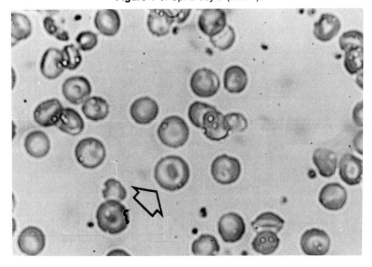

Figure 1-7. Target cell (*arrow*).

The normal range for RPI is 2–3. An RPI of less than 2 is seen in anemias in which decreased effective erythropoiesis is the predominant mechanism. If the RPI exceeds 3, the predominant mechanism is considered to be hemolytic (3–5).

The RPI correlates well with ferrokinetic measurements of effective erythropoiesis. In general, this index has been most useful in the diagnosis of the hypoproliferative anemias. The reticulocyte count or the corrected reticulocyte count is usually clearly elevated in the hemolytic anemias.

Use of the RPI assumes premature release of marrow reticulocytes resulting from increased erythropoietin in anemia. In renal failure, however, where production of erythropoietin is not consistent with the degree of anemia, use of this index may not be valid.

EXAMINATION OF THE MARROW

Marrow aspiration is an innocuous procedure in experienced hands. However, processing and interpretation of marrow specimens are time consuming and require experienced personnel. Examination of the marrow should, therefore, be performed only when preliminary evaluations suggest that such a study might provide useful additional information. Marrow examination is not helpful in a clear-cut case of iron deficiency anemia secondary to excessive menstrual bleeding or in a case of mild to moderate anemia associated with chronic renal failure. Furthermore, in general, examination of the marrow does not provide useful information in an obvious hemolytic state where the pathogenesis is otherwise apparent.

Table 1-5. **Correction Factor for Reticulocyte Production Index**

Packed Cell Volume (%)	Correction Factor
45	1.0
35	1.5
25	2.0
15	2.5

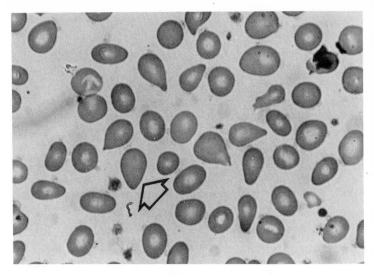

Figure 1-8. Teardrop cell (*arrow*).

Examination of the marrow does supply critical information in a number of specific instances. The presence of megaloblastic erythropoiesis or ring sideroblasts provides diagnostic confirmation. In patients with occult hypochromic, microcytic anemias, absence of iron on iron stain of aspirated material confirms the diagnosis of iron deficiency and distinguishes this disorder from hypochromic anemias associated with inflammatory disease. Etiology of anemia in disorders associated with marrow infiltration may only become apparent on examination of the bone marrow. A number of disorders can be evaluated adequately only by bone marrow biopsy. The latter include the pancytopenias and any disorder in which metastatic tumor or lymphoma may be present. Other indications for bone marrow biopsy are blood changes consistent with the diagnosis of myelofibrosis and failure to obtain adequate material by aspiration.

The normal myeloid/erythroid (M/E) ratio is approximately 3:1. When myelopoiesis is normal, this ratio reflects erythropoietic ac-

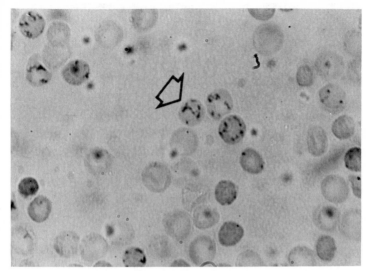

Figure 1-9. Reticulocyte (*arrow*) stained with new methylene blue.

tivity. In the hemolytic anemias, M/E ratio is often reversed, that is, values are greater than 1:1.

FERROKINETIC STUDIES

Understanding of erythrokinetics has been enhanced by iron turnover studies using the isotopically labeled iron, ^{59}Fe (6) (see Chapter 3). The measurements calculated in these studies are the plasma iron transport rate (PIT), a measure of the rate at which iron leaves the plasma; the red cell utilization (RCU), which measures the percent incorporation of radioactive iron into red cells; and the erythrocyte iron turnover rate (EIT), a measure of the rate at which iron moves from the marrow into circulating cells. PIT is calculated from the plasma iron clearance rate and the plasma iron level. RCU is the percentage of the tracer dose of ^{59}Fe that is measured in circulating cells within two weeks. EIT is the product of PIT and RCU.

Table 1-6. **Characteristic Ferrokinetic Changes**

Disorder	PIT (times normal)	RCU (%)[a]	EIT (times normal)
Increased erythropoiesis			
Hemolytic anemia (hereditary spherocytosis)	Increased (5.0)	60	Increased (3.0)
Ineffective erythropoiesis (thalassemia major)	Increased (10.0)	20	Increased (2.0)
Decreased erythropoiesis			
Severe renal disease	Normal (1.0)	30	Decreased (0.3)
Hypoplastic anemia	Decreased (0.7)	20	Decreased (0.2)

[a]Normal 80%–90%.

Using these measurements, total erythropoiesis may be divided into two components: effective erythropoiesis, resulting in the release of viable red cells into the circulation, and ineffective erythropoiesis, resulting in the formation of red cells that are destroyed within the marrow or shortly after release into the blood. Normally 10%–20% of erythropoiesis is ineffective. Characteristic ferrokinetic findings in disease states are shown in Table 1-6.

Two simple parameters provide essentially the same information obtained by ferrokinetic studies. The M/E ratio reflects total erythropoiesis, and the RPI correlates well with effective erythropoiesis. Some anemias are characterized by variable degrees of hemolysis and by increased ineffective erythropoiesis. These include megaloblastic anemias, thalassemias, and sideroblastic anemias.

DIFFERENTIAL DIAGNOSIS: CLASSIFICATION OF ANEMIA

The successful management of a patient with a lower than normal hemoglobin concentration requires precise definition of the nature and cause of the anemia. First, the physician must determine into which of a series of broad categories the patient fits. In achieving this aim consideration of several distinct but complementary classifications of anemia are helpful.

A pathophysiologic classification of anemia is based on the question of whether the condition is caused by increased destruction or loss of red cells, or by decreased production. The key to answering this question is the reticulocyte count. In the presence of anemia the normal bone marrow, supplied with all the building blocks required for formation of red cells accelerates their production to seven to eight times the normal rate. This increased erythropoiesis is reflected by the appearance of increased numbers of reticulocytes in the peripheral blood. Anemias that are caused primarily by increased destruction of mature red cells or by acute blood loss are therefore characterized by an increase in the reticulocyte count, which is roughly proportional to the degree of anemia. In contrast, when the anemia is caused by an inability of the bone marrow to produce adequate numbers of red cells, either because of bone marrow damage (as in aplastic anemia) or because of an inadequate amount of iron, vitamin B_{12}, or folic acid, the reticulocyte count is not increased and may be very low. Table 1-7 classifies anemias according to the reticulocyte count. The physician may occasionally be misled in the use of this classification. Patients with hemolytic anemia may, particularly after infections, undergo episodes of decreased bone marrow activity (aplastic crisis), under which circumstances the reticulocyte count is not elevated. Conversely, the patient with anemia caused by deficiency of an essential nutrient may manifest brief bursts of reticulocytosis when, in the course of the disorder, small amounts of the missing substance are made available to the marrow through diet or medication.

A second classification of anemia focuses on the size and hemoglobin content of the red cells. The red cell indices, MCV, MCH, and MCHC form the basis of this morphologic classification. Macrocytic anemias are characterized by an increased MCV. Such anemias may result either from a maturation defect (vitamin B_{12} and folate deficiency) or through the presence of large numbers of reticulocytes. In normochromic and normocytic anemias the red

Table 1-7. Pathophysiologic Classification of Anemia

Mechanism	Etiology	Disorder
Normal bone marrow response to anemia (elevated reticulocyte count)	Hemolytic anemia	Hemoglobinopathies
		Autoimmune hemolytic anemia
		Hereditary spherocytosis
		Hereditary nonspherocytic hemolytic anemia
		Paroxysmal nocturnal hemoglobinuria
	Anemia of acute blood loss	
	Overt bleeding	Gastrointestinal
		Genitourinary
		From wounds
	Covert bleeding	From fractures or contusions
		Into body cavities
Decreased red cell production by the bone marrow (low reticulocyte count)	Hypoproliferative disorders	
	Inadequate erythro-poietin response	Chronic disease
		Chronic renal insufficiency
		Hypometabolism
	Stem cell failure	Aplastic anemia
		Red cell aplasia
		Marrow infiltration

22

Impaired iron mobilization	Chronic disease
Disorders of erythrocyte maturation—disturbed hemoglobin synthesis	Iron deficiency
	Defective heme synthesis—sideroblastic anemias
	Defective globin synthesis—thalassemia
Abnormal nuclear maturation—disturbed DNA synthesis	Vitamin B_{12} deficiency
	Folic acid deficiency
	Congenital dyserythropoietic anemias

cells have a normal size and hemoglobin content, but not enough of them are present, as in aplastic anemia. Hypochromic microcytic anemias are characterized by a decreased MCV, MCH, and MCHC. Thus, the erythrocytes are small and poorly filled with hemoglobin. Hypochromic microcytic anemias are the result of inadequate formation of hemoglobin usually caused by a deficiency of an essential hemoglobin building block; iron deficiency and the thalassemias are characteristically hypochromic. (See Table 1-8 for a classification of anemias according to morphology.) Occasionally the red cell indices are such that an anemia does not fit into one of the three broad types—macrocytic, normocytic normochromic, and hypochromic microcytic—presented in the table. An example of this is normocytic microcytic anemia, which is encountered occasionally in patients with the anemia of chronic disease. How-

Table 1-8. **Morphologic Classification of Anemias**

Morphologic Classification	Anemia
Macrocytic anemia	Vitamin B_{12} deficiency
	Folic acid deficiency
	Refractory megaloblastic anemia
	Anemia of liver disease
	Hemolytic anemia
Normocytic normochromic anemia	Aplastic anemia
	Refractory anemia with hyperplastic marrow
	Hemolytic anemia
	Secondary anemia associated with chronic disease
Hypochromic microcytic anemia	Iron deficiency
	Thalassemia
	Unstable hemoglobins
	Sideroblastic anemia

ever, the three major groups listed account for the vast majority of anemias.

In addition to using these relatively well-established classifications of anemia, the physician should employ a very pragmatic, useful approach in determining its cause. This approach is based on statistical probabilities governing the cause of anemia in certain groups defined by age and sex. In infants and in women of childbearing age, the vast majority of anemias are caused by iron deficiency. If at the onset the physician considers the possibility of iron deficiency anemia and directs his or her attention to it, much needless further investigation can be averted. Similarly, with azotemia, one of the most common causes of anemia in elderly men, simply examining the levels of blood urea nitrogen or creatinine may obviate much further effort.

REFERENCES

1. Cartwright GE: *Diagnostic Laboratory Hematology*, ed 4. New York, Grune & Stratton, 1968, pp 28–119
2. Williams WJ, Schneider AS: Examination of the peripheral blood. In Williams WJ, Beutler E, Erslev AJ, et al (eds): *Hematology*, ed 2. New York, McGraw-Hill, 1977, pp 10–25
3. Hillman RS: Characteristics of marrow production and reticulocyte maturation in normal man in response to anemia. J Clin Invest 48:443–453, 1969
4. Ganzini A, Hillman RS, Finch CA: Maturation of the macroreticulocyte. Br J Haematol 16:119–135, 1969
5. Hillman RS, Finch CA: Erythropoiesis: normal and abnormal. Semin Hematol 4:327–336, 1967
6. Finch CA, Deubelbeiss JD, Cook PD, et al: Ferrokinetics in man. Medicine 49:17–53, 1970

SUGGESTED READING

Miale JB: *Laboratory Medicine: Hematology*. St. Louis, C.V. Mosby Co, 1977
Williams WJ, Beutler E, Erslev AJ, et al (eds): *Hematology*, ed 2. New York, McGraw-Hill, 1977
Wintrobe MM: *Clinical Hematology*. Philadelphia, Lea & Febiger, 1974

chapter 2

The Hypo-proliferative Anemias

The hypoproliferative anemias are disorders associated with diminished production of red cells not attributable to disturbances of maturation (Table 2-1). They are generally associated with normochromic normocytic red cell morphology without reticulocytosis. Characteristically, the reticulocyte count is low when adjusted for the degree of anemia. A Reticulocyte Production Index (RPI) of less than two is consistent with diminished effective red cell production (Table 2-1) (see Chapter 1).

The mechanisms for the hypoproliferative anemias are often complex. In anemia associated with chronic disease and in that seen in renal insufficiency, relative bone marrow failure is often

Table 2-1. **Hypoproliferative Disorders**

Inadequate erythropoietin response
    Chronic disease
    Chronic renal insufficiency
    Hypometabolism

Stem cell failure
    Aplastic anemia
    Red cell aplasia
    Marrow infiltration

Impaired iron mobilization
    Chronic disease

present. In this situation, the marrow does not possess the normal reserve required to compensate for a modest reduction in red cell survival. The mild hypoproliferative anemia seen in systemic disease, which is overshadowed by the underlying disease, usually requires minimal diagnostic evaluation. However, the physician must be alert to contributing causes for anemia such as iron loss resulting from bleeding or nutritional folate deficiency.

ANEMIAS WITH INADEQUATE ERYTHROPOIETIN RESPONSE

Chronic Disease

Anemia caused by chronic disease is second only to iron deficiency anemia in overall incidence (Table 2-2). It is the most frequent cause of anemia in hospitalized patients.

Anemia usually develops within two months after the onset of illness. It is customarily mild and eclipsed by the manifestations of the underlying disease although occasionally the anemia may be the presenting finding. The degree of anemia tends to correlate with the activity of the underlying disorder and with the severity of such signs and symptoms as fever and inflammation.

Levels of hemoglobin range from 8–12 g/dl and the anemia is usually normocytic and normochromic. However, some degree of hypochromia is frequently present in the course of the disease, particularly in rheumatoid arthritis. The reticulocyte count is generally normal or decreased with an RPI of less than two. Iron studies characteristically reveal decreased levels of serum iron with normal or decreased total iron binding capacity and decreased transferrin saturation. The bone marrow shows increased storage iron.

Three pathogenetic mechanisms have been implicated in the anemia of chronic disease: a mild reduction in red cell survival, impaired marrow response to anemia, and impaired mobilization of iron from iron stores. The bases for these mechanisms are uncertain. Impaired marrow response to anemia is associated with erythropoietin secretion that is inadequate for the degree of anemia.

Table 2-2. Conditions Commonly Associated with Anemia of Chronic Disease

Chronic inflammatory disease
Rheumatoid arthritis
Chronic infections
Chronic obstructive lung disease
Tuberculosis
Subacute bacterial endocarditis
Osteomyelitis
Chronic fungal disease
Malignant disease

Impaired iron mobilization or a reticuloendothelial iron blockade is largely responsible for the results of routine iron studies.

A number of secondary events may contribute to the anemia of chronic disorders, including marrow infiltration with chronic disease caused by cancer, folate deficiency with anorexia and inanition, and blood loss, particularly with involvement of the gastrointestinal tract. Diseases such as cancer or rheumatoid arthritis are also sometimes associated with abnormalities of heme synthesis that result in a sideroblastic anemia.

Chronic Renal Insufficiency

Chronic azotemia is consistently accompanied by anemia. The predominant history and findings usually can be attributed to known underlying renal disease. Anemia is, however, usually insidious in onset. It may ultimately be severe and associated with pallor, palpitations, and dyspnea on exertion.

The degree of azotemia and the severity of anemia are only roughly correlated. However, anemia progresses with worsening of kidney failure. Ultimately the hemoglobin stabilizes between 5 and 10 g/dl. In the absence of complications it is normocytic and normochromic. Routine iron studies generally show normal results.

The major mechanism responsible for the anemia of chronic

renal disease is deficient production of erythropoietin by the kidney. Uremia itself also appears to inhibit marrow responsiveness to erythropoietin. Another pathogenetic factor in uremia is decreased red cell survival.

Many complications of chronic renal disease and of long-term hemodialysis may contribute to anemia. These factors include iron deficiency caused by chronic bleeding associated with platelet dysfunction of uremia, impaired iron utilization seen with chronic disorders, particularly in renal disease with an inflammatory component such as chronic pyelonephritis; and folate deficiency. The latter may have a nutritional basis in a patient with anorexia or may be caused by loss of folate to the dialysis bath during hemodialysis.

Hypometabolism

Anemia commonly accompanies hypofunction of the pituitary gland or deficiencies of hormones of the target glands (e.g., thyroid, adrenal, and androgen deficiencies). The most frequent anemia in this group is that associated with hypothyroidism. Patients now rarely present with obvious myxedema. The disease is usually insidious and when the patient presents with fatigue and anemia the underlying diagnosis may not be apparent. Anemia is mild with hemoglobin usually greater than 10 g/dl in women and 12 g/dl in men; it is usually normocytic and normochromic but may be slightly macrocytic. Menorrhagia is a frequent complication of myxedema and may result in associated iron deficiency anemia.

Male patients with hypogonadism frequently have hemoglobin levels and hematocrits in the normal female range. Androgens increase production of erythropoietin. Anemia of hypopituitarism probably results from hormone deficiencies of the target glands.

ANEMIA OF STEM CELL FAILURE

Aplastic Anemia

The term aplastic anemia is used to designate a disorder in which pancytopenia is associated with severe marrow hypoplasia that cannot be attributed to an ongoing systemic disease process. Aplasia involving only erythropoiesis is referred to as pure red cell aplasia.

Known causes of aplastic anemia include a variety of drugs, ionizing radiation, and infectious hepatitis (Table 2-3). Radiation therapy, drugs used for cancer chemotherapy, and industrial hydrocarbons, such as benzene, produce regular and predictable suppression of hematopoiesis. Another group of chemical agents, largely drugs, result in idiosyncratic marrow aplasia. These include chloramphenicol, phenylbutazone, and anticonvulsants. Aplastic anemia resulting from viral hepatitis is often severe and associated with a high fatality rate. Fanconi's anemia is a rare form of aplastic anemia associated with multiple congenital anomalies. No etiology can be found for approximately 50% of cases of aplastic anemia. Pure red cell aplasia frequently appears to be part of an autoimmune disorder and 50% of the incidences are associated with a thymoma.

The onset of symptoms in most patients is insidious. Initial signs and symptoms may be secondary to thrombocytopenia or to anemia. Ecchymoses, petechiae, and mucosal bleeding are common signs. Symptoms may include fatigue, dyspnea on exertion, and palpitation. Infection associated with granulocytopenia is a less frequent presenting problem.

Blood counts characteristically show hemoglobin levels less than 9 g/dl, a white cell count of less than 2000/mm^3 due predominantly to granulocytopenia, and a platelet count of less than 70,000/mm^3. The reticulocyte count is markedly depressed. The anemia is normocytic and normochromic and no morphologic red cell changes are seen. The bone marrow is acellular.

Marrow Infiltration

Replacement of normal hematopoietic elements is a consistent feature of certain primary hematologic disorders, including leukemia, myelofibrosis, multiple myeloma, and, at times, lymphoma (Table 2-4). Anemia is usually overshadowed by other features of the primary disorder.

Table 2-3. **Causes of Aplastic Anemia**

Idiopathic

Secondary

    Chemical and physical agents
        Ionizing radiation
        Chemicals (industrial hydrocarbons, benzene solvents)
        Chemotherapeutic agents (alkylating agents, antimetabolites)
        Drugs[a]
            Antimicrobials (chloramphenicol)
            Anticonvulsants [methyl phenylethylhydantoin (Mesantoin), trimethadione (Tridione)]
            Gold compounds
            Phenylbutazone

    Viral infections (hepatitis)

Familial (Fanconi's anemia)

[a]Some of those with 20 or more reported cases listed.

Table 2-4. **Causes of Marrow Infiltration**

Neoplasms

    Hematologic malignancies
        Leukemia
        Malignant lymphomas
        Myeloma

    Metastatic cancer
        Carcinoma of the breast, prostate, lung, and gastrointestinal tract
        Neuroblastoma

Myelofibrosis

    Idiopathic

    Secondary to other myeloproliferative disorders or toxic exposure (e.g., irradiation)

Granulomatous disease

Gaucher's disease

Cancer without bone marrow metastases may cause anemia by the same mechanisms as other chronic disorders. When cancer metastasizes to the marrow, disturbed hematopoiesis most frequently results in anemia or in anemia and thrombocytopenia. Leukoerythroblastosis (i.e., the presence of immature granulocytes and nucleated red cells) is seen less commonly. Cancers particularly prone to metastasize to bone marrow include neuroblastoma and malignant tumors of the breast, prostate, and gastrointestinal tract, and small cell carcinoma of the lung.

DIAGNOSTIC EVALUATION

In the anemias associated with inadequate marrow response to erythropoietin, particularly in chronic disease and in renal failure, anemia will respond if the underlying disorder is treated successfully. However, contributing causes for the anemia, including blood loss and folate deficiency, may be present that require specific therapy. Chronic blood loss may make diagnosis particularly confusing when it is associated with a chronic inflammatory disease such as rheumatoid arthritis, in which hypochromia may be accompanied by abnormal iron metabolism even in the absence of blood loss.

The anemias of stem cell failure, and aplastic anemia in particular, must be differentiated from other causes of pancytopenia (Table 2-5). Aplastic anemia is largely a diagnosis of exclusion that in most cases can be accomplished by bone marrow biopsy. Primary hematopoietic disorders are associated with characteristic marrow morphology. In pancytopenia associated with hypersplenism, systemic lupus erythematosus, and some cases of preleukemia, the marrow shows normal or increased cellularity rather than aplasia. However, diseases such as paroxysmal nocturnal hemoglobinuria (PNH) and occasionally acute leukemia may present with hypocellular marrows. Marrow hypocellularity is not uncommonly seen in hairy cell leukemia.

The evaluation of the hypoproliferative anemias proceeds with the following:

Table 2-5. Causes of Pancytopenia

Aplastic anemia (see Table 2-3)
Marrow infiltration (see Table 2-4)
Megaloblastic anemias—B_{12} or folate deficiency
Disorders involving the spleen
      Congestive splenomegaly—portal hypertension
      Lymphomas
      Infiltrative disorders—Gaucher's disease
      Chronic infection—tuberculosis
      Primary splenic panhematopenia
Systemic lupus erythematosus
Paroxysmal nocturnal hemoglobinuria
Disseminated infection—atypical mycobacteria
Pregnancy (rare)

1. Hematologic evaluation, with attention to red cell morphology, red cell indices and the RPI, and bone marrow studies.
2. Studies of iron metabolism, including serum iron and total iron binding capacity and examination of aspirated bone marrow for stainable iron. The use of serum ferritin determination and measurement of free erythrocyte protoporphyrin are discussed in Chapter 3.
3. Studies of iron turnover using isotopically labeled iron. These studies have enhanced understanding of erythrokinetics. Although they are occasionally used to clarify difficult diagnostic problems, in practice hypoproliferative anemia can be diagnosed and its pathogenesis appreciated by simple laboratory tests, including red cell indices, reticulocyte count, and routine iron studies.

LABORATORY STUDIES

Hematologic Tests

GENERAL FEATURES

Blood cell morphology is generally normal with the most commonly encountered hypoproliferative anemias. Anemia alone characterizes those disorders associated with diminished response to erythropoietin whereas bone marrow failure is characterized by pancytopenia. Anemia is severe in advanced renal failure and in full-blown aplastic anemia but is generally mild in chronic disease and hypometabolism. Unexplained changes in blood cell morphology or suddenly worsening anemia require a search for a complicating disorder. Hypochromic microcytic red cell morphology and indices may develop in a patient with occult blood loss. The earliest change in a developing folate deficiency may be the appearance of circulating hypersegmented neutrophils.

PERIPHERAL BLOOD

Blood cell measurements

Red cell indices are generally normal. The adjusted or absolute reticulocyte count is not elevated and may be decreased. The general range of hemoglobins in the hypoproliferative disorders is shown in Table 2-6.

Morphology

Red cells are normocytic normochromic. Some degree of hypochromia may be present in chronic disease, particularly in chronic inflammatory disease such as rheumatoid arthritis. Burr cells may be seen with renal failure. Immature granulocytes and nucleated red cells and megakaryocyte fragments may be seen with bone marrow infiltration.

RETICULOCYTE PRODUCTION INDEX

The Reticulocyte Production Index (RPI) generally correlates well with effective erythopoiesis (1–3) (see Chapter 1 and Table 1-5).

BONE MARROW

Bone marrow studies in the anemias with inadequate erythropoietin response do not show any diagnostic changes and generally demonstrate normal cellularity and a normal M:E ratio. The latter

Table 2-6. Characteristic Hematologic Findings in Hypoproliferative Disorders

Disorder	Hemoglobin (g/dl)	RBC Morphology	Other changes
Chronic disease	8–12	Normal hypochromia or microcytosis	
Renal failure	5–10	Normal, may be burr cells	
Hypometabolism	> 9	Normal or slight macrocytosis	
Aplastic anemia	< 9	Normal	Pancytopenia
Marrow infiltration	Variable, > 9 with cancer	Normal, may be nucleated red cells; poikilocytosis with myelofibrosis	May be thrombo-cytopenia or pancytopenia; may be immature granulocytes

finding in the presence of anemia is consistent with an apparently inadequate erythropoietic response to anemia. In the anemia associated with stem cell failure, a needle biopsy is required to confirm the diagnosis of aplastic anemia, to demonstrate marrow fibrosis, and often to diagnose infiltrative disorders such as metastatic carcinoma and lymphoma.

Other Useful Tests

SERUM IRON AND TOTAL IRON-BINDING CAPACITY (TIBC)

Purpose

Serum iron studies in chronic disease often resemble those seen in iron deficiency anemia and differ from those seen in other hypoproliferative anemias (4) (see Table 2-7 and Chapter 3). These studies along with evaluation of marrow iron stores are helpful in diagnosing iron deficiency anemia caused by chronic blood loss, which frequently complicates these other disorders.

For sections on *Principle, Procedure, Specimen,* and *Interpretation,* see Chapter 3. Results of serum iron studies in hypochromic anemia and in the hypoproliferative anemias are shown in Tables 2-3 and 2-7.

STAINABLE BONE MARROW IRON

For sections on *Purpose, Principle, Procedure,* and *Specimen,* see Chapter 3 (5).

Interpretation

Unless chronic bleeding supervenes, the hypoproliferative anemias are associated with normal to increased marrow iron stores, which distinguish hypoferremia caused by chronic disease from iron deficiency anemia, in which marrow iron is depleted. Absent storage iron in the marrow in one of the hypoproliferative anemias is consistent with complicating iron deficiency.

Table 2-7. Iron Measurements in Iron Deficiency and in Hypoproliferative Anemias

Disorder	Serum Iron	Total Iron-binding Capacity	% Saturation	Bone Marrow Storage Iron
Iron deficiency	Decreased	Increased	Decreased (often < 16%)	Decreased
Hypoproliferative anemias				
Chronic disease	Decreased	Normal or decreased	Usually decreased (usually > 16%)	Normal or increased
Chronic renal insufficiency	Normal	Normal	Normal	Normal
Aplastic anemia	Usually increased	Normal	Usually increased	Usually increased

REFERENCES

1. Hillman RS: Characteristics of marrow production and reticulocyte maturation in normal man in response to anemia. J Clin Invest 48:443–453, 1969

2. Ganzini A, Hillman RS, Finch CA: Maturation of the macroreticulocyte. Br J Haematol 16:119–135, 1969

3. Hillman RS, Finch CA: Erythropoiesis: normal and abnormal. Semin Hematol 4:327–336, 1967

4. Beutler E, Robson MJ, Buttenweiser BS: A comparison of the plasma iron, iron binding capacity, sternal marrow iron and other methods in the clinical evaluation of iron stores. Ann Intern Med 48:60–82, 1958

5. Beutler E: Peripheral blood, bone marrow, and urine iron stains. In Williams WJ, Beutler E, Erslev AJ, et al: *Hematology*, ed 2. New York, McGraw-Hill, 1977, pp 1589–1590

chapter 3

Hypochromic Microcytic Anemias

Hypochromic microcytic red cells seen in the blood film of an anemic patient suggest a defect in the rate of hemoglobin synthesis. Such a defect may arise because insufficient iron is present, because of hereditary abnormalities in globin synthesis, such as the thalassemias or the unstable hemoglobins (see Chapter 9), or as a result of inhibition of heme synthesis by toxic materials such as lead. It may occur as a consequence of neoplastic disorders or as a hereditary or idiopathic disorder in which increased numbers of sideroblasts are present in the bone marrow. The most common types of hypochromic anemia are listed in Table 3-1.

Table 3-1. Causes of Hypochromic Anemia

Iron deficiency

Thalassemias
    Alpha-thalassemias
    Beta-thalassemias

Sideroblastic anemias
    Hereditary (sex linked)
    Acquired
        Drug induced (e.g., lead, isoniazid—INH)
        Leukemia or preleukemia
        Idiopathic

Chronic disorders
    Chronic infections
    Chronic inflammatory states
    Neoplastic diseases

Iron deficiency is the most common cause of anemia, which ranks among the most common of all diseases of humans. In infants and children a negative iron balance may occur as a result of inadequate dietary intake of iron. In adults, iron deficiency may be the result of pregnancy or of blood loss, and since losses of iron are normally very small, dietary intake plays at most a contributory role in the etiology of the disease. Identification of the cause of iron deficiency represents a particularly important responsibility of the physician since it may be the first sign of a malignant lesion of the gastrointestinal or genitourinary tract.

DIAGNOSTIC EVALUATION

Evaluation of the hypochromic microcytic anemias proceeds with the following:

1. Hematologic evaluation, with attention to red cell morphology and red cell indices and, occasionally, bone marrow study.
2. Serum iron and total iron-binding capacity, which reflect iron stores and help to distinguish iron deficiency from other causes of microcytic, hypochromic anemia.
3. Examination of aspirated bone marrow for stainable iron, which is the most direct assessment of iron stores.
4. Determination of serum ferritin, a blood test for quantitating iron stores.
5. Measurement of free erythrocyte protoporphyrin, of particular value as a screening test for distinguishing iron deficiency from thalassemia minor.
6. Hematologic response to therapy, which confirms the diagnosis of iron deficiency.

LABORATORY STUDIES

Hematologic Tests

GENERAL FEATURES

In well-developed iron deficiency anemia, hypochromia, microcytosis, and anisocytosis are usually present. However, no morphologic abnormalities of the red cells may be present in mild iron deficiency. Hypochromia and microcytosis are a uniform finding in the thalassemias, and the reductions in MCV and MCHC are generally greater than those observed in iron deficiency anemia of the same degree. Microcytosis with significant elevations of the red cell count to over six million per mm^3 are common in thalassemia minor. Stippled red cells are commonly seen on the blood film in thalassemia but are unusual in iron deficiency. Hypochromia is often present in patients with sideroblastic anemia, but it is by no means a universal finding. Overall decreases in the size of red cells and in the hemoglobin concentration are best determined by measuring indices with automated cell-counting equipment.

PERIPHERAL BLOOD

Blood cell measurements

The MCV and MCHC are decreased, and the reticulocyte count is modestly decreased, normal, or modestly increased. However, indices are often normal with hemoglobin over 12 g/dl.

Morphology

Hypochromia and microcytosis are present. Other changes are noted in Table 3-2.

Table 3-2.   **Prominent Findings in the Blood Smear in Hypochromic Anemia**

	Anisocytosis and Poikilocytosis	Basophilic Stippling	Dimorphism
Iron deficiency	Variable	No	No
Thalassemia minor	No	Yes	No
Sideroblastic anemias			
Hereditary	Yes	Yes	Yes
Acquired	Variable	Yes	Yes
Chronic disease	No	No	No

BONE MARROW

Erythroid hyperplasia is often present, but it is not as prominent as it is in the hemolytic anemias. The only specific finding in this group is decreased or absent stainable storage iron in iron deficiency anemia.

Other Useful Tests

SERUM IRON AND TOTAL IRON-BINDING CAPACITY (TIBC)

Purpose

Serum iron and TIBC determinations are particularly useful in mild iron deficiency anemia, in which decreased serum iron levels precede changes in red cell morphology or in red cell indices, and in distinguishing iron deficiency anemia from other microcytic hypochromic anemias (1, 2).

Principle

All transport iron in the plasma is bound in the ferric form to the specific iron-binding protein, transferrin. Serum iron refers to this transferrin-bound iron. Total iron-binding capacity, the concentration iron necesssary to saturate the iron-binding sites of transferrin, is a measure of transferrin concentration. Saturation of transferrin is calculated by the following formula:

$$\% \text{ transferrin saturation} = \frac{\text{serum iron } (\mu g/dl)}{\text{TIBC } (\mu g/dl)} \times 100$$

Normal mean transferrin saturation is approximately 30%. Unsaturated iron-binding capacity (UIBC) is the difference between TIBC and serum iron.

Procedure

Serum iron is freed from transferrin by acidification of the serum and is then reduced to the ferrous form. After the protein has been precipitated, the filtrate is reacted with a chromogen such as Ferrozine and the color formed is measured. The colorimetric determination of TIBC involves addition of iron to serum followed by removal of excessive, unbound iron by absorption on an absorbant or an ion exchange resin; the bound iron is then released from transferrin, reduced, and its concentration is measured as in the serum iron test. A radiometric method for TIBC is based on the determination of UIBC by adding ^{59}Fe ammonium citrate to serum and measuring its uptake. Serum iron is then measured colorimetrically and TIBC = serum iron + UIBC. The TIBC can also be determined by measuring transferrin by immunodiffusion.

Specimen

A specimen of serum should be drawn in the morning.

Interpretation

The representative normal range of values for serum iron is 60–180 μg/dl for men with values 10 μg/dl lower for women; for TIBC, 250–410 μg/dl; and for percent saturation, 20%–50%. Serum iron is low and percent saturation is characteristically reduced in both iron deficiency anemia and the anemia of chronic disease. Although the value for percent saturation is often reduced to levels less than 16% in iron deficiency anemia and is more frequently greater than 16% in chronic disease, values overlap in the two conditions. The TIBC is increased or normal in 90% of severe uncomplicated iron deficiency anemias and is decreased or normal in the microcytic anemia of chronic disease. Serum iron is increased in the sideroblastic anemias, thalassemias, and in other iron loading disorders such as hemochromatosis (Table 3-3).

Notes and precautions

Because of diurnal variations in serum iron levels (maximum, 7–10 a.m.) and the fact that stated ranges are for a.m. normal levels, specimens should be drawn in the morning. Patients should not be receiving iron therapy.

Table 3-3. Serum Iron, Iron-Binding Capacity, and Storage Iron in Hypochromic Anemias

Cause of Hypochromic Anemia	Serum Iron	TIBC	% Saturation	Bone Marrow Storage Iron
Iron deficiency	↓	↑[a]	↓	↓
Thalassemias	↑–N	↓–N	↑–N	↑
Sideroblastic anemias	↑–N	↓–N	↑–N	↑
Chronic disease	↓	↓–N	↓	↑–N

[a] The TIBC is occasionally normal in iron deficiency.

STAINABLE BONE MARROW IRON

Purpose

The most direct means for assessing body iron stores is by histo-chemical examination of aspirated bone marrow for storage iron (2, 3).

Principle

Iron is stored as ferritin, in which it is complexed to the protein apoferritin, and as hemosiderin, which is made up of ferritin aggregates. Ferritin is too small to be seen by light microscopy. Hemosiderin is the stainable form of storage iron that appears blue with an acid ferrocyanide solution used in the Prussian-blue reaction. Iron is stored in reticuloendothelial cells. Iron granules are formed in developing normoblasts. Normoblasts that contain one or more particles of stainable iron are known as sideroblasts.

Procedure

The bone marrow aspirate is stained using the Prussian-blue reaction. Search for sideroblasts requires a counterstain such as basic fuchsin.

Specimen

Either sectioned bone marrow fragments or particle smears are used.

Interpretation

Normally, hemosiderin granules are seen in reticuloendothelial cells in every third or fourth oil-immersion field. With reduced iron stores, either no hemosiderin granules or only a few are seen in the entire preparation. With increased iron stores, hemosiderin granules are seen in every oil-immersion field, often deposited in clumps. The appraisal of reticuloendothelial iron preparations is extremely helpful in the differential diagnosis of anemia (Table 3-3). Since iron from breakdown of red cell heme cannot be excreted and is diverted to the storage compartment, increased

45

amounts of iron are generally present in bone marrow of anemic patients who are not iron deficient. An exception may exist in myeloproliferative disorders in which absent bone marrow iron stores may be found without other evidence for iron deficiency; this may result from impaired storage function. Since stainable marrow iron may occasionally not be seen in healthy subjects, the presence of such iron is more diagnostic than its absence. When storage iron is present in the bone marrow, anemia cannot be a result of iron deficiency unless the patient has been treated with parenteral iron.

Normally, 20%–40% of red cell precursors are sideroblasts. Although a sideroblast count is not ordinarily necessary for the diagnosis of iron deficiency anemia, it may be useful when an inadequate number of marrow particles was obtained and in patients who have received parenteral iron. Loss of sideroblasts from the marrow is seen in iron deficiency anemia, after acute blood loss when reticuloendothelial stores have not yet been depleted, and in chronic inflammatory disease. The most important application of sideroblast counts is in the diagnosis of a sideroblastic anemia, characterized by the presence of ring sideroblasts. These are normoblasts that contain iron granules surrounding the nucleus over at least three-fourths of the nuclear circumference.

Notes and precautions

Some practice is required to distinguish stainable reticuloendothelial iron from artifacts. When a patient has received iron by the parenteral route, either as an iron carbohydrate complex, such as iron dextran (Imferon), or in the form of blood transfusions, histochemically stainable iron stores may be seen in the marrow in the presence of iron deficiency anemia.

SERUM FERRITIN

Purpose

The iron storage compound ferritin normally circulates in the plasma in minute amounts (4). The test for serum ferritin was developed to provide a quantitative and less invasive test for iron stores than the histochemical examination of aspirated bone marrow, particularly in children.

Principle

Ferritin is a complex of the protein apoferritin and iron. It appears to serve principally as an iron storage compound. The largest quantities of ferritin are found in the liver and reticuloendothelial cells. Ordinarily, serum ferritin concentration closely reflects the amount of stored iron.

Procedure

Reliable estimation of serum ferritin levels has been achieved with a sensitive radioimmune method using a sandwich technique. Ferritin is removed from the serum by solid-phase antiferritin antibodies, and radioactively labeled antiferritin antibodies are then permitted to bind to the removed ferritin.

Specimen

Serum is obtained.

Interpretation

The normal concentration of serum ferritin varies in a broad range from 10 ng/ml–1000 ng/ml. In iron deficiency anemia, serum ferritin is diminished and appears to be a relatively sensitive and reliable indicator of the presence of iron deficiency. Levels of serum ferritin may be low in iron deficiency without anemia, while elevated levels are common in iron overload states, including sideroblastic anemia.

Notes and precautions

Sufficient experience has not been gained with this relatively new technique to establish clearly its role in the estimation of body reserves. Levels of serum ferritin are elevated with inflammatory disease. When iron deficiency and inflammatory disease coexist, levels of serum ferritin may be in the normal range.

FREE ERYTHROCYTE PROTOPORPHYRIN (FEP)

Purpose

Levels of FEP are elevated in anemias associated with failure of iron incorporation into heme. With the advent of rapid micro methods for measuring FEP in recent years, this test is playing a growing diagnostic role in these disorders (5, 6).

Principle

When insufficient iron is available for developing erythroblasts, some protoporphyrin that was destined to be converted to heme accumulates as FEP. This substance is elevated both with depleted iron stores and in conditions associated with an internal block in iron utilization, as seen with certain chronic disorders and sideroblastic anemias.

Procedure

Free erythrocyte protoporphyrin is extracted from red cells with ethyl acetate/acetic acid and is quantitated fluorometrically.

Specimen

Whole blood is collected in anticoagulant. There is also a spot test for blood specimens collected on filter paper.

Interpretation

Normally FEP is less than 100 μg/dl packed red cells. Elevated levels are seen in iron deficiency, in chronic disease states associated with decreased tranferrin saturation, and in acquired idiopathic sideroblastic anemia. Marked elevation of FEP is seen in sideroblastic anemia secondary to lead intoxication with FEP values of about 1000 μg/dl packed red cells. In microcytic anemias associated with abnormal globin synthesis rather than abnormal heme synthesis, such as thalassemia minor, FEP levels are normal. Since iron deficiency anemia and thalassemia minor are the first and second most common causes respectively of hypochromic microcytic anemia, measurement of FEP promises to be particularly valuable as a screening test to distinguish these two disorders.

RESPONSE TO THERAPY

In the final analysis, the correctness of the diagnosis of iron deficiency depends on demonstration of an adequate response to iron therapy. Treatment usually consists of the oral administration of a ferrous iron salt, such as ferrous sulfate, in a dosage of 0.06–0.12 g iron three times a day. Under some circumstances the parenteral administration of iron may be preferred. Although reticulocytosis and a significant rise in hemoglobin concentration of the blood may occur as early as the third or fourth day after treatment, particularly in children, a reticulocyte response is often not observed for 7 or 8 days, and the hemoglobin concentration in the blood may not rise significantly during the first 10 days of treatment. Thereafter, however, restoration of the hemoglobin level to normal should be rapid and essentially complete by the sixth week after institution of therapy, regardless of how severe the anemia was initially. Infection, inflammatory disease, or neoplastic disease may prevent an adequate response, and continued bleeding may blunt the apparent therapeutic effect. However, the most common cause of failure to respond is an incorrect diagnosis.

REFERENCES

1. Sunderman TW: Serum iron, iron binding capacity. Proficiency Test Service Monthly Report. Philadelphia, Instititute of Clinical Science, October, 1978

2. Beutler MJ, Robson BS, Buttenweiser BS: A comparison of the plasma iron, iron binding capacity, sternal marrow iron and other methods in the clinical evaluation of iron stores. Ann Intern Med 48:60–82, 1958

3. Beutler E: Peripheral blood, bone marrow, and urine iron stains. In Williams WJ, Beutler E, Erslev AJ, et al (eds): *Hematology*, ed 2. New York, McGraw-Hill, 1977, pp 1589–1590

4. Lipschitz DA, Cook JD, Finch CA: A clinical evaluation of serum ferritin as an index of iron stores. N Engl J Med 290:1213–1216, 1974

5. Langer EE, Haining RG, Labbe RF, et al: Erythrocyte protoporphyrin. Blood 40:112–128, 1972

6. Stockman JA III, Laurence S, Weiner GE, et al: The measurement of free erythrocyte porphyrin (FEP) as a simple means of distinguishing iron deficiency from beta-thalassemic trait in subjects with microcytosis. J Lab Clin Med 85:113–119, 1975

chapter 4

Megaloblastic Anemias

Megaloblastic anemias are disorders resulting from deficiencies of coenzyme forms of folate and vitamin B_{12}. These coenzymes are necessary for a number of metabolic processes in humans, including DNA synthesis. The megaloblastic morphologic changes associated with defective DNA synthesis are seen in those tissues with rapid cell turnover—hematopoietic tissues and mucosal linings. The metabolic abnormalities responsible for damage to the central nervous system in B_{12} deficiency are unclear.

Pertinent data regarding the characteristics and body turnover of B_{12} and folate are given in Table 4-1. Because the minimum daily requirement of B_{12} is readily available in the diet, B_{12} deficiency rarely occurs on a nutritional basis. The very large B_{12} stores in relation to requirements account for the slow development of B_{12} deficiency over a period of years. On the other hand, because of the relatively narrow margin between requirements of folic acid and amounts obtained in the diet, a nutritional folate deficiency is not rare, and because of more limited folate stores, megaloblastic anemia can develop in a few months.

Pernicious anemia (PA) is the only primary disorder resulting from isolated malabsorption of B_{12} in adults. The pathogenetic lesion is severe gastric atrophy of unknown etiology with failure to secrete intrinsic factor necessary for B_{12} absorption. Autoantibodies to both parietal cells and to intrinsic factor, which are usually formed in this disease, appear to be secondary phenomena. Causes of secondary B_{12} malabsorption associated with megaloblastic anemias

51

Table 4-1. Some Characteristics of Vitamin B₁₂ and Folate

Characteristic	Vitamin B_{12}	Folate
Parent form	Cyanocobalamin	Pteroylglutamic acid (folic acid)
Molecular weight	1355	441
Natural forms	Methylcobalamin, deoxy-adenosyl-cobalamin, hydroxo-cobalamin	Reduced, methylated, or formyl-ated pteroylpolyglutamates
Foods	Animal origin only (liver, meat, fish, dairy produce)	Yeast, liver, green vegetables, nuts, cereals, fruit
Effect of cooking	Little or no effect	May destroy completely
Adult daily requirements	1–2 micrograms	100 μg
Normal daily intake	3–30 micrograms	600–700 μg
Body stores	Average 5 mg (4 years' supply)	6–20 mg (2–4 months' supply)
Site of absorption	Ileum	Duodenum and jejunum
Mechanism	Gastric intrinsic factor	Deconjugation, reduction, and methylation

are given in Table 4-2. As shown in the table, folate deficiency occurs in a large variety of states and may coexist with B_{12} deficiency in intestinal malabsorption.

Special studies, including radiography and intestinal biopsy, may be required to diagnose diseases of the small bowel. However, in most patients with typical clinical findings (Table 4-3), the diagnosis can be confirmed by other readily available tests. Conditions of folate deficiency that have a clinically apparent underlying cause include chronic alcoholism, megaloblastic anemia of pregnancy, relative folate deficiency in chronic hemolytic disorders, and the interference with DNA synthesis caused by antimetabolite therapy. Few supplementary laboratory studies are required to establish these diagnoses.

DIAGNOSTIC EVALUATION

Evaluation of megaloblastic anemias proceeds in the following logical sequence:

1. Hematologic evaluation with attention to blood and marrow morphology to establish the presence of a megaloblastic anemia.
2. Determination of the broad etiologic classification of the anemia based on the type of vitamin deficiency by means of blood B_{12} and folate levels (Table 4-2).
3. Determination of the cause of the deficiency by the presence of achlorhydria on gastric analysis in B_{12} deficiency associated with clinically apparent PA (Table 4-2), or, in other cases, by ascertaining the presence of B_{12} malabsorption and the role of intrinsic factor in the presence of such malabsorption by means of the Schilling test.
4. Confirmation of the type of vitamin deficiency by following the hematologic response to therapy.
5. Determination of serum lactic dehydrogenase (LDH), a simple ancillary procedure, which may help to establish the diagnosis of megaloblastic anemia and to follow the response to therapy. Serum LDH is often markedly elevated in megaloblastic anemia.

Table 4-2. Etiologic Classification of Megaloblastic Anemias

B_{12} deficiency

 Dietary deficiency (rare)

 Lack of intrinsic factor
  Adult PA
  Postgastrectomy
  Juvenile PA (rare)

 Diseases preventing ileal absorption
  Regional enteritis
  Extensive ileal resections; bypass procedure
  Familial selective B_{12} malabsorption (rare)
  Para-aminosalicylic acid therapy (rare)

 Competition for B_{12} by small bowel organisms
  Bacterial overgrowth—blind loops, diverticulae, strictures
  Fish tapeworm

Folate deficiency

 Dietary deficiency—partial cause in alcoholism

 Markedly increased requirements
  Megaloblastic anemia of pregnancy
  Megaloblastic anemia complicating chronic hemolytic states
  Neoplastic diseases

 Intestinal malabsorption in diffuse disease of jejunal mucosa[a]
  Gluten-induced enteropathy—nontropical sprue
  Tropical sprue

 Intestinal malabsorption induced by drugs
  Anticonvulsants—diphenylhydantoin, phenobarbital, primidone
  Other drugs—oral contraceptives, glutethimide, isoniazid

 Drug-induced block in folate metabolism with methotrexate and pyrimethamine (Daraprim)

No deficiency—no response to B_{12} or folate

 Antimetabolites other than folate antagonists—6-mercaptopurine, 5-fluorouracil, cystosine arabinoside, hydroxyurea

 Inherited disorders of DNA synthesis—orotic aciduria, deficiencies of enzymes needed for folate metabolism (rare)

[a]Associated with variable degree of B_{12} malabsorption and deficiency.

Table 4-3. **Clinical Features of Megaloblastic Anemia**

Feature	B_{12} Deficiency	Folate Deficiency
Etiology		
Poor diet	Rare	Common
Primary intestinal malabsorption	Rare in isolated deficiency	Common
Absent intrinsic factor	Yes, in PA	No
Age	PA rare under 35 years	All ages
Symptoms		
Insidious onset	Very common	Common
Weak, tired, exertional dyspnea	Common	Common
Sore tongue	Common	Common
Severe diarrhea	Uncommon	Common
Steatorrhea	No	Common
Paresthesias, mental symptoms	Yes (30% in PA)	No
Signs		
Marked weight loss (20 lbs)	Uncommon	Common
Glossitis	Common	Common
Decreased senses of position and vibration	Yes (< 10% in PA)	No

LABORATORY STUDIES

Hematologic Tests

GENERAL FEATURES

The diagnosis of megaloblastic anemia is contingent on the finding of megaloblastic erythropoiesis in the bone marrow. However, megaloblastic anemias are usually easily distinguished from other macrocytic anemias by findings in the peripheral blood (Table 4-4). The hematologic findings in megaloblastic anemias caused by folate deficiency are identical to those of B_{12} deficiency. Although the most striking morphologic changes occur in red cell precursors, all hematopoietic elements are affected and a variable degree of pancytopenia is present. Megaloblastic erythropoiesis results from the combination of impaired DNA synthesis and unimpaired ribonucleic acid synthesis.

Blood cell measurements

Pancytopenia is present, with MCV greater than 100 femtoliters and a decreased reticulocyte count.

Morphology

Oval macrocytes are seen, poikilocytosis is often marked, and polymorphonuclear leukocytes have hypersegmented nuclei, that is, greater than five lobes (often an early finding preceding red cell changes) (Figure 4-1).

BONE MARROW

Bone marrow is hypercellular with marked erythroid hyperplasia and with megaloblastic erythropoiesis characterized by red cell precursors that show a fine primitive nuclear pattern persisting alongside a relatively mature cytoplasm with some degree of orthochromia. Giant bands and metamyelocytes and large megakaryocytes are also present.

56

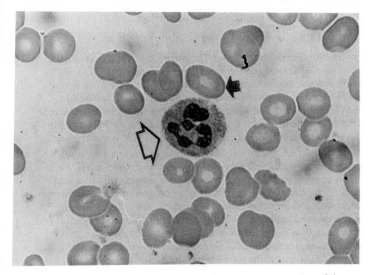

Figure 4-1. Polymorphonuclear leukocyte with hypersegmentation of the nucleus (open arrow) and oval macrocyte (solid arrow) in a case of PA.

Other Useful Tests

B$_{12}$ AND FOLATE BLOOD DETERMINATIONS

Purpose

Blood levels of B$_{12}$ and folate can provide valuable and rapid confirmation of the etiology of a megaloblastic anemia (1, 2).

Principle

Traditional test methods are microbiologic assays that depend on B$_{12}$ or folate growth requirements of a test organism. Antibiotics interfere with these assays. More recent procedures that are more rapid and do not show antibiotic interference are radioassays based on competitive protein-binding principles.

Procedure

The microbiologic assay for B$_{12}$ uses either *Euglena gracilis* or *Lactobacillus leishmanii* as the test organism, and the assay for

Table 4-4. Peripheral Blood Findings in Macrocytic Anemias

Type of Finding	Megaloblastic Anemia (Folate or B_{12} Deficiency or Metabolic Block)	Nonmegaloblastic Macrocytic Anemia[a]		
		Due to Accelerated Erythropoiesis (Acute Posthemorrhagic Anemia; Hemolytic Anemia)	Etiology Unknown	
			Myelofibrosis with Myeloid Metaplasia	Chronic Liver Disease; Hypothyroidism
Red cell morphology	Oval macrocytes, poikilocytosis	Round macrocytes, no poikilocytosis	Oval macrocytes, poikilocytosis	Round macrocytes, no poikilocytosis
White cell morphology	Hypersegmented polymorphonuclear leukocytes	Normal or left shift	Normal or variable number of immature neutrophils	Normal
White cell count	Decreased	Normal or elevated—under 30,000	Decreased or elevated to counts of 50,000	Normal, may be decreased in liver disease
Platelet count	Decreased	Normal or elevated	Low, normal, or elevated	Normal
Reticulocyte count	Decreased	Normal or elevated	Normal, decreased, or slightly elevated (e.g., 3%)	Normal or decreased

[a]This group of disorders does not always present with macrocytic anemia; the anemia may be normocytic.

folate uses *Lactobacillus casei*. Radioassay for B_{12} depends on the competition of the patient's serum and ^{57}Co-labeled B_{12} for the binder, intrinsic factor. Test methods for folate use the radioisotope ^{125}I or ^{3}H and a folate binder found in milk.

Red cell folate requires measurements of folate levels in whole blood and in serum and determination of the packet cell volume (PCV). A hemolysate is prepared for the whole blood assay by making a 1:21 dilution of whole blood in a 1% ascorbic acid solution. Red cell folate is then calculated by the formula:

$$\text{Red cell folate } (\mu g/l \text{ cells}) = \frac{\text{whole blood folate} - \left[\text{serum folate} \times \left(1 - \dfrac{PCV}{100} \right) \right]}{\dfrac{PCV}{100}}$$

Specimen

Vitamin B_{12} is measured in the serum. Folate is measured in serum and hemolysate, and red cell folate is calculated from the measurements.

Interpretation

Representative normal values by radioisotope techniques (Table 4-5) are somewhat higher than those obtained by microbiologic assay. A representative lower normal limit for serum B_{12} by the microbiologic assay is 160 ng/l and for red cell folate, 166 $\mu g/l$. The stated normal range for serum folate is the same by both techniques. Because serum levels of folate can change abruptly with changes in diet, red cell folate is a better index of tissue folate stores, and both serum and red cell folate are measured.

As indicated in Table 4-5, because B_{12} and folate levels show certain patterns in combination and occasionally overlap in each of the two deficiency states, both determinations are ordinarily performed in a given case. In typical B_{12} deficiency, serum B_{12} is less than 100 ng/l, and levels of RBC folate may be decreased with serum folate at normal to elevated levels. The discrepancy between

Table 4-5. **B_{12} and Folate Levels in Healthy and Deficient Subjects[a]**

Subject	B_{12} Serum ($\mu g/l$)	Folate	
		Serum ($\mu g/l$)	Red cells ($\mu g/l$)
Healthy subjects	300–900	5–21	200–700
B_{12} deficiency	< 200	> 3 > 21 in 25% of cases	< 140–400
Folate deficiency	> 200 in 90% of cases	< 3	< 140

[a]Values given are representative for radioisotope techniques. Somewhat lower levels are obtained with microbiologic assays.

the two folate values is attributable to a block in transfer of folate from the serum to the red cells in B_{12} deficiency. The usual folate deficiency shows low serum and red cell folates with normal B_{12} levels, but occasionally serum B_{12} may also be depressed.

Notes and precautions

In the case of serum folate, inadvertent hemolysis before separation of serum from the clot causes a false elevation of the test value.

More extensive use of the radioisotope assay for B_{12} has revealed technical problems that result in higher values for serum cobalamin than the true values (3, 4). In fact, an estimated 20% of patients with B_{12} deficiency may have been misdiagnosed as having normal B_{12} levels with the radioisotope assay. On the average, only 29% of the binders in commercial assay kits consist of intrinsic factor. The remainder consist of a protein referred to as R protein that binds with biologically inactive cobalamin analogs as well as true cobalamin in human plasma. New kits appear to have resolved this problem by use of an agent that blocks the nonspecific binding by R proteins. Purified intrinsic factor binders are also being developed; intrinsic factor is a highly specific binder for the biologically active cobalamin.

GASTRIC ANALYSIS FOR HYDROCHLORIC ACID (HCL)—THE AUGMENTED HISTALOG TEST

Purpose

Achlorhydria is an essential element for the diagnosis of adult PA. It reflects the gastric atrophy found in this condition (5). Gastric HCl is found only in a rare inherited childhood variant of PA.

Principle

Modern tests use maximal doses of either histamine or betazole hydrochloride (Histalog) to stimulate gastric secretion, and the pH is measured with a pH meter. The augmented Histalog test has replaced the test with histamine in many institutions because the cardiovascular side effects of histamine, such as hypotension tachycardia, are minimal or absent with Histalog.

Procedure

After an overnight fast, the patient is intubated with a nasogastric tube and the stomach contents are aspirated by continuous suction. After 15 minutes, Histalog is injected intramuscularly in a dose of 1.7 mg/kg. Fractional samples are collected over the ensuing two hours and their acidity is determined by a pH meter.

Specimen

Specimens of the gastric aspirant are collected every 15 minutes.

Interpretation

Achlorhydria is defined as a gastric secretion with a pH persistently above 3.5 that fails to fall more than 1.0 unit with maximal stimulation by histamine or Histalog. A less acceptable term used in some standard texts is that of anacidity, which defines the critical pH as 6.0.

When earlier techniques for assaying gastric acid were employed using submaximal stimulation and relying on the relatively insensitive color change seen with Töpfer's reagent to determine the presence of HCl or free acid, the finding of achlorhydria was fairly common in healthy persons and especially in aging individuals. With modern tests, such as the augmented Histalog test, such "physiologic" achlorhydria is rare regardless of the patient's age, and the only disease state other than PA in which achlorhydria occurs with any regularity is gastric carcinoma. *The presence of HCl rules out the diagnosis of adult PA.*

Notes and precautions

Histalog can cause allergic reactions such as urticaria and acute asthma and is therefore contraindicated in allergic individuals. Although the augmented Histalog test is generally well tolerated, as with all manipulations it is best delayed in a severely anemic, elderly patient. If necessary, testing for achlorhydria can be accomplished after the inception of therapy since achlorhydria in PA is irreversible.

TEST OF B_{12} ABSORPTION—THE SCHILLING TEST

Purpose

The Schilling test is used to measure B_{12} absorption (6). If absorption is found to be impaired, the test is used to determine whether malabsorption is caused by a lack of intrinsic factor, as found in PA, or by direct interference with intestinal absorption, as seen in diseases that have a primary effect on the small bowel.

Principle

A small physiologic oral dose of radioactive B_{12} is administered, followed by a large parenteral flushing dose of nonlabeled or cold B_{12}, and the amount of labeled B_{12} excreted in the urine is measured over a 24-hour period. The parenteral flushing dose of cold B_{12} is administered to saturate B_{12} binding sites, thereby leading to urinary excretion of absorbed, labeled B_{12}, which would otherwise be retained. If the results indicate diminished absorption of B_{12}, the test is repeated with intrinsic factor given with the oral dose of radioactive B_{12}. Correction of the test results to normal by intrinsic factor correlates with the diagnosis of PA, whereas failure to correct it is in keeping with intestinal malabsorption.

Procedure

The most commonly used isotopes for labeling B_{12} are ^{57}Co and ^{58}Co. At zero hour the patient empties the bladder, ingests 0.5–2.0 µg of the labeled vitamin, and begins the 24-hour urine collection. Two hours later, 1000 µg cold B_{12} is injected intramuscularly. If the 24-hour urinary excretion of labeled B_{12} is below normal no less than three days after the test is completed, it is repeated, with the addition of an active intrinsic factor preparation to the oral dose of labeled B_{12}. Excretion of labeled B_{12} is again determined by measuring radioactivity of the 24-hour urine specimen.

Interpretation

Representative values for the Schilling test in healthy subjects and in those with PA and intestinal malabsorption are given in Table 4-6. Various techniques call for administration of 0.5–2.0 µg labeled B_{12}. The percent excretion varies inversely with the dose. With a test dose of less than 1.0 µg, the normal 24-hour excretion is generally greater than 7% of the test dose. In PA, B_{12} absorption is markedly reduced and is corrected toward normal when intrinsic factor is administered with the oral B_{12}. (The values shown for PA in Table 4-6 represent 60 subjects, 90% of whom excreted less than 4% of the test dose.) Excretion is usually reduced to a lesser degree in intestinal malabsorption and intrinsic factor has no effect.

Notes and precautions

The major source of error in test performance is incomplete urine collection. Results are invalidated by impaired renal function, which causes delayed renal excretion of B_{12}. When the diagnosis of PA is a strong likelihood, it is best not to perform the

Table 4-6. Schilling Urinary Excretion Test of B$_{12}$ Absorption

	Urinary Excretion of Radioactive B$_{12}$[a] (%)	
Condition	Oral B$_{12}$ Alone[b]	Oral B$_{12}$ with Intrinsic Factor[b]
Normal	20.8 (10.7–35.5)	
PA	2.2 (0–6.9)	15.0 (8–27.2)
Intestinal malabsorption	5.0 (3.8–7.0)	4.5 (1.3–6.7)

[a]B$_{12}$ dose, 0.66 μg.
[b]Mean values with range in parentheses.

Schilling test before an adequate period of B$_{12}$ therapy. Sufficient intestinal malabsorption develops in some patients with untreated PA to cause a blunted rise in excretion when the test is performed with intrinsic factor. Furthermore, the large parenteral flushing dose of B$_{12}$ eliminates the possibility of a therapeutic future trial.

LACTIC DEHYDROGENASE (LDH)

Purpose

Although serum LDH is not needed to diagnose an obvious megaloblastic anemia, the test can be helpful in the differential diagnosis of an obscure macrocytic anemia and can be used as ancillary evidence for response to therapy in a megaloblastic anemia.

Principle

Lactic dehydrogenase reversibly catalyzes the oxidation of lactic acid, with simultaneous reduction of nicotinamide-adenine dinucleotide (NAD) forming reduced nicotinamide-adenine dinucleotide (NADH) and pyruvate. The rate of increase in absorbance at 340 nm is directly proportional to the LDH activity when all other reactants are present in quantities that are not rate limiting.

$$\text{Lactic acid} + \text{NAD} \underset{}{\overset{\text{LDH}}{\rightleftharpoons}} \text{pyruvic acid} + \text{NADH}$$

NAD is nonabsorbing at 340 nm and NADH absorbs at 340 nm.

Lactic dehydrogenase is found in nearly all tissues. Those with particularly high levels of the enzyme include the red cells, heart, liver, and skeletal muscle. Each of these tissues has a characteristic LDH isoenzyme pattern. Lactic dehydrogenase consists of five isoenzymes based on electrophoretic mobility. The fraction with the greatest mobility (anodic) is called LDH_1 and that with the least anodic mobility is LDH_5. In disease states, the LDH isoenzyme pattern of the serum reflects that of the diseased tissue. Lactic dehydrogenase isoenzymes of erythrocytes are largely LDH_1 and LDH_2.

Procedure

Well-established and standardized spectrophotometric manual and automated methods that are available to routine laboratories are based on the principles previously described. Lactic dehydrogenase isoenzyme determinations are becoming widely available because of their particular usefulness in the diagnosis of myocardial infarction.

Specimen

Serum or heparinized plasma are acceptable (see also Chapter 5) for use as specimens.

Interpretation

The normal range is 95–200 U/l (international units) or 205–425 W/L units/ml (Wroblewski-LaDue). Serum LDH is markedly elevated in untreated megaloblastic anemia (Table 4-7). The only disease state that may be associated with elevations of the same magnitude is disseminated carcinomatosis because of widespread tissue destruction.

As shown in Table 4-7, in an obscure macrocytic anemia, serum LDH can help to differentiate megaloblastic anemia from other anemias. Although some rise in LDH is seen with hemolytic anemias, the values do not approach those ordinarily seen in

Table 4-7. Serum Lactic Dehydrogenase in Macrocytic Anemias[a]

Megaloblastic anemia	4–50 times normal	1200–7500 U/l (2500–15,000 W/L μ/ml)
Hemolytic anemia	1–4 times normal	300–1200 U/l (500–2500 W/L μ/ml)
Other macrocytic anemias	Normal	95–200 U/l (205–425 W/L μ/ml)

[a]U/l = international units; W/L = Wroblewski–LaDue units.

megaloblastic anemia. In the case of megaloblastic anemia with a relatively moderate rise in LDH, additional diagnostic help can be obtained from LDH isoenzymes. In the megaloblast and in serum of megaloblastic anemia, LDH_1 is greater than LDH_2 (7). Serum LDH returns to normal levels about two weeks after inception of appropriate therapy in a case of megaloblastic anemia.

Notes and precautions

Hemolyzed serum results in spurious elevation of LDH and serum should be separated from the clot as soon as possible.

RESPONSE TO THERAPY

Therapy of megaloblastic anemia must sometimes be started before adequate laboratory confirmation of etiology (8). In combined B_{12} and folate deficiencies as seen in intestinal malabsorption, etiology may be difficult to ascertain. Even an established case of PA may be complicated by other disease, such as infection, or by an inapparent iron deficiency resulting in an inadequate response to B_{12} therapy. Therefore, initial therapy in megaloblastic anemia should always be regarded as a therapeutic trial.

Table 4-8. The Relation of Peak Reticulocyte Count to the Degree of Anemia in Patients with Pernicious Anemia Treated with B_{12}[a]

Initial Red Cell Count (Cells $\times 10^{12}/1$)	Reticulocytes at Peak (%)
1.0	50–70
1.0–1.4	36–47
1.5–1.9	25–34
2.0–2.4	15–22
2.5–2.9	10–16
3.0–3.6	4–9

[a]Data from Chanarin I: *The Megaloblastic Anemias.* Philadelphia, F. A. Davis, 1969.

The earliest hematologic change, the resumption of normoblastic erythropoiesis, is completed within 72 hours of the inception of appropriate therapy. The most useful early parameter is the reticulocyte count, which peaks within the first 7–10 days. The magnitude of the peak response is proportional to the severity of the anemia (Table 4-8). Reticulocyte counts must be performed daily during this period since, if performed less frequently, the peak level is easily missed. Blood counts are taken initially every three days; they return to normal in approximately six weeks. Levels of LDH return to normal about two weeks after inception of appropriate therapy.

Because of the close interrelationship between B_{12} and folate, a therapeutic dose of either agent produces a significant hematologic response in a deficiency of the other. Therefore, therapy in megaloblastic anemia should consist of physiologic doses of B_{12} or folic acid parenterally for the first 10 days. The daily dose should not exceed 10 μg for B_{12} or 200 μg for folic acid.

REFERENCES

1. Mollin DL, Anderson BB, Burman JF: The serum vitamin B_{12} level: its assay and significance. Clin Hematol 5:521–546, 1976

2. Rothenberg SP, Da Costa M: Folate binding proteins and radioassay for folate. Clin Hematol 5:569–587, 1976

3. Kolhouse FJ, Kondo H, Allen NC, et al: Cobalamin analogues are present in human plasma and can mask cobalamin deficiency because radio isotope dilution assays are not specific for true cobalamin. N Engl J Med 299:785–792, 1978

4. Cooper BA, Whitehead VM: Evidence that some patients with pernicious anemia are not recognized by radio dilution assay for cobalamin in serum. N Engl J Med 299:816–818, 1978

5. Cannon, DC: Examination of gastric and duodenal contents. In Davidsohn I, Henry JB (eds): *Todd-Sanford Clinical Diagnosis by Laboratory Methods*, ed 15. Philadelphia, W. B. Saunders Co, 1974, pp 887–904

6. Maslow WC, Donnelly WJ, Koppel DM, et al: Observations on the use of Co^{60} labeled vitamin B_{12} in the urinary excretion test: Clinical implications of the radioisotope technique. Acta Haematol 18:137–147, 1957

7. Winston RM, Warburton FG, Stott A: Enzymatic diagnosis of megaloblastic anemia. Br J Haematol 19:587–592, 1970

8. Herbert V: Megaloblastic anemias—mechanisms and management: Clinical differential diagnosis; therapeutic trial. DM (Aug) 1965, pp 19–23

chapter 5

Disorders Associated with Accelerated Erythrocyte Turnover

Accelerated erythrocyte turnover in the absence of blood loss is a characteristic of hemolysis. A wide variety of hereditary and acquired diseases associated with hemolysis (Table 5-1) will be discussed in succeeding chapters. In general, diagnosis of hemolysis requires evaluation of the various phases of erythrocyte turnover (Figure 5-1), including bone marrow production phase, circulating phase, and final removal of senescent or damaged cells. Although the actual mechanisms for each phase are not known, their sequence and elapsed time have been determined allowing normal ranges to be established.

Erythropoiesis derives from a marrow stem cell that requires approximately five days to progress from erythroblast to marrow reticulocyte. The daily production of red cells is estimated at 3×10^9 cells/kg and normally equals the rate of red cell destruction (1%/day). Marrow reticulocytes expel the nucleus as they pass through marrow sinusoids into the peripheral blood to become circulating reticulocytes, subsequently requiring one or two days to shed the reticular network to become mature erythrocytes. The spleen briefly sequesters a small percentage of reticulocytes and then rereleases them into the circulation. Mature red cells circulate for 120 days and are finally sequestered in the spleen by unknown mechanisms. Splenomegaly, therefore, would be expected to alter red cell circulation

Table 5-1. **Diseases of Accelerated Erythrocyte Turnover**

Etiologic Basis of Hemolysis	Classification of Disorder	Cause of Disorder
Hereditary	Red cell membrane defects	Hereditary spherocytosis, hereditary elliptocytosis
	Red cell enzyme defects	Glucose-6-phosphate dehydrogenase (G-6-PD) deficiency
		Pyruvate kinase deficiency
		Glutathione stabilizing enzyme deficiency
		Other deficiencies of the pentose pathway
	Red cell hemoglobin defects	Amino acid substitutions: HbS, HbC, etc.
		Alpha-chain production defects: alpha thalassemia, HbH
		Beta-chain production defects: beta thalassemia
Acquired	Infection	Bacterial: *Clostridium perfringens*
		Protozoal: malaria
		Viral: immune mechanisms—mycoplasma, infectious mononucleosis
	Physicochemical	Burns
		Benzene derivatives
	Mechanical	Heart valve prosthesis (aortic)
		Ulcerative colitis

Table 5-1. **Diseases of Accelerated Erythrocyte Turnover** (*Continued*)

Etiologic Basis of Hemolysis	Classification of Disorder	Cause of Disorder
Acquired		Hemolytic—uremic syndrome
		Disseminated intravascular coagulation
	Drugs	Interaction with G-6-PD deficiency
		Immune complexes
	Antibody	Alloantibody: incompatible transfusion; erythroblastosis fetalis
		Autoantibody: idiopathic, secondary to lymphocytic neoplasms, associated with collagen diseases, associated with viral infection, secondary to drugs
	Membrane defects	Paroxysmal nocturnal hemoglobinuria

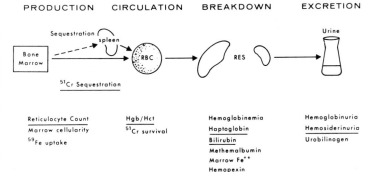

Figure 5-1. Laboratory evaluation of phases of red cell production and breakdown. The most useful tests for each function are underlined.

and survival. Red cells with defective membranes or with membranes damaged by physicochemical or immune mechanisms are removed more rapidly than normal by the spleen as well as by the other parts of the reticuloendothelial (RE) system including Kupffer's cells in liver sinusoids. The spleen removes marginally damaged red cells, the liver removes more severely damaged red cells, and intravascular hemolysis occurs with the most severe cell damage. There are a limited number of conditions so damaging to the red cell as to cause almost certain intravascular hemolysis. Commonly encountered causes are summarized in Table 5-2.

Red cell destruction releases heme, globin, and iron. Heme is broken down into biliverdin, reduced to bilirubin by biliverdin reductase in the reticuloendothelial system, conjugated to soluble mono- and diglucuronides in the liver, and excreted in the feces as urobilin, urobilinogen, and stercobilinogen. Minimal amounts of the soluble urobilinogen are reabsorbed from the portal circulation and excreted in the urine. Heme iron is taken up by the reticuloendothelial cells and reappears in marrow synthesis of new red cells or is stored in the reticuloendothelial cells as ferritin or hemosiderin. The globin peptide chains are degraded to component amino acids that return to the metabolic pool. Accelerated red cell turnover results in increased amounts of all breakdown products, many of which can be measured with relative ease.

When intravascular hemolysis occurs, free hemoglobin (Hb) is released into the bloodstream; it is bound by the alpha$_2$ globulin, haptoglobin (Hp). The Hp:Hb complex is then metabolized directly by the reticuloendothelial system. If the binding capacity of haptoglobin is exceeded, hemoglobinuria results. Other plasma proteins that bind free hemoglobin include transferrin and albumin. Oxidation of the ferrous ion of the albumin-heme complexes produces the brown pigment, methemalbumin.

DIAGNOSTIC EVALUATION

Accelerated erythrocyte turnover can be determined by evaluation of marrow production, calculation of circulating red cell survival, and measurement of breakdown products of cell destruction. Increased marrow production is estimated by the following:

1. Hematologic findings, which categorize the anemia by red cell indices as normochromic and establish accelerated release to the peripheral blood with the reticulocyte count. Bone marrow aspiration that includes stains for marrow iron is useful in documenting accelerated marrow erythroid production and breakdown. Where the cause of a normochromic anemia is clearly hemolysis (e.g., in hemoglobinopathies), marrow aspirate may be unnecessary.

2. Plasma and urinary pigments. With increased destruction of red cells, levels of each of the degradation products increase and can be measured. Breakdown products commonly measured in acute hemolysis are bilirubin, total and fractionated, and plasma and urine hemoglobin. In less acute or chronic compensated hemolysis, urine hemosiderin and serum methemalbumin measure long-term red cell degradation. Determination of bilirubin in compensated hemolytic anemia is of limited usefulness. Increased plasma bilirubin increases fecal pigments but tests for urobilin and fecal urobilinogen are unsatisfactory and unnecessary. Urine urobilinogen, which is increased in hemolysis, is also increased in ineffective erythropoiesis and in liver disease, and, therefore, the test for this substance is now outmoded (Table 5-3).

3. Serum haptoglobin, which is easily measured, is a useful test in the absence of intravascular hemolysis when its consumption would be immediately predictable.

4. Radioisotope tracer studies, which are usually limited to ^{51}chromium (^{51}Cr), which estimates survival of circulating red cells and site of cell sequestration and destruction, and to ^{59}iron (^{59}Fe), which is incorporated into precursor erythrocytes and evaluates rate of production, site of production, rate of red cell release, and site of sequestration. ^{51}Chromium red cell survival studies are not always available or necessary. They are helpful in quantitating rate of accelerated turnover ($T^{1/2}$ or half-life) and they may be of use in evaluating therapy. Testing requires three weeks but abbreviated tests of one hour are also performed. Tests for ^{51}Cr red cell survival can include sequestration studies to determine the site of red cell destruction, which is helpful in evaluating the potential benefit of splenectomy.

5. Ferrokinetics (^{59}Fe), a test that is not commonly available, is used to evaluate red cell turnover as a function of iron incorporation into heme. It should be combined with sequestration studies to determine

Table 5-2. Causes of Intravascular Hemolysis[a] and Diagnostic Tests for Identification

Disease	Mechanism	Diagnostic Test
Antibody		
Alloantibody		
ABO incompatible transfusion	Anti-A, anti-B	Recheck blood groups and clerical work
Anti-Kidd (anti-Jk[a])	Delayed hemolysis	Antibody screening with enzyme-treated red cells
Anti-Kell, anti-Duffy[a], anti-Lewis[a]	Current transfusion	Antibody screen
Antipenicillin	IgG antibody	DAT; test vs. drug-treated red cells
Autoantibody—cold autoimmune hemolytic anemia (mycoplasma)	Anti-I	Cold agglutinin titer; DAT
Infections		
Clostridium perfringens	Hemolysin	Blood cultures
Escherichia coli sepsis	Hemolysin	Wound cultures
Cholera	Hemolysin	Stool cultures
Malaria	Mechanical	RBC smear

Inherited RBC defects		
Glucose-6-phosphate dehydrogenase (G-6-PD) deficiency	Drug interaction	G-6-PD assay
Hemoglobinurias		
Paroxysmal nocturnal hemoglobinuria (PNH)	C' sensitive RBC membrane	Acid hemolysis sucrose lysis
Paroxysmal cold hemoglobinuria (PCH)	IgG antibody	Donath-Landsteiner test
Physicochemical agents		
Third-degree burns	Heat damage to red cell membrane	Red cell morphology
Prosthetic valves	Mechanical	Red cell morphology
Cardiac bypass surgery	Mechanical	Pump-hemoglobin
Distilled water-prostate resection	Osmotic hemolysis	Urine sediment
Snake bites	Lecithinase	History

[a]Causes that are most likely to be encountered, not single case reports.

75

Table 5-3. Urine and Serum Pigments in Accelerated Red Cell Turnover

Pigment	Normal Range	Significance
Bilirubin, serum	0.5–2.0 mg/dl	Limited; in nonjaundiced patients, < 3.0 mg/dl; in jaundiced patients fractionation may not be diagnostic
Indirect bilirubin, serum	< 0.5 mg/dl	Increased early in hemolysis
		Nonhemolytic elevation in hereditary disorders of conjugation (Crigler-Najjar syndrome, Gilbert's disease)
Hemoglobin, plasma	≤ 10 mg/dl	Significant above 50 mg/dl
		Cherry-red plasma > 150 mg/dl
		Binds to haptoglobin transferrin, or albumin
Hemoglobin, urine	None present	Appears after haptoglobin saturation
		Hematuria must be excluded
		Myoglobinuria gives false-positive dip-stick test
Methemalbumin, serum	None present	Qualitative determination in haptoglobin electrophoresis
		Spectrophotometric qualitative test (Schumm test) less readily available
Hemopexin	80–100 mg/dl	Radial immune diffusion measurement
		Not readily available and requires 24–28 hours
Urobilinogen, fecal or urine		No longer used
Urobilin, fecal		Not used

sites of production, marrow or extramedullary, and is helpful if splenectomy is being considered. This study requires three to four weeks. Since ^{59}Fe has a longer half-life than ^{51}Cr, ^{59}Fe studies should follow chromium studies.

6. Ancillary screening tests, as summarized in Table 5-4, are used to document the cause of accelerated erythrocyte turnover once its presence has been established. These tests are discussed at greater length in subsequent chapters.

LABORATORY STUDIES

Hematologic Tests

GENERAL FEATURES

Increased red cell turnover stimulates increased marrow production and leads to premature release of marrow reticulocytes before they are stripped of nuclear fragments or their reticular network. These cells are seen on Wright-stained peripheral smears as polychromatophilic macrocytes. Nucleated red cells may also be seen. With a competent bone marrow, the reticulocyte count is persistently elevated, differing from acute blood loss, in which reticulocytosis is of brief duration and usually less than 5%. Reticulocytosis varies with severity and duration of hemolysis. Marrow turnover may increase four to six times permitting reticulocyte counts as high as 60%–70%. Chronic hemolysis may deplete marrow levels of folic acid, diminishing production so that reticulocytosis is inadequate for the degree of hemolysis.

The spleen may be enlarged as a result of increased phagocytosis and in some cases, particularly hereditary hemolytic anemias, the liver is also enlarged. Depending on the rate of red cell destruction and the ability of the liver to conjugate and excrete the degradation products, variable degrees of jaundice may be present.

PERIPHERAL BLOOD

Blood cell measurements

Anemia can be severe (Hb 2 g/dl) to mild (Hb 11.5 g/dl). Mean corpuscular volume (MCV) is 80–110μ; reticulocytes produce a mild macrocytosis. MCV greater than 115μ suggests macrocytic

Table 5-4. Common Screening Tests for Causes of Accelerated Erythrocyte Turnover

Etiologic Basis of Hemolysis	Classification of Disorder	Test
Hereditary	Red cell membrane defects	Red cell morphology, osmotic fragility
	Red cell enzyme defects	Glucose-6-phosphate dehydrogenase (G-6-PD) screening, pyruvate kinase screening tests
	Red cell hemoglobin defects	Hemoglobin electrophoresis, Heinz body test, HbA_2 and HbF quantitation
Acquired	Infection—protozoal	Red cell morphology, malarial smears
	Physicochemical—burns	Red cell morphology—spherocytes
	Mechanical—intravascular fibrin, prosthetic valves	Red cell morphology—fragments
	Drugs—interaction with enzyme defect	G-6-PD screening
	Antibody	
	Alloantibody or autoantibody	Direct antiglobulin test
		Serum antibody screening; cold agglutinin titer, Donath-Landsteiner test
	Drug-induced antibody	Antibody screening with drug-treated cells
	Miscellaneous membrane defects—PNH	Acid hemolysis test or sucrose lysis test

anemia or, rarely, secondary folate depletion. MCV less than 70μ in a normochromic anemia suggests hemolysis is due to hemoglobinopathy or paroxysmal nocturnal hemoglobinuria (PNH).

Morphology

Morphology generally includes polychromatophilia, macrocytes, and nucleated red cells. Specific morphology is variable depending on etiology or red cell turnover:

1. Spherocytes—hereditary spherocytosis, autoimmune hemolytic anemia.
2. Target cells—hemoglobinopathies, jaundice, postsplenectomy.
3. Cell fragments—hemolytic uremic syndrome, disseminated intravascular coagulation (DIC), prosthetic valves.
4. Microspherocytes—HbC disease, ABO erythroblastosis, burns.

BONE MARROW

Bone marrow is hypercellular with marked normoblastic erythroid hyperplasia reversing the M/E ratio from the normal 3:1 or 4:1 to 1:2. Dyssynchronous nuclear and cytoplasmic maturation creates "megaloblastoid" cells without giant metamyelocytes or other stigmata of megaloblastic dyscrasias. If folic acid or vitamin B_{12} are relatively depleted by prolonged rapid turnover, a true megaloblastic cell population may appear; marrow exhaustion with aplasia can eventually result. Special staining of particle smears with ferroferricyanide (Prussian blue) shows increased iron in marrow histiocytes, termed marrow siderosis. Stainable iron seen in mitochondria of orthochromic normoblasts produces a ring effect present only when ineffective erythropoiesis is present. In hemolysis if normoblasts contain granules they are larger and cover the nucleus. Absence of stainable iron in hemolysis suggests PNH.

Other Useful Tests

SERUM BILIRUBIN, TOTAL AND FRACTIONATED

Purpose

Increases in indirect bilirubin in the jaundiced patient support the diagnosis of hemolysis (1).

Principle

Hyperbilirubinemia indicates increased red cell destruction, failure of liver conjugation, or block of excretory pathways. In hemolysis, an increased bilirubin load is presented to the liver faster than conjugation can proceed so that non-water-soluble (indirect) fraction of bilirubin is increased. In liver failure or obstructive jaundice, conjugation does occur, and hyperbilirubinemia is predominantly direct.

Procedure

Bilirubin is measured by an internationally standardized test generally using the Evelyn-Malloy method or a modification. Bilirubin is coupled with a diazo dye and the color is quantitated spectrophotometrically at one minute. The quick reacting fraction is considered to be conjugated or direct bilirubin. The total bilirubin is measured after the addition of alcohol, and the indirect fraction is calculated by subtracting the amount of direct bilirubin from the total.

Interpretation

Normal ranges for total bilirubin are 0–1.5 mg/dl, and for indirect bilirubin, less than 0.3 mg/dl. Levels of total bilirubin above 2.5 mg/dl are usually associated with clinical jaundice. The level depends on the ability of the liver to compensate. Initially more than half the bilirubin will be indirect or unconjugated fraction. If liver function is adequate, after several days the rate of glucuronide conjugation is increased so that direct and indirect fractions are nearly equal, and bilirubin fractionation is no longer diagnostic.

In well-compensated hemolytic anemia, levels of total bilirubin may be less than 3 mg/dl and no clinical jaundice is seen. Thus, bilirubin levels should not be used to exclude the diagnosis of accelerated red cell turnover.

In hemolytic disease of the newborn, lipid-soluble, indirect-fraction bilirubin is deposited in the striate nucleus producing kernicterus. In the newborn, a shift in conjugation from indirect to direct bilirubin usually occurs at 7–10 days as liver function matures.

Notes and precautions

Misleading elevations of indirect bilirubin can be seen in hereditary disorders of conjugation (Crigler-Najjar syndrome, Gilbert's disease) and secondary to steroids found in breast milk that interfere with conjugation of bilirubin.

PLASMA, HEMOGLOBIN

Purpose

Qualitative assessment of plasma hemoglobin is usually satisfactory in acute intravascular hemolysis (1). Quantitation is useful in sera where other pigments (e.g., bilirubin) make interpretation of plasma color uncertain.

Principle

Massive red cell injury results in intravascular hemolysis, seen macroscopically as cherry-red plasma. Free hemoglobin can be quantitated by a modified benzidine reaction.

Procedure

A modified benzidine reaction oxidizes a colorless dye to blue in the presence of hemoglobin, as shown in the following reactions:

1. $Hb\text{-}Fe^{++} + 2H_2O_2 \longrightarrow Hb\text{-}Fe^{+++} + O_2 + 2H_2O$

2. $O_2 + \underset{\text{(colorless)}}{\text{benzidine}} \longrightarrow \underset{\text{(blue)}}{\text{benzidine}}$

The color is measured spectrophotometrically. The test lacks accuracy below 30 mg/dl but free hemoglobin at that level is not clinically important; the method also measures methemalbumin. Quantitation is not available in all hospital laboratories.

Specimen

Five milliliters of blood is collected in heparin or EDTA rather than a clot to prevent mechanical hemolysis of red cells during clot formation, allowing more accurate measurement. Blood must be drawn atraumatically and plasma should be separated within one to two hours.

Interpretation

The normal level of plasma hemoglobin is less than 10 mg/dl. At low levels test variability is great, and, thus, the test is only reliable above 50 mg/dl, which is the threshold for visual estimation. Free hemoglobin levels less than 30 mg/dl are technically inaccurate, and may be seen with difficult venapuncture, mechanical destruction of red cells by vacutainer tubes, or during clotting of specimen. Hemoglobinemia above 150 mg/dl results in hemoglobinuria. At levels above 200 mg/dl plasma becomes clear cherry red.

Notes and precautions

Orthotolidine (o-tolidine) is substituted for benzidine as a result of federal regulations controlling potentially carcinogenic agents.

OTHER SERUM PIGMENTS—METHEMALBUMIN, HEMOPEXIN

Purpose

The presence of hemoglobin degradation products corroborates the diagnosis of hemolysis (2, 3). Their presence usually indicates chronic or continuing hemolysis.

Principle

Free hemoglobin dissociates into $\alpha\beta$ dimers, which bind to plasma proteins, haptoglobin, transferrin, and albumin. Ferrous iron of hemoglobin bound to albumin oxidizes to ferric iron of methemalbumin giving a distinctive rusty appearance to serum. Free hemoglobin in the presence of chloride ion produces hematin, which is bound by the protein hemopexin. Increases in methemalbumin or decreases in hemopexin imply hemolysis.

Procedure

Methemalbumin is qualitated during measurement of haptoglobin using electrophoresis on agar. It can also be qualitatively measured by the Schumm test, in which an intense chromogen of methemalbumin develops following the introduction of ammonium sulfide after the addition of ether. Quantitative measurement uses the shift in spectral bands of hemoglobin with the addition of sodium dithionite.

Quantitation of hemopexin is not generally available. It can be measured by radial immunodiffusion or qualitatively estimated by immunoelectrophoresis. It usually parallels levels of haptoglobin, but occasionally haptoglobin is normal while hemopexin is decreased (e.g., in thalassemia).

Specimen

Serum or plasma are satisfactory specimens.

Interpretation

Methemalbumin is not present in the normal patient; hemopexin has a normal range of 80–100 mg/dl. Methemalbumin clears within four or five days of the cessation of hemolysis. Levels of hemopexin less than 40 mg/dl indicate hemolysis.

URINE HEMOGLOBIN AND HEMOSIDERIN

Purpose

Hemoglobinuria indicates concurrent or recent hemoglobinemia above the excretion threshold of 150 mg/dl (1). It is usually seen as cloudy, smoky, dark-red, or cola-colored urine. In the absence of detectable hemoglobin, hemosiderin indicates ongoing hemolysis.

Principle

Qualitative analysis of free hemoglobin is made by peroxidase reaction of o-tolidine or benzidine, which produces a blue color. This reaction is the basis of Hemastix. Hemoglobin, even in undetectable hemolysis, deposits heme in renal epithelial cells, where it is oxidized to hemosiderin.

Procedure

Spectrophotometric assays of free hemoglobin are tedious and not generally available in hospital laboratories. Dip-stick tests and examination of the urine sediment for red cells are usually satisfactory to identify the pigment. Methodology for the dip-stick test is based on peroxidase reduction and conversion of o-tolidine to a blue color graded 0–3+. Hemosiderin is detected in urinary sediment with the Prussian-blue reaction.

Specimen

Fresh random urine is used. Urine that has been allowed to stand permits hemolysis of any red cells present, allowing hematuria to be confused with hemoglobinuria.

Interpretation

In the normal patient, no hemoglobin or hemosiderin is detectable. Other causes of a positive Hemastix reaction are hematuria or myoglobinuria. Urinary sediments that contain significant numbers of red cells usually produce some free hemoglobin in hypotonic or alkaline urines. Myoglobinuria cannot be distinguished from hemoglobinuria by Hemastix and is identified by electrophoresis (it migrates in hemoglobin C zone) or by solubility in 80% ammonium sulfate (hemoglobin precipitates). Hemosiderin granules must be intracellular to have significance.

Notes and precautions

Prussian-blue, positive granules can be seen in urinary sediments if distilled water is not used. The granules are not intracellular, however, in hemoglobinuria.

SERUM HAPTOGLOBIN

Purpose

Absence of haptoglobin indicates hemolysis, liver failure, or, rarely, an hereditary variant (1).

Haptoglobin is an alpha$_2$ globulin produced in the liver that binds free hemoglobin on a molecule-for-molecule basis. The entire Hp:Hb complex is metabolized in the reticuloendothelial system, a normal mechanism of regulating the renal threshold of hemoglobin. With intravascular hemolysis haptoglobin is completely saturated; excess hemoglobin is then bound by other serum proteins, hemopexin, transferrin, and albumin, before spilling into the urine as hemoglobinuria. Absence of haptoglobin implies saturation and degradation as in hemolysis, or, alternatively, failure of production (i.e., liver failure). Hp^o is a genetic variant found in some black individuals that does not bind hemoglobin; however, it is of no clinical significance.

Haptoglobin is an acute-phase reactant, increasing three to four times in inflammation, infection, or tissue necrosis (e.g., pneumonia or myocardial infarction). Such increases may mask increased binding of hemoglobin in hemolysis.

Procedure

Haptoglobin is usually measured by one of three techniques: semiquantitatively, by residual hemoglobin-binding capacity using electrophoresis on agar or cellulose membranes; quantitatively, by residual hemoglobin binding capacity measured spectrophotometrically; or by quantitation of antigen by radial immunodiffusion, a haptoglobin-antihaptoglobin immune precipitin reaction. Both spectrophotometric and electrophotometric measurements depend on development of blue color in modified benzidine reactions using H_2O_2–o-tolidine reduction by heme-Fe^{++}.

Electrophoretic evaluation is semiquantitative since the patient's serum, possibly with some binding of heme by haptoglobin already, is incubated with increasing amounts of a known hemoglobin solution (0, 25, 50, 100, and 200 mg/dl) until binding capacity is exceeded and heme binds to transferrin. After incubation of hemoglobin solutions and patient serum, the mixtures are inoculated on agar or cellulose and a short-term electrophoresis separates the plasma proteins into albumin and alpha$_1$, alpha$_2$, beta, and gamma globulins. The H_2O_2–o-tolidine dye reaction stains proteins bearing heme, permitting identification of bound haptoglobin, free or transferrin-bound hemoglobin, and methemalbumin. When haptoglobin residual binding capacity has been exceeded, a second zone of transferrin-bound heme appears, and haptoglobin is reported as the level at which residual binding capacity is exceeded. With increased destruction of red cells, haptoglobin is already saturated in vivo so that the transferrin band appears with the lowest concentrations of added heme.

Spectrophotometric methods quantitate color development based on the peroxidase reaction of Hb:Hp complexes after the addition of known concentrations of hemoglobin to the patient's serum. Radial immunodiffusion is slow requiring 24–48 hours to the end point of immune precipitation. Newer nephelometric techniques require minutes (macromolecular nephelometers) to hours (micromolecular or laser nephelometers).

Specimen

Fresh serum is obtained atraumatically. To avoid extraneous hemolysis serum should not be allowed to remain on red cells. Testing specimens with macroscopic hemoglobinemia is superfluous.

Interpretation

The normal range for haptoglobins is 40–180 mg/dl. Haptoglobin by electrophoresis is reported by zones. Less than 25 mg/dl of haptoglobin is consistent with hemolysis, while greater than 200 mg/dl is consistent with inflammation and not helpful in the diagnosis of hemolysis.

Spectrophotometric results may be falsely high if the serum contains peroxidases or other oxidants that increase development of color.

Molecular sites for hemoglobin binding are not those for antibody binding by antihaptoglobin. With radial immunodiffusion false elevations of haptoglobin may appear because haptoglobin

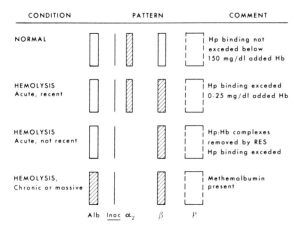

Figure 5-2. Schematic electrophoretic patterns of haptoglobin binding by electrophoresis.

bound to hemoglobin retains antigenic determinants for antibody. Thus saturated Hp:Hb complexes are also measured if they have not been removed by the reticuloendothelial system. This method is most useful in excluding Hp°. Electrophotometric methods permit visual identification of methemalbumin, free hemoglobin in untreated patient serum, and replacement by unbound hemoglobin in single-episode hemolysis (Figure 5-2).

Haptoglobin is decreased or absent in liver failure, after recent massive transfusion due to removal of senescent transfused red cells, and in some blacks who genetically lack binding sites on the haptoglobin molecule.

DIRECT ANTIGLOBULIN TEST (DAT)—DIRECT COOMBS TEST

Purpose

Detection of globulin adsorbed to the patient's red cells suggests immune mechanisms may be an underlying cause of hemolysis (1, 2) (see Chapter 14).

Principle

Antihuman globulin reagent produced in rabbits agglutinates human red cells that are coated with human globulin. Broad-spectrum reagents agglutinate cells coated both with gamma globulin (IgG, IgM) or beta globulin (complement).

Procedure

Patient red cells are centrifuged with antiglobulin reagent and agglutination is graded 0–4+. Adsorbed globulin must be eluted and tested for activity against red cells before it is classified as antibody.

Specimen

Using the red cells from EDTA specimens prevents nonspecific absorption of complement in specimens with strong but not pathologic cold agglutinins. Specimens must be maintained at 37 C until cells and serum have been separated.

Interpretation

Weakly positive results (±) are not usually clinically significant and eluates are usually not successful. Strongly positive tests (2–4+) due to antibody do not correlate with the degree of hemolysis. Common causes of nonantibody globulin attached to red cells are multiple myeloma and Keflin therapy.

A negative DAT does not exclude hemolysis if red cell destruction has been massive and complete, as in incompatible transfusions.

Notes and precautions

Refrigeration of blood specimens containing cold agglutinins causes false-positive results or exaggerates true positives by the resultant cold absorption of the agglutinin and complement.

RADIOACTIVE CHROMIUM SURVIVAL AND SEQUESTRATION

Purpose

Radioactive chromium survival and sequestration provides objective information regarding red cell survival and site of red cell destruction or sequestration (4).

Principle

Radioactive labels are attached to the patient's red cells (^{51}Cr) or incorporated into them at the time of synthesis (^{59}Fe). Radioactive labels have included DF^{32}P, ^{3}H, and ^{51}Cr to study red cell survival and sequestration. ^{59}Iron or glycine ^{14}C have been used to measure synthetic rate. These tests are not generally available except in hospitals with well-developed nuclear medicine departments. The two labels used most often are ^{51}Cr and ^{59}Fe. For ^{51}Cr several well-described protocols are available for tagging the cells, collecting the samples from the patient for counting, and plotting the counts against time. ^{59}Iron is used to determine plasma iron clearance and turnover, as well as red cell utilization and site of production.

Procedure

Red cells from the patient or from the potential donor unit are incubated with 50 μCi ^{51}Cr, which binds to the cell membrane and the beta chains of hemoglobin (4–6). Ascorbic acid oxidizes chromium to prevent further tagging and the labeled sample is injected into the patient. Serial blood samples of equal volume are drawn in the first 60 minutes for the abbreviated test, followed by frequent sampling during the first 48 hours and then over a three-week period for the complete test. Samples are counted and the counts are plotted against time so that a straight line is achieved on linear, semilog or log-log paper and the half-life is determined. ^{51}Chromium elutes from the red cell at a rate of 0.5%–1.2% daily, so that corrections derived from published charts are calculated before plotting (6). Beginning on day 2 and periodically over a 14-day period, external counting is performed over the patient's precordium, liver, and spleen to determine the site of red cell destruction.

Specimen

Counts can be made on whole blood samples collected in heparin or on the packed cells and plasma separately. The minimum volume is 3 ml with all specimens of equal volume for accurate counting.

Interpretation

[51]Chromium red cell survival has a normal half-life of 25–32 days, but each laboratory must determine its own normal range. For sequestration studies spleen:liver ratios are calculated. The normal range is 1.0–1.5, the range for hypersplenism is 1.5–2.0, for hemolytic anemia, greater than 3; and for hereditary spherocytosis, 4–5. Excessive sequestration in the liver suggests severe red cell damage either by the ^{51}Cr label or by complement lysis. Splenic sequestration occurs in hypersplenism or when red cells are marginally damaged as with IgG antibodies.

Notes and precautions

The ^{51}Cr testing should be performed first if it is to be combined with ^{59}Fe studies because of the much shorter half-life of the [51]Cr. The patient's blood volume must remain stable for the two to three weeks of the test. Other gamma-emitting labels used in nuclear medicine for lung scans, brain scans, and so forth must not be given until the ^{51}Cr study is completed.

Procedure

In ferrokinetics 10 μCi of injected ^{59}Fe binds to unsaturated transferrin (4, 7). It is transported to the marrow and incorporated into maturing erythrocytes. Serial blood samples are drawn over the first two hours and sporadically over the next 10 days to two weeks. External body counting is done over the precordium, which acts as the baseline, and over the liver, spleen, sacral and sternal marrow, and other bones as indicated. External counts are plotted against days for each organ site. The hematocrit is monitored to assess plasma iron turnover.

Specimen

The patient's anticoagulated blood samples should be of equal volume for accurate counting.

In healthy individuals ^{59}Fe is cleared rapidly by incorporation into red cells. Splenic uptake gradually increases reflecting blood flow; liver radioactivity is much less because of a lesser blood flow. Sacral and sternal bone marrow reflect initial uptake, with gradual decrease as red cells containing radioactive hemoglobin are released. Increasing splenic uptake is consistent with hemolysis; initial high levels of radioactivity that remain constant correlate with blood flow as in hypersplenism.

Plasma iron turnover measures plasma iron clearance in relation to hematocrit. The normal range is 0.4–0.8 mg/dl/24 hr. Plasma iron turnover is increased with rapid red cell turnover or marrow hyperplasia. Red cell utilization of ^{59}Fe can be 90% in healthy individuals. The normal range is 0.3–0.7 mg/dl/24 hr. Decreased utilization is present in hemolysis, ineffective erythropoiesis, or aplasia.

INEFFECTIVE ERYTHROPOIESIS

Anemia may result from accelerated erythrocyte turnover or from ineffective production. In many cases, ineffective erythropoiesis follows prolonged accelerated turnover. Gross abnormality in red cell maturation may result in destruction within the marrow and has been equated with intramedullary hemolysis. Disease processes in which ineffective erythropoiesis is frequent are listed in Table 5-5.

DIAGNOSTIC EVALUATION

In ineffective erythropoiesis, maturation and release of red cells is slowed although survival of cells released may be normal. Intramedullary destruction of red cells releases bilirubin and RBC lactic dehydrogenase (LDH_1, LDH_2). The increased bilirubin is conjugated and excreted into the gut, where it is converted to stercobilin.

91

Table 5-5.	**Causes of Ineffective Erythropoiesis**
	Uremia
	Megaloblastic anemias
	Thalassemia major
	Sideroblastic anemia (sideroachrestic anemia)
	Myeloid myelosis (pancytopenia with hypercellular marrow)
	Polycythemia vera
	Erythroleukemia (Di Guglielmo syndrome)

Reticulocytes are released slowly to the peripheral blood, and iron uptake in the production of heme is abnormal. Splenomegaly may often be seen in the neoplastic diseases but is not a direct consequence of ineffective erythropoiesis.

LABORATORY STUDIES

Hematologic Tests

PERIPHERAL BLOOD

Blood cell counts

Anemia is modest (Hb, 8–11 g/dl). Mean corpuscular volume is 80–110μ. Reticulocyte count is usually less than 2% and, for the degree of anemia, is relatively inadequate. Corrected reticulocyte counts calculated for the degree of anemia are rarely needed in the diagnosis, are often misleading in evaluating prognosis, and give a relatively simple technical procedure more complexity than it deserves.

Morphology

Red cell morphology is usually normal.

BONE MARROW

Bone marrow cellularity is normal to increased, which allows differentiation from erythroid hypoplasia, in which cellularity is decreased. Iron stains of the marrow show increased iron deposition in developing normoblasts in certain diseases. Iron deposition is in the mitochondria that surround the nucleus producing ring sideroblasts as in sideroachrestic anemia.

Other Useful Tests

LACTIC DEHYDROGENASE, PLASMA

Purpose

Increased red cell breakdown either peripherally or within the marrow releases metabolic products, which include LDH. Specific isoenzyme fractions (LDH_1, LDH_2) are associated with red cells. A marked increase in LDH_1 in the absence of myocardial infarction suggests increased red cell destruction.

Principle

Lactic dehydrogenase has multiple molecular forms with varying electrical charge that allows these forms to separate when migrating in an electrical field. Plasma is electrophoresed to spread isoenzymes into five zones in the supporting medium, usually cellulose or agar gel. LDH_1 and LDH_2 are found in large amounts in heart muscle and red cells. LDH_5 is found in large quantities in the liver.

Procedure

Plasma is inoculated onto the supporting medium and electric current is applied. The substrate is spread over the surface of the agar, and the isoenzymes present in the plasma cause localized zones of color development, that can be measured by fluorescent or reflective spectrophotometry. The total LDH is quantitated spectrophotometrically and then divided by proportions determined electrophoretically into LDH_1, LDH_2, LDH_3, LDH_4, and LDH_5.

Specimen

Five milliliters of blood are collected in heparin atraumatically. Anticoagulated specimens prevent mechanical hemolysis, which can result during clot formation. Hemolysis in the specimen must be avoided to prevent false elevations of LDH_1.

Interpretation

The normal ranges for the lactic dehydrogenase isoenzymes are:

LDH_1 ⎫	myocardial or red cell	18%–33%
LDH_2 ⎭		28%–40%
LDH_3		18%–30%
LDH_4		6%–16%
LDH_5—hepatic		2%–13%

In ineffective erythropoiesis, LDH_1 usually exceeds LDH_2, a reversal of the normal pattern.

PLASMA AND FECAL PIGMENTS

Ineffective release of red cells may lead to increased rate of destruction in the marrow detectable only with radiolabeled precursors of hemoglobin that would permit one to distinguish these pigments from the normal ones. These tests are not commonly available in most laboratories.

FERROKINETICS

Ferrokinetics using ^{59}Fe may be available in hospitals with active nuclear medicine departments. Iron uptake from plasma is accelerated with early increase in radioactivity over the sternum. Since iron is poorly incorporated into heme, radioactivity measured in released peripheral red cells is low, rising only slowly. The procedure was described earlier in this chapter. Iron utilization is subnormal in either erythroid hypoplasia or ineffective erythropoiesis, and the underlying cause is diagnosed in part by bone marrow cellularity. $^{59}Chromium$ survival of released red cells is usually normal.

REFERENCES

1. Davidsohn I, Henry JB: *Todd-Sanford Clinical Diagnosis by Laboratory Methods*, ed 15. Philadelphia, W. B. Saunders Co, 1974

2. Dacie JV, Lewis SM: *Practical Hematology*, ed 4. New York, Grune & Stratton, 1968, pp 208–214

3. Kawai T: *Clinical Aspects of the Plasma Proteins.* Philadelphia, J. B. Lippincott Co, 1973, pp. 42–44

4. Kniseley RM, Korst DR, Nelp WB, et al: The blood. In Wagner HN Jr (ed): *Principles of Nuclear Medicine.* Philadelphia, W. B. Saunders Co, 1969, pp 437–441

5. International Committee for Standardization in Hematology: Recommended methods for radioisotopic erythrocyte survival studies. Am J Clin Pathol 58:71–80, 1972

6. Mollison PL: *Blood Transfusion in Clinical Medicine*, ed 5. London, Blackwell Scientific, 1972, p 20

7. Erslev AJ: Erythrokinetics. In Williams WJ, Beutler E, Erslev AJ, et al: *Hematology*, ed 1. New York, McGraw-Hill, 1972, pp 1389–1391

chapter 6

Hereditary Erythrocyte Membrane Defects

Hereditary spherocytosis and hereditary elliptocytosis (ovalocytosis) are hereditary abnormalities of the red cell shape. It is generally believed that they are caused by an inherited defect of the red cell membrane, and many proposals have been made concerning their nature. Nonetheless, the cause of these disorders is not known.

HEREDITARY SPHEROCYTOSIS (HS)

Hereditary spherocytosis is probably the most common type of hereditary hemolytic anemia among individuals of Northern European origin, but it occurs in all races throughout the world. The inheritance is that of an autosomal dominant disorder. Therefore it is to be expected that one of the patient's parents will be affected and that each of the patient's children will have a 50% chance of inheriting the disorder.

The chronic hemolytic state in HS may vary widely in severity, ranging from an asymptomatic compensated hemolysis to a moderately severe chronic anemia. The age at diagnosis depends on the severity of the hemolytic process; the more severe forms of the disease are diagnosed early. Clinical manifestations are most often first noted in children or adolescents. Typical complaints include mild jaundice and nonspecific manifestations of anemia such as weakness. Because of an increased turnover of bilirubin, patients with this condition have a high incidence of gallstones. Some patients give a history of intermittent jaundice, dark urine, and weakness, often triggered by an infection. Patients in whom an aplastic crisis occurs may have symptoms of rapidly developing anemia with lessening jaundice. The most consistently positive physical finding is splenomegaly, which may be marked. A variable degree of jaundice is frequently seen, and slight scleral icterus is usually present.

The most consistent and therapeutically most important feature of hereditary spherocytosis is the clinical cure by splenectomy of hemolytic anemia. Red cell life span after this procedure is restored to normal or near normal.

HEREDITARY ELLIPTOCYTOSIS

Hereditary elliptocytosis exists in several genetically distinct forms. Although hemolytic anemia is present in at least one form of the disorder, approximately 90% of patients with this abnormality show no clinical evidence of hemolysis. In patients with hemolytic anemia, splenectomy has usually been found to relieve the hemolysis. Hereditary elliptocytosis, like HS, is inherited as an autosomal disorder. Elliptocytes are readily identified on the stained blood film (Figure 6-1). Since this generally represents a benign anomaly, hereditary elliptocytosis should only be incriminated as the cause for anemia when evidence for hemolysis, such as an elevated reticulocyte count, is found. Aside from the red cell morphology, no characteristic laboratory findings are seen in this disorder. *The tests discussed in this chapter pertain only to the diagnosis of HS.*

DIAGNOSTIC EVALUATION

Since hereditary spherocytosis is inherited as an autosomal dominant disorder, attempted confirmation of this mode of inheritance by family studies is an important part of the diagnostic

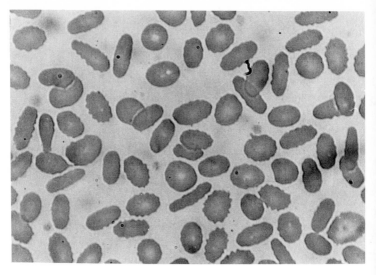

Figure 6-1. Elliptocytes.

evaluation. Sometimes examination of the blood of family members reveals the presence of laboratory stigmata of HS even when no history of anemia, jaundice, or gallstones can be elicited. This finding is not surprising since the expression of HS may be very mild in some affected individuals. Occasionally even careful examination of the parents of an affected individual fails to reveal the presence of HS. Although this finding should cause the physician to consider the possibility that the diagnosis of HS is incorrect, the disorder can arise as a new mutation; well-documented cases of HS have occurred without a positive family history.

The uniform success of splenectomy in abolishing hemolysis is in itself a diagnostic clinical feature of HS. If significant hemolysis persists after splenectomy in a patient presumed to have hereditary spherocytosis, the presumptive diagnosis is incorrect.

Evaluation of a patient presumed to have hereditary spherocytosis proceeds with the following:

1. Hematologic evaluation, with attention to red cell morphology and, at times, a bone marrow study.
2. Osmotic fragility test to confirm the presence of spherocytosis.
3. Antiglobulin test (see Chapter 5) to rule out an autoimmune hemolytic anemia as a cause for spherocytosis.
4. Autohemolysis test, which may be of some value in atypical cases in which the diagnosis is in doubt.
5. Determination of serum bilirubin to confirm the presence of unconjugated hyperbilirubinemia attributable to hemolysis as the cause for jaundice.

LABORATORY STUDIES

Hematologic Tests

GENERAL FEATURES

The central morphologic finding in HS is the presence of spherocytes on the peripheral blood film. Spherocytes appear as slightly smaller than normal, densely staining red cells with diminished or absent central pallor. The increased intensity of staining is caused in part by the fact that the spherical cell is thicker. In addition, the mean corpuscular hemoglobin concentration is generally somewhat increased. The appearance of red cells varies greatly in different parts of the blood film, even when it is well prepared. Since this phenomenon may result in errors, particularly by inexperienced observers, the diagnosis of HS should not be based on the appearance of the blood film alone.

PERIPHERAL BLOOD

Blood cell measurements

Hemoglobin levels frequently range between 9 and 12 g/dl mean corpuscular volume and MCH are usually in the normal range but may be elevated in the presence of prominent reticulocytosis. Characteristically the MCHC is often elevated to as high as 37 g/dl (normal, 26–34 g/dl). The general range for reticulocytes is 10% ±

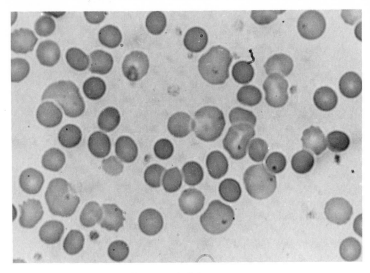

Figure 6-2. Spherocytes.

5%. However, reticulocyte counts may be markedly elevated to levels of greater than 50%.

Morphology

The spherocyte has the characteristic appearance of a small, densely staining red cell with diminished or absent central pallor (Figure 6-2). However, in mild forms of the disease, these cells may not be present in large numbers. Improper technique in preparation of the smear may result in the appearance of artifactual spherocytes to the eyes of an inexperienced observer. Prominent macrocytosis and polychromasia with very high reticulocyte counts may be present.

BONE MARROW

The typical bone marrow finding is erythroid hyperplasia. However, in the presence of an aplastic crisis, erythroid hypoplasia may be seen. With complicating folate deficiency, which may super-vene in any severe chronic hemolytic anemia, megaloblastic eryth-ropoiesis may be found.

Other Useful Tests

OSMOTIC FRAGILITY TEST

Purpose

The osmotic fragility test is necessary to confirm the morpho-logic findings of spherocytosis (1).

Principle

The osmotic fragility of red cells is basically a measurement of the extent of redundancy of the red cell membrane. In a hypotonic medium, red cells fill with water until the osmotic pressure inside the cell is reduced to that outside the cell. The red cell membrane is normally sufficiently redundant so that the volume of the cell can increase to about 1.8 times the resting volume before becoming a perfect sphere. Once a cell reaches this volume (the critical hemolytic volume), further entry of water produces lysis. A cell that is spherocytic in the resting state has less membrane redundancy than a cell that is normally biconcave. For this reason, less water can enter before the cell lyses.

Procedure

Tests should be carried out on freshly drawn blood and on blood that has been incubated for 24 hours. The osmotic fragility test is performed by adding small volumes of blood to tubes containing buffered salt solutions with osmolarity equivalent to those of 0.15%–0.9% sodium chloride (NaCl) solution. A control tube contains distilled water. After standing at room temperature for one hour, the tubes are centrifuged and the percentage of hemolyzed cells is estimated by measuring the amount of hemoglobin released into the supernatant solution.

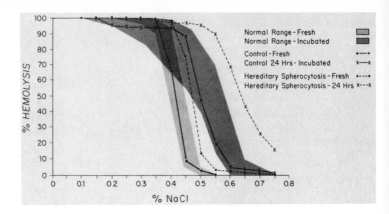

Figure 6-3. Osmotic fragility of normal erythrocytes and those from a patient with hereditary spherocytosis. The osmotic fragility is normal in fresh cells from some patients with hereditary spherocytosis, although it is usually increased. The osmotic fragility of normal cells is increased by autoincubation, but that of cells from patients with hereditary spherocytosis is increased to a greater extent than normal. (Reprinted with permission from Beutler E: Osmotic fragility. In Williams WJ, Beutler E, Erslev A, et al (eds): *Hematology,* ed 2. New York, McGraw-Hill, 1977, pp 1609–1610.)

Specimen

Heparinized or defibrinated blood is used.

Interpretation

The normal range of values for the osmotic fragility test is presented in Table 6-1 and in Figure 6-3. Increased osmotic fragility of the erythrocytes is the basic diagnostic feature of HS; unless abnormal osmotic fragility is demonstrated, the diagnosis cannot be considered to be established. However, it is not uncommon in mild forms of the disease to find minimal increase in osmotic fragility on freshly drawn blood. In such cases the incubated fragility is of particular diagnostic importance. Since increased osmotic fragility merely reflects the presence of spherocytes, this finding does not distinguish HS from autoimmune hemolytic disease with spherocytosis, in which osmotic fragility is also increased. In the latter

Table 6-1. **Normal Values for Osmotic Fragility Tests**

NaCl (%)	Lysis (%)	
	Fresh	Incubated
0.20		95–100
0.30	97–100	85–100
0.35	90–99	75–100
0.40	50–95	65–100
0.45	5–45	55–95
0.50	0–6	40–85
0.55	0	15–70
0.60	0	0–40
0.65	0	0–10
0.70	0	0–5
0.75	0	0

disorder, however, the increase of fragility that occurs with incubation is much less. Increased resistance to hemolysis is characteristic of thalassemia, in which an increase of the surface:volume ratio of the red cell is present.

Notes and precautions

Reporting osmotic fragility as percent saline concentrations for beginning and completion of hemolysis is an inadequate representation of test results. Osmotic fragility is best appreciated when reported graphically (see Figure 5-1).

AUTOHEMOLYSIS TEST

Purpose

The primary usefulness of the autohemolysis test is to assist in the diagnosis of atypical cases of HS (2, 3). While it has also been used in the differential diagnosis of hereditary nonspherocytic hemolytic anemia, the availability of specific enzymatic assays has made the autohemolysis test obsolete for this purpose.

Principle

When red cells are incubated in their own serum, hemolysis occurs gradually. Although the exact mechanism of lysis is probably quite complex, it seems likely that inability to maintain cation gradients plays an important role especially in hereditary spherocytosis.

Procedure

The autohemolysis test is carried out by incubating sterile blood with and without the addition of glucose for 48 hours and measuring the amount of hemoglobin released into the plasma.

Specimen

Defibrinated whole blood or whole blood anticoagulated with heparin or EDTA is used as a specimen.

Interpretation

Autohemolysis is normally less than 3.5% at the end of 48 hours without added glucose and less than 0.6% with added glucose. Autohemolysis in the absence of added glucose is generally greatly increased in HS; this increase is prevented to a large extent by the addition of glucose.

REFERENCES

1. Beutler, E: Osmotic fragility. In Williams WJ, Beutler E, Erslev AJ, et al (eds): *Hematology*, ed 2. New York, McGraw-Hill, 1977, pp 1609–1610

2. Selwyn JG, Dacie JV: Autohemolysis and other changes resulting from the incubation in vitro of red cells from patients with congenital hemolytic anemia. Blood 9:414–438, 1958

3. Beutler E: Autohemolysis. In Williams WJ, Beutler E, Erslev AJ, et al (eds): *Hematology*, ed 2. New York, McGraw-Hill, 1977, pp 1610–1611

Hereditary Erythrocyte Disorders of the Main Glycolytic Pathway: Pyruvate Kinase Deficiency

Since the mature erythrocyte does not contain mitochondria, it must depend entirely on glycolysis for the energy needed for such vital functions as maintenance of membrane integrity and operation of the cation pump. About 90% of glycolysis occurs by way of the anaerobic Embden-Meyerhof pathway, in which glucose is broken down to lactate in a series of enzyme-catalyzed reactions through phosphorylated intermediates. The important products of this pathway are adenosine triphosphate (ATP), the major high-energy compound in erythrocytes with a net yield of two moles of ATP for each mole of glucose metabolized, and reduced nicotinamide-adenine dinucleotide (NADH), an essential coenzyme for the reduction of methemoglobin. The principal phosphorylated intermediate via a simple shunt off this pathway is 2,3-diphosphoglycerate (2,3-DPG), which alters the affinity of hemoglobin for oxygen and plays an essential role as a regulator of oxygen delivery to the tissue (Figure 7-1). (Details of the hexose monophosphate pathway are shown in Figure 8-1.)

About 10% of glycolysis occurs via the hexose monophosphate (HMP) shunt, which bypasses the early steps of the main glycolytic

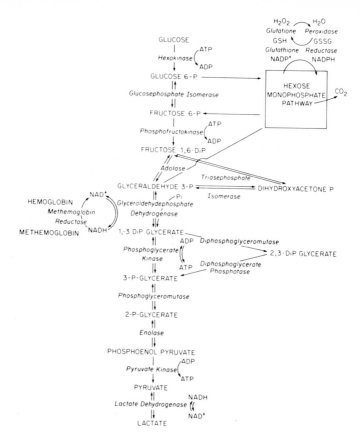

Figure 7-1. Glucose metabolism of the erythrocyte. (Reprinted with permission from Beutler E: Energy metabolism and maintenance of erythrocytes. In Williams WJ, Beutler E, Erslev AJ, et al (eds): *Hematology,* ed 2. New York, McGraw-Hill, 1977, pp 177–190.)

pathway. This route generates reduced NAD phosphate (NADPH). NADPH is required for reduction of glutathione, which is essential for the protection of hemoglobin and red cell enzymes from oxidative damage (see Figure 8-1).

HEREDITARY NONSPHEROCYTIC HEMOLYTIC ANEMIA (HNSHA)

Hereditary spherocytosis was fully described as a clinical entity at about the turn of the century. In subsequent years, cases were recorded that were characterized by a hereditary hemolytic state first observed during infancy or childhood in which spherocytes were not present in the peripheral blood film in any significant numbers and in which osmotic fragility of the red cells was normal. This group of disorders came to be designated as hereditary nonspherocytic hemolytic anemia (HNSHA). Dacie described different patterns for results with the autohemolysis test that separated some of these disorders on the basis of correction of increased autohemolysis by glucose and ATP.

Prominent causes of HNSHA are pyruvate kinase (PK) deficiency, a relatively common deficiency of the main glycolytic pathway (Table 7-1). However, HNSHA is now known to be a heterogeneous group of disorders. Included in this group, along with deficiencies of the main pathway, are the unstable hemoglobins and disorders of the pathways of the HMP shunt and glutathione metabolism (Table 7-2).

Table 7-1. **Erythrocyte Enzymes of the Main Glycolytic Pathway with Deficiencies Clearly Associated with Hemolytic Anemia**

Hexokinase
Glucose-phosphate isomerase
Phosphofructokinase
Aldolase
Triosephosphate isomerase
Diphosphoglycerate mutase
Phosphoglycerate kinase
Pyruvate kinase

Table 7-2. Erythrocyte Disorders Associated with Hereditary Nonspherocytic Hemolytic Anemia

Disorder	Example	Comments
Deficiencies of the main glycolytic pathway	PK deficiency	Relatively common cause
Unstable hemoglobins	Hemoglobin Zurich	
Deficiencies of the HMP shunt pathway	Exceptional G-6-PD variants	See Chapter 8
Deficiencies of glutathione metabolism	Some cases of hereditary glutathione deficiency	See Chapter 8

Most patients with HNSHA manifest only the hemolytic state, often associated with splenomegaly. Patients with triosephosphate isomerase deficiency, phosphoglycerate kinase (PGK) deficiency, and aldolase deficiency manifest neurologic disorders as well.

DISORDERS OF THE
EMBDEN-MEYERHOF PATHWAY:
PYRUVATE KINASE DEFICIENCY

Pyruvate kinase deficiency is the most common of the red cell enzyme deficiencies involving the main glycolytic pathway and can serve as the prototype for the remainder, which are quite rare. Like almost all disorders of the main pathway, PK deficiency shows an autosomal recessive mode of inheritance; the exception is PGK deficiency, which is inherited as a sex-linked disorder.

Pyruvate kinase deficiency is usually first detected in infancy or later in childhood with anemia or jaundice and with splenomegaly of slight to moderate degree. The severity of the anemia and of the clinical manifestations varies widely from case to case. Any of the characteristic features of chronic hemolytic anemia may be found, including jaundice, splenomegaly, and an increased incidence of gallstones; in patients with severe anemia aplastic crises have been observed. In severe forms of PK deficiency, splenectomy appears to be beneficial.

DIAGNOSTIC EVALUATION

HNSHA is a useful classification conceptually in the diagnostic evaluation of the red cell enzyme deficiencies. As in other autosomal recessive disorders, the family history is usually negative unless siblings are affected. However, biochemical studies of family members often reveal the hereditary nature of a disorder. Laboratory studies must ascertain the presence of a nonspherocytic anemia. In the case of a specific red cell enzyme deficiency, the diagnosis must ultimately be established by biochemical assay.

Evaluation of these disorders proceeds with the following:

1. Hematologic evaluation, with a search for spherocytes in particular on evaluation of the blood film and supravital stains for Heinz bodies.
2. Screening tests for HS, particularly the osmotic fragility test and occasionally the autohemolysis test.
3. Hemoglobin electrophoresis to rule out the hemoglobinopathies (see Chapter 9); heat stability test or isopropanol stability test to rule out hemoglobin variants with unstable hemoglobin.
4. Screening tests for glucose-6-phosphate dehydrogenase (G-6-PD) deficiency (see Chapter 8) and for PK deficiency.
5. Appropriate quantitative red cell enzyme assays.
6. Ancillary tests, which are part of the diagnostic evaluation of any chronic hemolytic anemia, including *Coombs test* to rule out an autoimmune hemolytic process and determination of serum bilirubin.

LABORATORY STUDIES

Hematologic Tests

GENERAL FEATURES

No pathognomonic hematologic findings are present in PK deficiency or in any of the other glycolytic red cell enzyme deficiency states. Hematologic findings are compatible with chronic hemolytic anemia and their prominence is proportional to the severity of the anemia. The single most important morphologic criterion for this group of disorders is a negative one, that is, the absence of significant spherocytosis.

PERIPHERAL BLOOD

Blood cell measurements

In PK deficiency, levels of hemoglobin range from 5–12 g/dl and MCV may be moderately increased. Reticulocytosis is proportional to the severity of the anemia, up to 15%, but may be more markedly increased, up to 54% after splenectomy.

Morphology

Cells are normocytic normochromic or, when in association with reticulocytosis, macrocytic with polychromatophilia; poikilocytosis may be seen. Rare, irregularly contracted, densely staining red cells may be present.

Supravital stain for Heinz bodies

A search for Heinz bodies is used to screen for anemias associated with oxidative denaturation of hemoglobin or red cell inclusions associated with unstable hemoglobins (see Chapter 9).

Other Useful Tests

OSMOTIC FRAGILITY TEST

Purpose

The principal utility of the osmotic fragility test is in the diagnosis of HS.

For sections on *Principle*, *Procedure*, and *Specimen*, see Chapter 6.

Interpretation

Osmotic fragility is clearly increased in HS and in autoimmune hemolytic anemia with spherocytosis. However, even in such cases, osmotic fragility of unincubated blood is often normal and incubation is required to demonstrate the abnormality. Although increased osmotic fragility is sometimes reported in HNSHA, such increases have been minimal and not of the magnitude seen with spherocytic anemias.

AUTOHEMOLYSIS TEST

Purpose

The autohemolysis test can occasionally be useful in confirming the diagnosis of hereditary spherocytosis.

For sections on *Principle*, *Procedure*, *Specimen*, and *Interpretation*, see Chapter 6.

HEAT STABILITY TEST AND ISOPROPANOL STABILITY TEST

Purpose

The heat stability and isopropanol stability tests are used to screen for the unstable hemoglobins.

For sections on *Principle*, *Procedure*, *Specimen*, and *Interpretation*, see Chapter 9.

FLUORESCENT SCREENING TEST FOR PK DEFICIENCY

Purpose

The fluorescent test is a biochemical screening test for PK deficiency [1].

Principle

Pyruvate kinase catalyzes the phosphorylation of adenosine diphosphate (ADP) to ATP by phosphoenolpyruvate (PEP):

$$PEP + ADP \xrightarrow[\text{Mg + K}]{\text{PK}} pyruvate + ATP$$

This reaction is coupled to the NADH-dependent conversion of pyruvate to lactate:

$$Pyruvate + NADH + H^+ \xrightleftharpoons{\text{LDH}} lactate + NAD^+$$

The loss of fluorescence of NADH as it is oxidized to NAD is observed under ultraviolet light.

Procedure

The blood sample is centrifuged, the plasma and buffy coat are aspirated, and a suspension of the red cells is added to a buffered hypotonic screening mixture that also lyses the red cells but not the white cells. The screening mixture provides PEP, ADP, NADH, and $MgCl_2$. It is spotted on filter paper immediately after mixing and every 15 minutes thereafter. The paper is examined under illumination with long-wave ultraviolet light after the spots are thoroughly dry. The patient's sample is compared with that of a healthy control subject.

Interpretation

The first spot should fluoresce brightly. With the normal sample, fluorescence disappears at the end of 15 minutes of incubation. In contrast, in PK-deficient samples, fluorescence fails to disappear even at the end of 45 or 60 minutes.

Notes and precautions

False-negative results may be observed if the patient has been transfused recently enough so that large numbers of transfused cells are still circulating.

Red Cell Enzyme Assays

Most of the quantitative assays of red cell enzyme activity use spectrophotometric techniques that depend on the absorption of light of the reduced pyridine nucleotide, NADPH, or NADH at 340 nm (2). The reactions involved in these procedures are linked to pyridine nucleotide, and the rate of oxidation or reduction of the pyridine nucleotide is measured with the spectrophotometer. Reduction results in the formation NADPH or NADH with an increase in optical density at 340 nm; oxidation results in formation of NADP or NAD with a decrease in optical density at 340 nm.

In practice it is often enough to know whether the activity of the enzyme in question is markedly deficient. Slight deviations from normal are not likely to be of clinical importance. For this reason, a number of screening techniques for the detection of enzyme deficiencies have been developed that are useful for the laboratory that does not have resources required for quantitative assays. Instead of measuring the rate of oxidation or reduction of pyridine nucleotide by spectrophotometer, fluorescence visible to the naked eye is used as an indicator. Reduced pyridine nucleotides fluoresce when illuminated with long-wave ultraviolet light while no such fluorescence occurs with oxidized pyridine nucleotides. In addition to the screening procedure for PK described previously, screening tests are available for glucose-phosphorate isomerase, triosephosphate isomerase, and for the HMP shunt enzymes, G-6-PD and glutathione reductase (see Chapter 8). Measurement of red cell reduced glutathione (GSH) is discussed in Chapter 8. Hereditary GSH deficiency resulting from deficiency of the enzymes of GSH synthesis is associated with marked reduction of red cell GSH.

REFERENCES

1. Beutler E: A series of screening procedures for pyruvate kinase deficiency, glucose-6-phosphate dehydrogenase deficiency and glutathione reductase deficiency. Blood 28:553–562, 1966
2. Beutler E: *Red Cell Metabolism: A Manual of Biochemical Methods*, ed 2. New York, Grune & Stratton, 1975

Hereditary Disorders of the Hexose-Monophosphate Shunt Pathway: Glucose-6-Phosphate Dehydrogenase Deficiency

Glucose-6-phosphate dehydrogenase (G-6-PD) catalyzes the first step in the hexose monophosphate (HMP) oxidative shunt pathway resulting in the reduction of NADP to NADPH (Figure 8-1). NADPH is required as a cofactor for red cell glutathione reductase to maintain glutathione in the reduced state (GSH). The important functions of GSH in the red cell appear to include the detoxification of low levels of hydrogen peroxide, which may form spontaneously or as a result of drug administration, and maintenance of the integrity of the red cell by reducing oxidized sulfhydryl groups of hemoglobin, membrane proteins, and enzymes that may become oxidized.

GLUCOSE-6-PHOSPHATE DEHYDROGENASE DEFICIENCY

G-6-PD deficiency results from the inheritance of any one of a large number of abnormalities of the structural gene that codes the amino acid sequence of the enzyme G-6-PD. Normal G-6-PD, designated as B, represents the most common type of enzyme

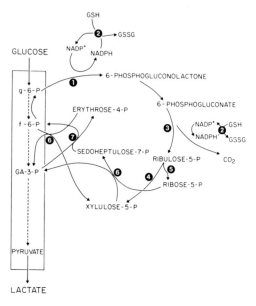

Figure 8-1. The hexose monophosphate pathway of the erythrocyte: (*1*) glucose-6-phosphate dehydrogenase, (*2*) glutathione reductase, (*3*) phosphogluconate dehydrogenase, (*4*) ribulose phosphate epimerase, (*5*) ribose phosphate isomerase, (*6*) transketolase, and (*7*) transaldolase. (Reprinted with permission from Beutler E: Energy metabolism and maintenance of erythrocytes. In Williams WJ, Beutler E, Erslev AJ, et al (eds): *Hematology,* ed 2. New York, McGraw-Hill, 1977, pp 177–190.)

encountered in all population groups that have been studied. Among Africans a variant of G-6-PD, G-6-PD A, is also present. This type migrates more rapidly on electrophoresis than the normal B enzyme. Approximately 20% of American black males carry this variant. About 11% of American black males have a G-6-PD variant that has the same electrophoretic mobility as G-6-PD A but is unstable and deteriorates as the red cell ages. This variant, G-6-PD A−, is the most common clinically significant type of abnormal G-6-PD among the American black population; their red cells contain only 5%–15% of the normal amount of enzyme activity.

Among white populations, by far the most common variant is G-6-PD Mediterranean. This variant is found frequently in Syrians, Sicilians, Greeks, Sephardic Jews, and Arabs. Several variants appear to be common in Asian populations.

Since the gene determining the structure of G-6-PD is carried on the X chromosome, inheritance of G-6-PD deficiency is sex linked. For this reason, the effect is fully expressed in affected males and is never transmitted from father to son but only from mother to son. In females, only one of the two X chromosomes in each cell is active. Consequently females who are heterozygous for G-6-PD deficiency have two populations of red cells, deficient and normal cells. The ratio of deficient to normal cells may vary greatly. Some heterozygous females appear to be entirely healthy whereas others are fully affected. The normal variability of expression of G-6-PD deficiency in heterozygotes is the result of certain features of the X-chromosome inactivation process.

The most common clinical manifestation of G-6-PD deficiency is that of a self-limited episode of drug-induced hemolysis in an otherwise apparently healthy individual beginning one to three days after administration of an oxidant drug is initiated (Table 8-1). Heinz bodies appear in the red cells and the concentration of hemoglobin begins to decline rapidly. As hemolysis progresses Heinz bodies disappear from the circulation, presumably as the erythrocytes that contain them are removed by the spleen. In severe cases, abdominal or back pain may occur. The urine may turn dark or even black. Within four to six days the reticulocyte count is generally increased except in instances in which the patient has received a drug for treatment of an active infection. In the A− type of deficiency, the hemolytic anemia is self limited because the young red cells produced in response to hemolysis have nearly normal levels of G-6-PD and are relatively resistant to hemolysis. Although acute hemolytic episodes have been associated most often with administration of drugs, such episodes may also follow a variety of infections including pneumonia, typhoid, and infectious hepatitis. Such episodes have also been associated with diabetic

117

Table 8-1. **Drugs and Chemicals that have Clearly Been Shown to Cause Clinically Significant Hemolytic Anemia in Glucose-6-Phosphate Dehydrogenase**

Acetanilid
Methylene blue
Nalidixic acid (NegGram)
Napthalene
Niridazole (Ambilhar)
Nitrofurantoin (Furadantin)
Pamaquine
Pentaquine
Phenylhydrazine
Primaquine
Sulfacetamide
Sulfanilamide
Sulfapyridine
Sulfamethoxazole (Gantanol)
Thiazolesulfone
Toluidine blue
Trinitrotoluene (TNT)

Table 8-2. **Clinical Features of Glucose-6-Phosphate Dehydrogenase Variants**

G-6-PD Variant	Clinical Features
Episodic hemolytic anemia with drug administration or infection	Usual manifestation in A − and Mediterranean variants
Favism	Occurs especially in Mediterranean children; not seen in A − type of deficiency
Neonatal icterus	Observed in infants with Mediterranean and Chinese variants; rare in newborn blacks
Hereditary nonspherocytic hemolytic anemia	Seen with rare variants; occasionally seen in Mediterranean type of defect

acidosis. Other stresses that may result in acute hemolytic anemia in individuals who are G-6-PD deficient are exposure to fava beans and the neonatal state; these are associated with severe G-6-PD enzyme deficiency. The rare cases presenting as hereditary non-spherocytic hemolytic anemia are also associated with markedly deficient G-6-PD activity (Table 8-2).

OTHER ENZYME DEFECTS IN THE HEXOSE MONOPHOSPHATE SHUNT

Deficiencies of other enzymes in the HMP shunt and glutathione metabolism are comparatively rare (Table 8-3).

Hereditary GSH deficiency of the red cell results from a deficiency of either of the two enzymes of GSH synthesis, gamma-glutamyl cysteine synthetase or GSH synthetase. In some cases the clinical manifestation of these deficiencies is similar to that of G-6-PD; others present with a chronic hemolytic anemia. Some variants with GSH synthetase deficiency also lack GSH synthetase in the tissues. Patients with this condition excrete large amounts of oxoproline (pyroglutamic acid) in the urine and suffer from a progressive neurologic disorder.

Partial deficiency of glutathione reductase (GR) is a "nondisease." Low levels of GR are found in patients with dietary riboflavin

Table 8-3. **Erythrocyte Enzyme Deficiencies of the Hexose Monophosphate (HMP) Shunt Pathway and of Glutathione Metabolism Clearly Associated with Hemolytic Anemia**

G-6-PD

GSH deficiency secondary to deficiency of:
    Gamma-glutamyl cysteine synthetase
    GSH synthetase

Glutathione reductase (only total deficiency)

deficiency. Glutathione reductase is a flavin enzyme that requires the cofactor flavin-adenine dinucleotide (FAD); GR activity is impaired with FAD deficiency. Virtually total absence of GR was reported only once, and this severe deficiency produced a single hemolytic episode in an otherwise hematologically healthy person.

Glutathione peroxidase deficiency does not appear to cause hemolytic anemia. Many hematologically healthy persons have levels of this enzyme as low as or lower than those found in persons in whom hemolysis was attributed to a deficiency of the enzyme.

DIAGNOSTIC EVALUATION

The diagnosis of the previously mentioned disorders depends on their clinical presentation. Evaluation of the rare variants that present as hereditary nonspherocytic hemolytic anemia (HNSHA) is discussed in Chapter 7. In patients who present with neonatal icterus, fetal-maternal Rh or ABO incompatibility must be ruled out.

The most common type of G-6-PD deficiency presents as an acute hemolytic anemia. In such cases a careful history regarding ingestion of drugs is important. Other causes of episodic anemia include PNH (see Chapter 10) and some of the unstable hemoglobins (see Chapter 9). When the hemolytic nature of the episodes is less apparent and in particular in cases associated with infection, differential diagnosis includes an aregenerative crisis that may occur in any of the severe hereditary anemias. The following studies are used to confirm the diagnosis of G-6-PD deficiency.

LABORATORY STUDIES

Hematologic Tests

GENERAL FEATURES

The clinical and hematologic findings in subjects who are G-6-PD deficient are normal in the absence of hemolysis. Blood counts and red cell morphology are not remarkable. The changes that will be described are those associated with a hemolytic episode after a stress, for example, after drug ingestion.

Heinz bodies develop in the erythrocytes immediately preceding and in the early phases of hemolysis (see Chapter 9). If the hemolytic anemia is very severe, red cell fragmentation and spherocytic cells may be seen in the stained film. As the level of hemoglobin falls, reticulocytosis occurs and polychromasia is seen on the stained smear; these morphologic changes are not striking. No consistent changes occur in platelets or in white cells.

BONE MARROW

Bone marrow study reveals erythroid hyperplasia consistent with acute hemolysis.

Other Useful Tests

FLUORESCENT SCREENING TEST FOR GLUCOSE-6-PHOSPHATE DEHYDROGENASE

Purpose

The fluorescent screening test is highly reliable for the detection of both severe and mild types of G-6-PD deficiency in males not undergoing hemolysis (1).

Principle

In the presence of G-6-PD and NADP, glucose-6-phosphate is oxidized through 6-phosphogluconate in the reaction:

$$\text{Glucose-6-P} + \text{NADP}^+ \xrightarrow{\text{G-6-PD}} \text{6-phosphogluconate} + \text{NADPH} + \text{H}^+$$

Since phosphogluconate dehydrogenase (6-PGD) is present in virtually all hemolysates, further reduction of NADP occurs in the reaction:

$$\text{6-Phosphogluconate} + \text{NADP}^+ \xrightarrow{\text{6-PGD}} \text{ribulose-5-P} + \text{NADPH} + \text{H}^+$$

When mildly G-6-PD-deficient hemolysates are incubated with G-6-P and NADP, a small amount of NADPH is formed. In the presence of oxidized glutathione (GSSG), provided in the screening mixture, NADPH is reoxidized in the glutathione reductase reaction:

$$GSSG + NADPH + H^+ \xrightarrow{GR} 2\ GSH + NADP^+$$

Thus, the screening test measures, in effect, the difference between approximately twice the G-6-PD activity and the glutathione reductase activity.

Procedure

Whole blood is added to a buffered screening solution containing saponin, G-6-P, $NADP^+$, and GSSG. After incubation for 5–10 minutes at room temperature, the mixture is spotted on filter paper, allowed to dry, and observed for fluorescence.

In patients with the A− variant of G-6-PD who have recently undergone hemolysis, the test may be modified by centrifuging the blood sample in a microhematocrit tube and using the bottom 10% of the red cell column for the test. These are the older, most enzyme-deficient cells.

Specimen

Blood collected in heparin EDTA or acid citrate dextrose (ACD) solution is satisfactory. Blood that is several weeks old, and even spots of blood collected on filter paper and dried, may be used.

Interpretation

With normal blood the dried spot is brightly fluorescent. Deficient samples show little or no fluorescence.

No false-positive or false-negative tests are observed. However, in patients with the A− variant of G-6-PD with ongoing or acute hemolysis, since most enzyme-deficient cells have been removed from the circulation, the remaining young cells and reticulocytes have normal or near normal G-6-PD activity. Diagnosis of G-6-PD deficiency under these circumstances can be accomplished either by repeating the screening test in two or three weeks or by means of the modification of the screening test noted previously. In severe G-6-PD deficiency of the Mediterranean or similar types in which even very young cells have very low levels of G-6-PD, a screening test suffices for diagnosis, even in the presence of a severe hemolytic reaction, provided that the patient has not been transfused.

ASCORBATE CYANIDE TEST

Purpose

Since G-6-PD is linked to the X chromosome, it is subject to X inactivation in females (2). Therefore, females who are heterozygous for G-6-PD deficiency have varying proportions of red cells that are G-6-PD deficient. If the proportion of deficient cells is large enough, heterozygotes can be detected by the same fluorescent screening test used for males who are G-6-PD deficient. When the proportion of deficient cells is relatively low, however, the ascorbate cyanide test is probably the most sensitive screening procedure for the heterozygous state.

Principle

Hydrogen peroxide is generated from the coupled oxidation of ascorbate and oxyhemoglobin. When catalase is inhibited with cyanide, the glutathione-dependent system is required to prevent peroxidative damage to hemoglobin. Since this system is compromised in G-6-PD deficiency, hemoglobin is oxidized by hydrogen peroxide and brown hemoglobin degradation products appear. Because the cells are not lysed during the test, even a relatively small proportion of enzyme-deficient red cells imparts the characteristic brownish color of G-6-PD deficiency.

Procedure

Two milliliters of whole blood is well oxygenated to a bright red color by gentle swirling. The specimen is then added to an ascorbate-glucose reagent, cyanide reagent is added, and the mixture is incubated at 37 C with intermittent mixing for three hours.

Specimen

Whole blood is used.

Interpretation

Normal blood remains red, whereas samples that are G-6-PD deficient turn brown. For the reasons mentioned, this test is valuable in screening for G-6-PD heterozygotes, but it lacks the specificity of the fluorescent screening test. Positive ascorbate cyanide test results are seen in GR and PK deficiency and in unstable hemoglobinopathies.

Red Cell Enzyme Assays

In males not undergoing hemolysis the G-6-PD fluorescent screening test is generally adequate for diagnosis (3). Quantitative enzyme assays are usually carried out in specialized research laboratories. In general, assays of the enzymes of the HMP shunt pathway are NADP or NADPH-linked reactions in which the rate of increase of optical density with the formation of NADPH or of decrease in optical density with the formation of NADP is 340 nm as measured by a spectrophotometer. The reactions involved in the quantitative G-6-PD assay are those discussed in the section on the fluorescent screening test for that enzyme. Quantitative assay for G-6-PD activity may reveal the presence of G-6-PD deficiency in a person who has recently undergone hemolysis. Since G-6-PD is normally an age-dependent enzyme, activity should be increased in a patient with reticulocytosis. No increase or normal or slightly lower G-6-PD activity in such a patient implies that G-6-PD deficiency is present. The G-6-PD assay is also helpful in detecting heterozygous females.

Measurement of GSH can be carried out by means of a test involving the reaction of GSH with dithiobisnitrobenzoic acid (DTNB) to give a yellow color that is measured colorimetrically at

412 nm. Red cells in hereditary glutathione deficiencies generally contain very little GSH. Moderate degrees of GSH deficiency may exist as a secondary manifestation of other red cell defects. The most common cause of modestly reduced red cell GSH level is G-6-PD deficiency.

REFERENCES

1. Beutler E, Mitchell M: Special modifications of the fluorescent screening method for glucose-6-phosphate dehydrogenase deficiency. Blood 32:816–818, 1968

2. Jacob H, Jandl JH: A simple visual screening test for G-6-PD deficiency employing ascorbate and cyanide. N Engl J Med 274:1162–1167, 1966

3. Beutler E: *Red Cell Metabolism: A Manual of Biochemical Methods*, ed 2. New York, Grune & Stratton, 1975

chapter 9

Disorders of Hemoglobin Synthesis

Hemoglobin is a tetrameric protein composed of globin and four heme groups. The globin is composed of two polypeptide chain pairs and each of the four polypeptides is associated with one heme group.

In hemoglobin A (HbA), the major normal adult hemoglobin, each chain of one polypeptide pair is designated as an alpha (α) and each of the other pair a beta (β) chain. Hemoglobin A is then depicted structurally as $\alpha_2\beta_2$. The two minor adult hemoglobins are HbA$_2$ and HbF. The beta chain is replaced by a delta (δ) chain in HbA$_2$ and by a gamma (γ) chain in HbF. Hemoglobin A$_2$ is depicted as $\alpha_2\delta_2$ and HbF as $\alpha_2\gamma_2$. The alpha chain has 141 amino acids; beta, gamma, and delta chains each have 147 amino acids. At birth, HbF is the predominant hemoglobin, but within the first year of life it is largely replaced, and hemoglobins are then present in the adult proportion of approximately 97% HbA, 2% HbA$_2$, and 1% HbF.

GENETICS

Each globin chain, that is, alpha, beta, gamma, and delta, has its own autosomal genetic locus. Most hemoglobin variants result from substitutions of a single amino acid. The most common variants, HbS and HbC, are beta-chain mutations (Table 9-1). These variants can appear in the heterozygous or homozygous state.

Table 9-1. Chemical Differences between Hemoglobin Variants caused by Beta-Chain Mutations

Hb	Position	Amino Acid Residue in HbA	Amino Acid Residue in Abnormal Hb
S	6	Glutamic acid	Valine
C	6	Glutamic acid	Lysine
D$_{Punjab}$[a]	121	Glutamic acid	Glutamine
E	26	Glutamic acid	Lysine

[a]Only common HbD variant.

Double or combined heterozygosity for the genes responsible for any of the hemoglobin variants is also seen. A minor hemoglobin that is formed by posttranscriptional modification of HbA is HbA$_{1c}$. This hemoglobin, formed by the addition of glucose to the N terminal of the HbA beta chains, is found in increased amounts in diabetes mellitus.

In the thalassemias, globin chains are structurally normal but are produced in inadequate amounts. The thalassemias are classified according to the chain affected, for example, alpha-thalassemia, beta-thalassemia, and delta-thalassemia. The beta-thalassemic disorders are classified as minor or major for the heterozygous and homozygous states respectively. The heterozygous beta-thalassemia minor is a common disorder. Combined or double heterozygous disorders involving the structural variants and the thalassemias are also seen; the commonest of these is sickle beta-thalassemia disease. The genetics of the alpha-thalassemias are more complex.

NOMENCLATURE

Early hemoglobin variants were differentiated primarily by their electrophoretic mobility and were assigned letter names. Later, when different hemoglobin variants were discovered with the same mobility, the new variant was distinguished by following the letter previously ascribed to that mobility with the place of discovery of the new variant. Finally, when the exact amino acid structure of a hemoglobin variant was determined, a simple designation was adopted that characterized the amino acid substitution by a superscript to the involved globin chain, for example, for HgS, $\alpha_2\beta_2^{6 \text{ glutamic acid} \rightarrow \text{valine}}$. Sickle cell anemia refers to the homozygote for HbS and the sickle cell trait is related to the heterozygote. The word disease is used for a homozygote with other hemoglobin variants, for example, homozygous HbC disease (HbCC); again trait refers to the heterozygotes, for example, HbC trait (HbAC). The word disease is also applied to the HbS double heterozygous states as with sickle cell-HbC disease. When letter designations are used for the hemoglobins in the heterozygous hemoglobinopathies, the first letter refers to the preponderant hemoglobin found in the red cell. Thus, HbAS indicates that HbA exceeds HbS in the red cell of that heterozygous variant.

CLINICAL DISORDERS

Disorders in hemoglobin synthesis can be divided into those caused by formation of abnormal globin chains resulting in structural hemoglobin changes (often referred to as the hemoglobinopathies) and the thalassemias, which are associated with suppression of normal globin-chain production, that is, decreased quantities of normal hemoglobin. Combinations of these two types of disorders are also seen (Table 9-2).

Hemoglobin Disorders Caused by Abnormal Globin Chains

Mutations involving the genes that direct formation of globin chains result in amino acid substitutions that may produce pronounced changes in the properties of hemoglobin. A functional classification of the abnormal hemoglobins based on these changes is shown in Table 9-2.

128

Of the mutant hemoglobins with decreased solubility, the one causing the most common clinically significant hemoglobinopathy is HbS. The heterozygous disorder resulting from this hemoglobin, the sickle cell trait, should generally be considered an entirely benign disorder although on rare occasions it may be responsible for hematuria. The homozygous disorder is a sickle cell disease, sickle cell anemia. This disorder is characterized by moderately severe hemolysis and by painful crises resulting from microinfarction of blood vessels. When the gene for HbS is inherited together with the gene for certain other abnormal hemoglobins, particularly for HbC (SC disease) or beta-thalassemia (S-thalassemia), sickle cell diseases very similar to sickle cell anemia result. Since the sickle cell gene occurs in approximately 9% of black Americans, the gene for HbC in 3%, and for beta-thalassemia in 1% of black Americans, these disorders are collectively quite common, affecting approximately 1 in 260 black Americans. Two other hemoglobins in this category are not rare, particularly in the heterozygous state: HbD, which is seen in blacks, and HbE, which is a common mutation in Asian populations. Both of these result in a mild hemolytic anemia even in the homozygous state. In HbE disease the anemia is hypochromic and associated with splenomegaly. Hypochromia is also found uniformly in the trait.

The remaining hemoglobinopathies are much less common. Those caused by formation of unstable hemoglobins are inherited as autosomal dominant disorders and are characteristically associated with chronic hemolysis. The anemia is often hypochromic. Some unstable hemoglobins are associated with increased oxygen affinity. In such cases, reticulocytosis may be greater than usually observed for the degree of anemia seen. Hemoglobins in which the essential functional change is increased oxygen affinity result in erythrocytosis. Hemoglobins that have decreased oxygen affinity are very rare.

A mutant hemoglobin that is unable to maintain heme iron in the reduced state and to bind oxygen, designated as HbM, results in hereditary methemoglobinemia. Methemoglobin has a brownish

Table 9-2. Functional Classification of Abnormal Hemoglobins

Type of Abnormality	Functional Abnormality	Clinical Disorder[a]	Examples
Qualitative (structural) abnormalities	None	No physiologic or clinical disorders	HbG$_{Philadelphia}$; most hemoglobin variants
	Aggregation of hemoglobin molecules	Hemolytic anemia	HbS, HbC
	Unstable hemoglobins[b] with increased susceptibility to oxidative denaturation and formation of inclusion bodies	Hemolytic anemia	Hb$_{Zurich}$ Hb$_{Köln}$
	Methemoglobinemia caused by mutations that prevent reduction of heme iron	Cyanosis	HbM
Abnormal[b] oxygen affinity	Increased oxygen affinity	Erythrocytosis	Hb$_{Chesapeake}$
	Decreased oxygen affinity	Cyanosis/anemia	Hb$_{Seattle}$
Quantitative abnormalities—thalassemias	Alpha-thalassemias with decreased alpha-chain production	Range from mild anemia with hypochromia to hematologic disease in newborn or to hydrops fetalis	Hb Barts, HbH

	Beta-thalassemias with decreased beta-chain production	Mild hypochromic anemia to severe hemolytic anemia	Beta-thalassemia minor Beta-thalassemia major (Cooley's anemia)
	Delta-beta-thalassemias with decrease of both delta- and beta-chain production	Thalassemia-type syndromes	Delta-beta-thalassemia
	Delta-thalassemias with decreased delta-chain production	No significant clinical or hematologic abnormality	Delta-thalassemia
Combined structural disorders with thalassemias (double heterozygotes)	Aggregation of hemoglobin molecule and suppression of normal hemoglobin chain	Disorder usually resembles that seen with structural variant alone but often milder	HbS-beta-thalassemia
Thalassemialike syndromes	Lepore syndromes resulting from delta-beta fusion chain caused by abnormal crossing over of genes for delta and beta; suppression of normal delta chains and beta chains	Clinical syndromes similar to those seen with β-thalassemia	Hb Lepore
	HPFH[c] results from failure to switch from gamma to beta- and delta-chain production after birth	No clinical or hematologic abnormality	HbF 15%–100%

[a]Homozygous states generally associated with more severe disorder than heterozygotes.
[b]Abnormal oxygen affinity frequently seen with unstable hemoglobins.
[c]Can be seen in combination with HbS, thalassemia, or HbC.

Table 9-3. **The Alpha-Thalassemias**

Genotype	Phenotype	Hematologic Findings
$\alpha\alpha\alpha\alpha$	Normal	Normal
$\alpha\alpha\alpha\alpha^{Th}$	Silent carrier	Normal
$\alpha\alpha\alpha^{Th}\alpha^{Th}$	α-thalassemia trait	Mild hypochromic anemia
		In newborn, Hb Barts; in adults, sometimes rare HbH inclusions in red cells after BCB[a] incubation
$\alpha\alpha^{Th}\alpha^{Th}\alpha^{Th}$	HBH disease	Hemolytic disease
		In newborn, increased Hb Barts; in adult, HbH present; many positive red cells after BCB incubation
$\alpha^{Th}\alpha^{Th}\alpha^{Th}\alpha^{Th}$	Hydrops fetalis	Stillborn, anemic macerated fetus
		Cord blood 100% Hb Barts

[a]*BCB*, brilliant cresyl blue.

color, and patients who inherit this hemoglobin have a cyanotic appearance. Like the unstable hemoglobins, hemoglobins with increased oxygen affinity and the HbMs are inherited as autosomal dominant disorders.

THE THALASSEMIAS

Alpha-thalassemia is a common disorder in Southeast Asia. Because the locus directing synthesis of the alpha chain is duplicated, each healthy individual has four alpha-chain genes, two for each set of chromosomes. Alpha-thalassemia results from the absence or a defect of one or more of these genes. The characteristics of the alpha-thalassemias are summarized in Table 9-3. The most serious clinical state results from absence of activity of all four alpha-chain genes. The absence of alpha chains is incompatible with life. The chains synthesized in fetal red cells form γ_4 tetramers designated as hemoglobin Barts. Hemoglobin Barts is unstable and its oxygen dissociation curve is shifted far left. When it is the only hemoglobin formed, fetal death results with a disorder known as hydrops fetalis. If one alpha-chain gene is functional, a less severe disorder occurs. At birth, fetal hemoglobin as well as hemoglobin Barts is present. In later infancy, childhood, and adulthood, the beta chains that are formed also form β_4 tetramers designated as hemoglobin H. The resulting disorder, HbH disease, is a moderately severe, chronic hemolytic anemia. If two normal alpha-chain genes are present, a mild hypochromic anemia designated as alpha-thalassemia minor is observed. The presence of three normal alpha chains does not result in a clinically detectable abnormality.

Beta-thalassemia is a common disorder, particularly among Mediterranean populations. It is the Mediterranean anemia first described by Thomas Benton Cooley and sometimes known by his name. When only one beta-thalassemic gene has been inherited, the clinical disorder designated beta-thalassemia minor results. This is a benign, hypochromic anemia in which the concentration of hemoglobin in the blood may be diminished to 10 or 11 g/dl but the RBC count is normal or, very frequently, elevated. In beta-thalassemia minor, the amount of hemoglobin A_2 is invariably increased because alpha chains that cannot find beta chains with which to combine may combine with delta chains. Slightly elevated levels of HbF are present in about 30% of patients with beta-thalassemia minor. Often, patients with thalassemia minor are mistakenly diagnosed as being iron deficient, because they have a hypochromic anemia (see Chapter 3). When two beta-thalassemic genes have been inherited, a very serious disorder of infancy and early childhood, thalassemia major, results. It is characterized by massive splenomegaly, extreme erythroid hyperplasia in the bone marrow, severe hemolytic anemia, and failure to thrive. In beta-thalassemia major, prominent elevation of HbF ranging from 30%–100% is found. With HbF values at lower levels in this range, the hemoglobin is distributed heterogeneously among the cell population, helping to distinguish the disorder from the benign condition designated as hereditary persistence of fetal hemoglobin (HPFH), in which a homogeneous distribution is seen.

Beta-thalassemia genes are not all the same. Some result in complete suppression of beta-chain synthesis and are designated as β^0 genes. Others, which permit some formation of normal beta chains, are designated as β^+ genes and result in milder clinical syndromes than the β^0 variants.

Often classified as beta-thalassemias, delta-beta-thalassemias are associated with suppression of both delta and beta chains. They are clinically similar to the beta-thalassemias. Heterozygotes present as thalassemia minor, often with prominent elevation of HbF. However, the homozygotes present as a clinically milder disease than is usually seen with beta-thalassemia major. The Lepore syndromes, which are often classified in this category, are caused by a mutant hemoglobin, Hb Lepore. This hemoglobin results from a crossover mutation; the hybrid globin chain consists partly of delta chains and partly of beta chains. Hemoglobin Lepore can be detected by electrophoresis.

DIAGNOSTIC EVALUATION

The development of practical procedures using readily available equipment and reagents has enabled the general laboratory clinician to perform a reasonably complete evaluation of the hemoglobin disorders. However, a complete family history, clinical evaluation, and family studies play a particularly important role in evaluating laboratory data with these disorders. For example, over 50 different variants behave like HbS on hemoglobin electrophoresis, although most of these are rare or clinically insignificant. Thus, when a serious discrepancy exists between family or clinical findings and laboratory results, more sophisticated studies including structural analysis of hemoglobin may be required.

Although solubility or turbidity tests have been widely used in screening for sickle cell trait they are not entirely satisfactory for genetic counseling because they fail to detect the genetically important carriers of HbC and of beta-thalassemia Evaluation of the hemoglobin disorders proceeds with the following:

1. Hematologic evaluation, with (1) attention to RBC morphology and (2) use of supravital stains to detect inclusion bodies.

2. Hemoglobin electrophoresis for the detection of globin-chain variants with altered electrophoretic mobility.

3. Tests of hemoglobin solubility as a means of distinguishing HbS from the electrophoretically similar HbD and less frequent variants; solubility tests and the sickling test to screen for sickle cell trait.

4. Alkali denaturation test for fetal hemoglobin and microchromatography for measuring HbA_2 to delineate the thalassemias.

5. The acid elution test (method of Kleihauer and Betke) to evaluate the distribution of HbF in red cells for the diagnosis of HPFH.

6. The heat stability test and isopropanol stability test for detecting unstable hemoglobins; the test for HbH inclusion bodies.

7. When indicated, spectrophotometric determinations for methemoglobinemia seen with HbMs, and measurement of oxyhemoglobin dissociation or $P_{50}O_2$ for detecting hemoglobins with altered oxygen affinity (see Chapter 13). Detailed structural analysis of globin chains using "fingerprinting" of tryptic digests by means of electrophoresis and chromatography and amino acid sequencing are performed by specialized laboratories.

LABORATORY STUDIES

Hematologic Tests

GENERAL FEATURES

Hematologic abnormalities associated with the hemoglobin disorders can be classified into (*a*) those associated with chronic hemolysis, (*b*) changes characteristic of a particular disorder, (*c*) findings seen after splenectomy or (in the case of sickle cell disease) findings related to splenic atrophy, (*d*) changes caused by folate deficiency that may accompany chronic hemolysis, and (*e*) those seen with aplastic crises, which may accompany infections. The most severe anemia and most striking morphologic changes are seen in the homozygous disorders. The heterozygous states may be normal or may show minimal hematologic abnormalities.

PERIPHERAL BLOOD

Blood cell measurements

Anemia is severe in the serious homozygous disorders, with characteristic ranges for hemoglobin of 5–8 g/dl in sickle cell anemia and 2.5–6.5 g/dl in thalassemia major. The heterozygotes may be hematologically normal, as in sickle cell trait, or show mild anemia, as in beta-thalassemia minor.

Morphology

See Table 9-4 and Figures 9-1 through 9-4.

BONE MARROW

Erythroid hyperplasia is proportional to the severity of the hemolysis. A prominent increase in iron deposition is often seen.

TESTS FOR RED CELL INCLUSIONS

Heinz bodies

Heinz bodies are particles of denatured hemoglobins that are attached to the cell membrane (see Figure 9-4). These are demonstrated with supravital dyes such as crystal violet. Heinz bodies are found in association with unstable hemoglobin disorders in splenectomized patients. They are also seen during acute drug-induced hemolysis.

Crystal cells of hemoglobin C disease

Crystal cells of HbC disease are present in as many as 10% of the circulating cells in patients with this disorder, but these tetrahedral crystals are rarely seen in blood films of nonsplenectomized patients. In such patients, crystal cells may be produced by hypertonic dehydration of red cells in a 3% NaCl buffer for 4–12 hours.

Table 9-4. Red Cell Morphology in Disorders of Hemoglobin Synthesis

Type of Change	Morphology
Changes secondary to hemolysis	Polychromatophilia, fine stippling, macrocytosis—all associated with reticulocytosis; nucleated red cells.
Changes associated with splenectomy or splenic atrophy	Basophilic stippling, Howell-Jolly bodies, target cells, Pappenheimer bodies, abnormal poikilocytes
Changes characteristic of specific disorders	
Sickle cell disorders	Sickle cells
HbC disorders	Target cells; hemoglobin crystals may be seen in splenectomized patients
Disorders caused by unstable Hb	Red cell inclusions with supravital stains—Heinz bodies, HbH inclusions
Thalassemia	Microcytosis, target cells, basophilic stippling

137

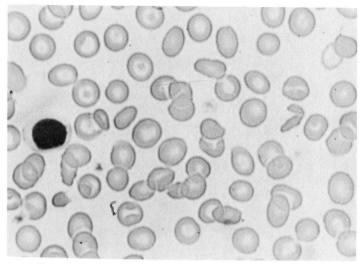

Figure 9-1. Beta-thalassemia. Note microcytosis and targeting.

Crystals are then seen in 50%–75% of red cells in HbCC disease; lower percentages are found with HbSC and other HbC variants.

Red cell inclusions in hemoglobin H disease

Red cell inclusions in HbH disease can be produced by incubating whole blood with brilliant cresyl blue (see section on tests for HbH inclusion bodies, later in chapter).

Other Useful Tests [1-3]

HEMOGLOBIN ELECTROPHORESIS

Purpose

Hemoglobin electrophoresis is the principal procedure used to detect and identify abnormal hemoglobins.

Principle

Electrophoresis is the movement of charged molecules in an electric field. Hemoglobins, like all proteins, are amphoteric; they

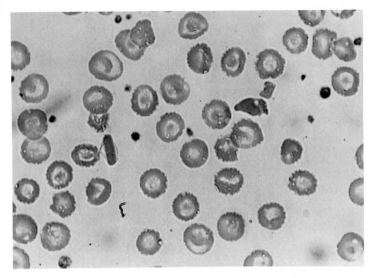

Figure 9-2. Hemoglobin C disease. Note targeting and crystal.

are charged positively or negatively depending on the pH of the suspending medium. In a basic solution with a pH of about 8, many hemoglobins have a negative charge and migrate toward the positive pole or anode. The relative speeds with which different hemoglobins migrate toward the anode are proportional to their net negative charges. Because HbS contains valine in place of the glutamic acid of HbS, HbS has a smaller negative charge and a slower anodal mobility than HbA in an alkaline medium. In an acid pH, hemoglobins are positively charged and their relative mobilities in relation to the anode are the reverse of that seen in an alkaline medium.

Procedure

Electrophoresis on cellulose acetate at pH 8.4–8.8 is the method of choice for initial electrophoretic testing in the general clinical laboratory. Although use of starch gel as a support medium gives excellent separation of hemoglobins, starch gel electrophoresis is a

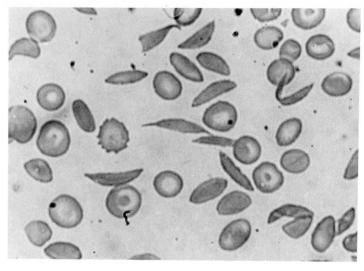

Figure 9-3. Sickle cell disease.

relatively slow, tedious procedure that is now used primarily by specialized laboratories.

Red cells are hemolyzed and subjected to electrophoresis on cellulose acetate for 15–30 minutes. A control hemolysate is run concurrently with the patient sample. Hemoglobins A, A_2, F, S, and C are most often included in controls. After the run, the membrane is stained and hemoglobins are identified by their positions. The hemoglobins can then be quantitated by elution and spectrophotometric assay or by scanning the membrane with a densitometer. Electrophoresis in citrate agar at pH 6.2 can be used to complement conventional cellulose acetate electrophoresis (see section on *Interpretation*). The procedure is basically the same as that described for cellulose acetate but requires a 45–90-minute run.

Specimen

Whole blood is used.

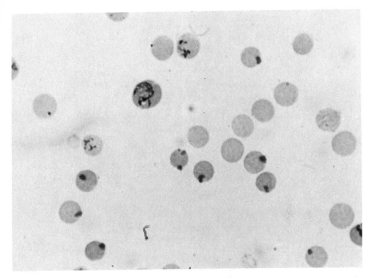

Figure 9-4. Heinz bodies.

Interpretation

The electrophoretic patterns of some hemoglobin variants are shown in Figure 9-5. Hemoglobins are often divided on the basis of their anodal electrophoretic mobility at an alkaline pH. Slow-moving hemoglobins include C, E, A_2, and O. Intermediate hemoglobins include D, G, S, and Lepore. Hemoglobins A and F are more anodal. Among the fast-moving hemoglobins are H, I, and Barts (Figure 9-6). When a prominent band is found in the HbS region on cellulose acetate electrophoresis at pH 8.6, its identity can be confirmed by electrophoresis on citrate agar at pH 6.2; the latter separates HbS from HbD and HbG. Citrate agar also differentiates HbC from HbS, O, E, and A_2 and provides sharp separation of hemoglobins F and A.

Notes and precautions

The main limitation of hemoglobin electrophoresis is its inability to detect amino acid substitutions that do not affect change.

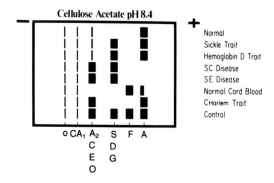

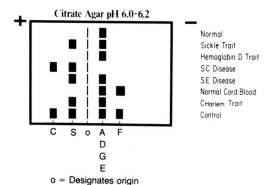

o = Designates origin

Figure 9-5. Comparison of various hemoglobin samples on cellulose acetate and citrate agar. (Modified with permission from Schmidt RM, Brosious BS: *Basic Laboratory Methods of Hemoglobinopathy Detection.* Publication No. (CDC) 77-8266. Atlanta, DHEW, 1976.)

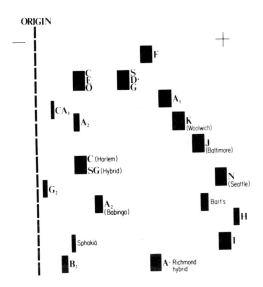

Figure 9-6. Relative mobilities of hemoglobins on cellulose acetate (TEB), pH 8.4. (Modified with permission from Schmidt RM, Brosious BS: *Basic Laboratory Methods of Hemoglobinopathy Detection.* Publication No. (CDC) 77-8266. Atlanta, DHEW 1976.)

Such variants are seen in particular among the unstable hemoglobins and with hemoglobins associated with altered oxygen affinity. Furthermore, as noted previously, different amino acid substitutions may lead to the same change in electrophoretic mobility.

THE SICKLE CELL TEST

Purpose

In most cases of sickle cell anemia, a few sickled red cells are readily observed on the routinely prepared stained blood smear. Such sickling is also seen with the double heterozygous sickle cell disorders such as SC disease or the S-thalassemias, in which HbS is the major hemoglobin component. However, in sickle cell trait and in some sickle cell disorders with a lesser propensity for sickling, various maneuvers are required to induce in vitro sickling.

143

Principle

When red cells containing HbS are deoxygenated, they sickle. Deoxygenation can be accomplished by mixing a drop of blood with a reducing agent on a slide and covering the preparation with a cover slip.

Procedure

The sickle cell test is performed by mixing the amount of blood that adheres to the end of an applicator stick with a drop of freshly prepared 2% sodium metabisulfite solution and covering the suspension with a cover slip. When sickle hemoglobin is present in the red cells, they begin to deform within 10 minutes, assuming crescent and holly-leaf shapes. The preparation is observed on the microscope within 30 minutes by means of the high dry objective.

Specimen

Venous or capillary blood is used.

Interpretation

The test results are positive for sickle cell traits and for all sickle cell disorders in which HbS is present in a concentration of 25% or greater. Sickling has also been described in other relatively rare variants including HbC_{Harlem}, HbI, and Hb Barts.

Notes and precautions

The most frequently encountered technical problem resulting in a false-negative test is outdated metabisulfite reagent that has lost its reducing power. With HbS disorders, test results may not become positive until the infant is one or two months of age because of the relatively high percentage of HbF in the red cells in infancy.

SOLUBILITY TEST FOR HbS

Purpose

Solubility tests have been used most widely in screening for sickle cell trait for the purpose of genetic counseling and as a means of differentiating HbS from HbD, which is electrophoretically identical at an alkaline pH.

Principle

The solubility test is based on the relative insolubility of reduced HbS compared to other hemoglobin variants and compared to HbA in a high-phosphate buffer solution.

Procedure

A solution of 1.24 M KH_2PO_4/1.24 M K_2HPO_4, containing saponin to lyse the red cells and sodium hydrosulfite (dithionite) to reduce the hemoglobin, is used. Blood is added and the solution is observed for turbidity by noting the patient's ability to read ruled black lines held behind the test tubes. Commercial kits are available (Sickledex).*

Specimen

Whole blood is used as a specimen.

Interpretation

Positive test results are indicated by a turbid suspension through which the ruled lines behind the test tube cannot be seen. Test results are positive for sickle cell trait and sickle cell disorders, and with rare exceptions (e.g., HbC_{Harlem}) they are negative with all other hemoglobins. The differentiation of sickle cell trait from sickle cell disease may not always be clear since it is based upon a quantitative difference in turbidity. The solubility test is inadequate as a means of screening for genetic counseling because it fails to detect the important carriers of HbC and beta-thalassemia.

Notes and precautions

In the presence of severe anemia, the blood sample usually used may not contain sufficient HbS to cause a turbid solution. With a

---

*Manufactured by Ortho Pharmaceutical Corp., Raritan, NJ.

hemoglobin level less than 7 g/dl, the sample size should be doubled. False-positive results may be seen with lipemic plasma.

ALKALI DENATURATION TEST FOR FETAL HEMOGLOBIN

Purpose

Measurement of fetal hemoglobin helps to diagnose and differentiate the thalassemias, to diagnose the double heterozygotes with combined thalassemia and a structural hemoglobin variant, and to diagnose the HPFH. Because the mobility of HbF is close to that of HbA on routine electrophoresis, measurement of HbF based on electrophoretic techniques has not been reliable.

Principle

A rapid and simple method for measuring HbF is based on the fact that it is more resistant to denaturation by a strong alkali than other hemoglobins.

Procedure

Alkali is added to a hemolysate and after one minute denatured hemoglobin is precipitated by the addition of ammonium sulfate. The filtrate contains HbF, which is quantitated spectrophotometrically.

Interpretation

The normal value for HbF is less than 2% (Table 9-5). Patients with beta-thalassemia minor may have elevated HbF levels of 2%–5%. Those with the less common delta-beta-thalassemia minor may show much higher levels. Patients with homozygous beta-thalassemia show levels of HbF ranging from 30%–100%. Levels in HPFH range from 15%–100%. Elevated Hb levels from 2%–5% have been reported in a large variety of hematologic conditions, including aplastic anemia, pernicious anemia, hereditary spherocytosis, myelofibrosis, leukemia, and metastatic disease with bone marrow involvement.

Specimen

Whole blood is used.

Notes and precautions

The alkali denaturation test is very sensitive at low levels of HbF. However, at levels greater than 10%, the method underestimates HbF, and accurate measurement requires special chromatographic techniques.

QUANTITATION OF HbA$_2$ BY CHROMATOGRAPHY

Purpose

Levels of HbA$_2$ are elevated in the commonest type of thalassemia minor. Quantitation of HbA$_2$ by routine electrophoresis on cellulose acetate has not been uniformly reliable.

Principle

The most accurate and rapid procedure generally available for measuring HbA$_2$ is a microchromatographic technique using anion exchange column chromatography to separate HbA$_2$ from HbA.

Procedure

Hemoglobin A$_2$ is separated from HbA by use of a column consisting of diethylaminoethyl (DEAE)-cellulose as the ion exchange resin. The resin is equilibrated with a tris(hydroxymethyl)aminomethane (TRIS)-phosphate buffer and the hemoglobin solution is applied. The more strongly charged HbA adheres to the ion exchange resin. Hemoglobin A$_2$ passes through and is quantitated spectrophotometrically. Commercial kits with disposable columns are available (HbA$_2$ Quik Column kit).*

Specimen

Whole blood is used.

---

*Manufactured by Helena Laboratories, Beaumont, TX.

Interpretation

The normal range of values for HbA$_2$ is 1.5%–3.5% (Table 9-5). With beta-thalassemia the range is 3.5%–8%. However, HbA$_2$ levels may not be elevated in the presence of coexisting iron deficiency.

Notes and precautions

A number of hemoglobin variants are eluted from the column under the usual test conditions. These include hemoglobins C, E, O, D, and, to a lesser extent, S. When a value greater than 8% is found, the presence of such a variant is likely. Hemoglobin A$_2$ may be separated and quantitated in the presence of HbS by eluting the two hemoglobins separately, using buffers with different pH for elution.

THE ACID ELUTION TEST FOR FETAL HEMOGLOBIN IN RED CELLS (METHOD OF KLEIHAUER AND BETKE)

Purpose

The acid elution test is a staining procedure used to differentiate HPFH from other states associated with high fetal hemoglobin levels.

Principle

When hemoglobin is precipitated inside the red cell and fixed with alcohol, the precipitates formed in the case of HbA and its variants can be solubilized in a buffered solution of citric acid. Hemoglobin F remains precipitated inside the cell.

Procedure

A blood smear is prepared in the usual manner and fixed in 80% ethanol. It is then treated with a citric acid-phosphate buffer, pH 3.3, which elutes HbA from the red cells. The blood film is then stained with eosin, which stains any residual precipitate.

Table 9-5. Hemoglobin Analysis in Beta-Thalassemic Disorders

Genetic Classification[a]	Clinical	HbA_2 (%)	HbF (%)	HbA (%)	Hemoglobin Variant (%)
Normal		1.5–3.5	< 2	97	0
Heterozygotes					
Beta-thalassemia	Thalassemia minor	3.5–8.0	< 5	> 90	0
Delta-beta-thalassemia	Thalassemia minor	1.5–3.5	4–30	Remainder	0
Delta-beta-Lepore	Thalassemia minor	< 1.5	2–14	Remainder	Hb Lepore ≈ 10
Homozygotes					
Beta-thalassemia°	Thalassemia major	Variable	Almost 100%	0	0
Beta-thalassemia+	Thalassemia major or intermedia	1.5–4.0	30–90	Remainder	0
Delta-beta-thalassemia	Thalassemia intermedia	0	100	100	0
Delta-beta-Lepore	Thalassemia major	0	75	0	Hb Lepore = 25
Double heterozygotes					
HbS beta-thalassemia+	Sickle cell thalassemia	3.5–8.0	8–15	≈ 20	HbS = 60–70
HbS beta-thalassemia°	Sickle cell thalassemia	3.5–8.0	8–15	0	HbS = 90

[a]Thalassemia° refers to genetic type with no production of beta chains; thalassemia+ refers to genetic type with reduced production of beta chains.

149

Specimen

Whole blood is used.

Interpretation

Smears from normal blood show little if any uptake of stain and cells appear as ghosts. A heterogeneous distribution of fetal hemoglobin is seen in newborn infants, with fetal-maternal transfusion, and in the thalassemias with elevated HbF. The only condition in which HbF is evenly distributed in nearly all of the red cells is HPFH.

Notes and precautions

The intensity of the staining often differs markedly from one part of the blood film to another and considerable experience may be required to interpret this procedure.

HEAT STABILITY TEST

Purpose

The heat stability test is used to detect unstable hemoglobins.

Principle

The unstable hemoglobins tend to precipitate within red cells. In vitro, such precipitation can be demonstrated when a hemolysate is exposed to heat.

Procedure

A buffered hemolysate is warmed to 50 C for three hours and then observed for the formation of a precipitate.

Specimen

Whole blood is used.

Interpretation

The appearance of a flocculent precipitate after about one hour generally indicates the presence of an unstable hemoglobin. However, since some normal samples also show some precipitate after this period of time, simultaneous specimens of healthy control subjects are run for comparison.

ISOPROPANOL STABILITY TEST

Purpose

The isopropanol stability test is used to detect unstable hemoglobins. It is easier to perform than the heat stability test.

Principle

Normal hemoglobin is somewhat unstable in isopropanol. The effect is accentuated with the unstable hemoglobins.

Procedure

A hemolysate is added to buffered isopropanol and incubated at 37 C. The preparation is observed for precipitation at intervals.

Specimen

Whole blood is used.

Interpretation

Unstable hemoglobins generally show turbidity within 5 minutes, while normal hemoglobins do not precipitate until 30–40 minutes. False-positive tests may be obtained with sickle hemoglobin, fetal hemoglobin, and methemoglobin.

TEST FOR HEMOGLOBIN H INCLUSION BODIES

Purpose

Hemoglobin H is an unstable hemoglobin that may be difficult to detect on routine electrophoresis. This test is particularly useful for the detection of HbH and may suggest the presence of other unstable hemoglobins.

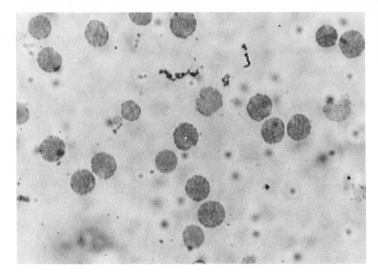

Figure 9-7. Hemoglobin H disease. Note golf-ball stippling.

Principle

Incubation of whole blood with brilliant cresyl blue causes denaturation of unstable hemoglobin, which precipitates in red cells resulting in diffuse stippling.

Procedure

Three to four drops of whole blood are incubated with 0.5 ml of a 1% solution of brilliant cresyl blue in citrate-saline solution. Blood films are made at 10 minutes, one hour, and four hours.

Specimen

Fresh whole blood is used.

Interpretation

Positive cells have a diffusely stippled pattern resembling a golf ball with the reticulum staining light blue (Figure 9-7). In HbH disease, 50% or more of the cells on the one-hour slide may be positive. In alpha-thalassemia trait an occasional cell may be positive. Results with other unstable hemoglobins are variable and a longer period of incubation is usually required for precipitation. The 10-minute slide is a control that shows the number of reticulocytes present.

REFERENCES

1. Miale JB: *Laboratory Medicine: Hematology*, ed 5. St. Louis, C. V. Mosby Co, 1977, pp 1026–1035 (appendix)
2. Schmidt RM, Brosious BS: *Basic Laboratory Methods of Hemoglobinopathy Detection*. HEW Publication No. (CDC) 77-8266. Atlanta, DHEW, 1976
3. Williams WJ, Beutler E, Erslev AJ, et al (eds): *Hematology*, ed 2. New York, McGraw-Hill, 1977, pp 1589–1604 (appendix)

chapter 10

Paroxysmal Nocturnal Hemoglobinuria

Paroxysmal nocturnal hemoglobinuria (PNH) is a relatively rare chronic hemolytic disorder. Its name implies that hemolysis is episodic and that hemoglobinuria is a major feature. However, the classic presentation of the passage of red urine in the morning on arising is not usually observed. More frequently, chronic hemolysis, often associated with leukopenia and thrombocytopenia, is the predominant feature of the disorder. Hemosiderinuria, not hemoglobinuria, is a constant feature.

Episodes of abdominal pain may be a prominent symptom. They may be associated with thrombosis of the portal, mesenteric, or hepatic vein. Some patients have severe, refractory headaches that may be caused by small vessel thrombosis. Thrombophlebitis may occur in the legs or in the arms and may lead to thromboembolism.

The cause of PNH is unknown. It often arises as a sequella of aplastic anemia and it seems to be caused by an abnormality of the cell membrane, but the nature of the underlying defect is not known. The red cells have a markedly increased sensitivity to lysis by complement, a defect that appears to be shared by other cells as well. The complement sensitivity of the erythrocytes forms the basis of two of the diagnostic tests of PNH, the sucrose hemolysis test and the acid hemolysis test.

DIAGNOSTIC EVALUATION

Depending on the predominant features of the presenting illness, PNH may need to be differentiated from other causes of chronic hemolytic anemia, pancytopenia, iron deficiency, and hemoglobinuria and myoglobinuria. Iron deficiency may result from loss of substantial amounts of iron in the urine in the form of hemosiderin.

Laboratory evaluation of this disorder proceeds with the following:

1. Hematologic evaluation with complete blood count and study of red cell morphology and bone marrow study.
2. Sucrose hemolysis test as a screening test for PNH.
3. Acid hemolysis test as a definitive diagnostic test for PNH.
4. Test for urine hemosiderin, since hemosiderinuria is a constant feature of PNH.
5. Tests for intravascular and extravascular hemolysis: test of serum for unconjugated bilirubin, hemoglobin, methemalbumin, and haptoglobin; urine test for hemoglobin.

LABORATORY STUDIES

Hematologic Tests

GENERAL FEATURES

Paroxysmal nocturnal hemoglobinuria most commonly presents as a chronic hemolytic anemia. The degree of anemia varies widely from borderline to severe, with hemoglobin levels of less than 6 g/dl. In addition to episodes of sleep-related rhythmicity in hemolysis associated with hemoglobinuria in some cases, patients with PNH suffer from irregularly recurring exacerbation in hemolysis, apparently precipitated by events such as infections, operations, and transfusions. The majority of patients with PNH exhibit neutropenia and thrombocytopenia at some stage in their disease. In fact, PNH can arise as a sequella of otherwise typical aplastic anemia. Because relatively large amounts of iron are often lost in the urine even in the absence of observable hemoglobinuria, patients with PNH are often iron deficient.

PERIPHERAL BLOOD

Blood cell measurements

The degree of anemia varies widely, with hemoglobin levels ranging from less than 6 g/dl to normal levels. The MCV may be somewhat increased with prominent reticulocytosis or indices may be consistent with iron deficiency anemia. The percent of reticulocytes may be markedly elevated; however, absolute reticulocyte count may be low for the degree of anemia. This discrepancy can be attributed to associated iron deficiency or to a bone marrow stem cell defect.

Morphology

No characteristic morphologic changes are seen. Macrocytosis and polychromatophilia may accompany prominent reticulocytosis. Iron deficiency may result in hypochromia and microcytosis.

BONE MARROW

Normoblastic hyperplasia is the most frequent finding with adequate numbers of megakaryocytes and myeloid elements. However, marrow cellularity may be decreased or the marrow may be aplastic. Stainable storage iron is often absent, even when obvious iron deficiency is not present.

Other Useful Tests

SUCROSE HEMOLYSIS TEST

Purpose

The sucrose hemolysis test is the most convenient screening test for PNH (1).

Principle

An isotonic sucrose solution of low ionic strength appears to enhance the binding of complement to the red cell membrane.

When a small amount of serum as a source of complement is added to such a solution, PNH cells are lysed whereas normal cells are not.

Procedure

A small amount of fresh, normal, type-compatible serum is added to a buffered sucrose solution. Washed red cells from the patient are added and the suspension is incubated for 60 minutes at room temperature.

Specimen

Whole blood is used.

Interpretation

Greater than 5% lysis is compatible with the diagnosis of PNH. Lysis usually amounting to less than 5% may be found in the megaloblastic anemias and in autoimmune hemolytic disease. A definitive diagnosis requires performance of the acid hemolysis test (see the following section).

Notes and precautions

When originally described it was suggested that the sucrose hemolysis test could be carried out using unbuffered sucrose solutions. However, this has proven unwise and may lead to false-negative results.

ACID HEMOLYSIS TEST

Purpose

The acid hemolysis test is required to make a definitive diagnosis of PNH (1).

Principle

A definitive diagnosis of PNH depends on demonstration of the following characteristics of in vitro hemolysis: it occurs with patient cells but not with control cells, it is enchanced by slightly acidifying the serum used, it is abolished by heat inactivating the serum at 56 C, and its potency is not restored to the heated serum by the addition of guinea pig complement. These characteristics of the hemolytic system can be demonstrated using Ham's acid hemolysis test.

Procedure

The acid hemolysis test is carried out using type-compatible blood from a healthy control subject and blood from a patient with PNH. Four serum preparations should be used from patient and control: unaltered serum, serum with a pH adjusted to 6.8 as measured by a pH meter, serum at pH 6.8 that has been heat inactivated to 56 C for three minutes, and heated serum to which guinea pig complement has been added. Red cells from patient or control subject are suspended in each of these types of serum.

Specimen

Whole blood is used.

Interpretation

Positive test results are those in which hemolysis of the patient's erythrocytes occurs in acidified serum and not in heated serum either with or without addition of guinea pig complement. Some hemolysis may be present in the unaltered serum but this is generally less than that observed in acidified serum. No hemolysis of control cells should occur in any of the tubes.

Notes and precautions

Erroneous test results can be obtained by either over- or under-acidification of serum. In the test as originally described, the pH of the serum was not verified with a pH meter since such instruments were not available. Careful adjustment of the pH of the serum to 6.8 ± 0.1 is necessary if reliable results are to be obtained.

TEST FOR URINE HEMOSIDERIN

Purpose

Urine hemosiderin is nearly always present in PNH and may be a valuable aid in making the diagnosis (2).

Principle

Even in the absence of discernible hemoglobinuria, chronic low-grade intravascular hemolysis is sufficient in PNH to lead to depletion of serum haptoglobin and to the presence of hemoglobin in the kidney, which is reabsorbed by the tubules. Tubules become heavily laden with iron, which is excreted in the urine as hemosiderin granules demonstrable with the Prussian-blue stain.

Procedure

The presence of hemosiderin in the urine is demonstrated by adding a drop of a mixture of equal parts of 4% hydrochloric acid and 4% potassium ferrocyanide to the sediment of a centrifuged urine specimen. The mixture is incubated at room temperature for 10 minutes with frequent agitation.

Specimen

A random urine specimen is used for testing urine hemosiderin.

Interpretation

Hemosiderin appears as blue particles. While considerable emphasis has been placed on the intercellular location of hemosiderin in urine, cells containing hemosiderin may have disintegrated in the urine and free hemosiderin may be the predominant form. Urine of healthy patients does not contain hemosiderin.

Ancillary Tests

Many other procedures have been described for the detection of PNH. The thrombin activation test, lysis of A cells in the presence of anti-A, and Ham's presumptive tests are all capable of detecting most patients with PNH. However, they are unnecessarily cumbersome and have been superseded by more recently developed procedures such as the sucrose hemolysis test. Quanitative testing of complement sensitivity may give more precise information regarding the size of the complement-sensitive population; however, it is too complex for routine clinical use. Red cell acetylcholinesterase activity and leukocyte alkaline phosphatase activity are diminished in PNH.

REFERENCES

1. Rosse WF: Studies for paroxysmal nocturnal hemoglobinuria. In Williams WJ, Beutler E, Erslev AJ, et al (eds): *Hematology*, ed 2. New York, McGraw-Hill, 1977, pp 1611–1613
2. Beutler E: Peripheral blood, bone marrow, and urine iron stains. In Williams WJ, Beutler E, Erslev AJ, et al (eds): *Hematology*, ed 2. New York, McGraw-Hill, 1977, pp 1589–1590

chapter 11

Acquired Hemolytic Anemias

Excluding the inherited (intrinsic) hemolytic anemias and PNH, a varied group of hemolytic anemias are caused by extrinsic factors such as chemical, physical, and infectious agents and circulating antibody (Table 11-1). Although older terminology grouped these extrinsic hemolytic anemias into a direct Coombs-positive category, only the antibody-associated anemias are actually in this group. When red cell enzyme deficiency and hemoglobinopathy have been excluded, antibody-induced hemolysis becomes the most frequently occurring hemolytic anemia. Antibodies can be produced in response to foreign red cell antigens (alloantibody), to self-antigens (autoantibody), or to drugs bound to red cell membrane or plasma proteins. Antibody can also be transfused passively from mother to fetus (erythroblastosis fetalis).

ALLOANTIBODIES CAUSED BY INCOMPATIBLE TRANSFUSION OF ERYTHROCYTES

Antibodies to red cell antigens foreign to the host result from previous transfusion (IgG, IgM), from previous pregnancy (IgG), from unknown causes spontaneously (IgM), or, rarely, from injections of red cells, an antiquated method of conferring immunity to infectious disease that is occasionally seen in immigrant populations (IgG). Antibody may be present without history of transfusion

Table 11-1. Hemolytic Anemias Caused by Extrinsic Factors

Category	Specific Agent

Infectious	Protozoa
	    Malaria
	Bacterial
	    Cholera
	Viral

Physicochemical	Burns
	Chemicals
	    Dose-related toxins, e.g.,
	       benzene, phenylhydrazine
	Drugs
	    Interaction with RBC enzyme
	      deficiency

Antibody-induced	Alloantibody
	    Incompatible transfusion
	    Erythroblastosis fetalis
	Autoantibody
	    Warm autoantibodies
	    Cold autoantibodies
	Paroxysmal cold hemoglobinuria (PCH)
	Drug-induced antibody
	    Toxic immune complexes—quinidine,
	      quinine
	    Haptens—penicillin type/cephalothin
	    Alpha methyldopa type

Miscellaneous	Paroxysmal nocturnal hemoglobinuria (PNH)

reaction. The immediate clinical significance of the antibody depends on whether transfusion has been given in the past two to three weeks (delayed transfusion reaction) or whether transfusion is being contemplated.

DIAGNOSTIC EVALUATION OF ALLOANTIBODIES

Diagnostic evaluation begins with a complete history regarding sources of exposure to red cell products, how recently exposure occurred, and any symptoms associated with the exposure. The immediate significance of antibody depends on whether transfusions are being given currently (transfusion reaction) or are being contemplated (compatible donor selection). In a logical sequence hematologic findings may be less important than:

1. Serum antibody screening, which should include several serologic techniques and temperature variations to detect both IgG and IgM antibodies.
2. Antibody identification combined with appropriate antigen typings of the patient's red cells.
3. Direct antiglobulin test if transfusions have been given in the previous three to six weeks or if autoimmune hemolysis is suspected.
4. Tests to evaluate acute hemolysis if transfusion reaction is suspected. Such tests include plasma/urine hemoglobin, serum haptoglobin, and serum bilirubin. If intravascular hemolysis has occurred, tests to monitor renal function are also performed.

LABORATORY STUDIES OF ALLOANTIBODIES

Hematologic Tests

GENERAL FEATURES

Hematologic tests are informative only if transfusions are currently being given. An abrupt fall in hemoglobin up to 14 days after transfusion, a failure to maintain hemoglobin levels after transfusion, or the appearance of jaundice suggests incompatible transfusion. Prolonged administration of incompatible blood can result in splenomegaly and lead to the mistaken diagnosis of autoimmune hemolytic anemia. Intravascular hemolysis may result with ABO-incompatible transfusion and with transfusion reactions caused by anti-Kell, anti-Duffy (anti-Fy^a), or anti-Kidd (anti-Jk^a or anti-Jk^b). The latter may cause intravascular hemolysis 10–14 days after transfusion. Intravascular hemolysis may be followed by disseminated intravascular coagulation (DIC).

PERIPHERAL BLOOD

Blood cell measurements

Variable anemia is present if transfusions are current; otherwise no symptoms occur. One unit of packed red cells should increase the hemoglobin 1.5 g/dl or the hematocrit 3% in an adult of average size.

Acute hemolysis may be associated with leukocytosis, sometimes with a left shift.

Morphology

Transfusions that are ABO incompatible are associated with microspherocytes. Disseminated intravascular coagulation can be associated with red cell fragmentation.

BONE MARROW

Bone marrow examination is usually not helpful. Prolonged transfusion with incompatible blood results in an increase in marrow iron.

Other Useful Tests

SERUM ANTIBODY SCREENING

Purpose

Serum antibody screening detects the presence of antibody to red cells (1).

Principle

Antibody to red cell antigens agglutinates or hemolyzes screening cells that have the antigen, providing the medium of the reaction and the temperature of reaction is appropriate. These tests are widely available although reliability of their interpretations is variable.

Procedure

The patient's serum is screened with commercially supplied red cells that have most of the 18 major antigen groups represented. Screening cells and serum are incubated at room temperature and at 37 C; this is followed by the antiglobulin reaction (indirect Coombs test) to detect IgM and IgG antibodies respectively. IgA antibodies are rarely detected in blood group serology. If antibody is strongly suspected laboratories in larger hospitals or reference laboratories automatically perform tests at 4 C or may use enzyme-treated red cells.

Specimen

Ten milliliters of serum are obtained fresh to conserve complement since some antibodies are complement dependent. If blood must be mailed to a reference laboratory, the serum should be separated from the cells to prevent spurious hemolysis. However, red cells must accompany the serum. The serum can be frozen if conditions do not appear optimal, for example, if it is being mailed to a hot climate, across the continent, or over a holiday.

Interpretation

Any degree of hemolysis or agglutination at any stage of the testing is considered positive and graded 0–4+. The antibody must then be identified to assess transfusion hazard and future availability of blood. Results of antibody screening may be negative despite previous reactions to transfusion or incompatible pregnancies, since antibodies may fade completely with time or are of such low titer that they are detectable only with enzyme-treated red cells or with cells homozygous for the antigen. Suspicious histories should be reported to the laboratory so that technologists can expand their testing beyond the routine screening procedures. Antigen-incompatible transfusions have diminished survival that is sometimes abrupt, as with anti-Jk^a. Antibody is found in 2%–3% of the previously transfused population, 2%–3% of the previously pregnant, and less than 1% of all others for a combined incidence of 5%–6%.

ANTIBODY IDENTIFICATION

Purpose

Antibody identification assesses current hazard to transfusion, predicts reliability of cross-match procedures, evaluates availability of blood (particularly under emergency circumstances), and detects multiple antibodies.

Principle

The availability and completeness of identification procedures vary in hospital laboratories, but every area usually has at least one reference laboratory available, and specimens with positive results on screening can be referred by the hospital blood bank. Depending on distance and complexity of the problem, results may require one to five days.

Procedure

Serum is tested with commercially available panels of 9 or 10 red cell samples for which all antigens are known, as provided on printed protocols. Serum is also tested with the patient's own cells and usually with samples of cord blood as well. Serum and cell samples are incubated at room temperature and at 37 C using the techniques described in the section on Diagnostic Evaluation. The presence of agglutination or hemolysis is noted and graded. Variability in strength of agglutination, temperature of reaction, or medium of reaction may indicate the presence of more than one antibody. Once antibody specificity is known, the patient's red cells are typed for the appropriate antigen.

166

Serum separated from the clot and a sample of the patient's red cells, either from the clot or from a separate anticoagulated (EDTA) tube, are used as specimens. If serum cannot be tested within 48 hours, it should be stored frozen to conserve complement.

Interpretation

Alloantibody agglutinates specific cells of the panel but not the patient's own. The pattern of reactive cell samples is compared with the protocol sheet to determine specificity. The patient's own cells should be negative for the particular antigen, and if they are not, the antibody specificity is not confirmed and must be re-evaluated.

IgG antibodies act at 37 C by indirect antiglobulin or by enzyme techniques. They usually follow previous transfusion or incompatible pregnancy. Three antibodies are particularly dangerous in transfusion since they cause intravascular hemolysis and/or DIC: anti-Kell, anti-Fy^a, and anti-Jk^a or anti-Jk^b. The Kidd antibodies may not be found during antibody screening but rapidly increase their titer with incompatible transfusions and may cause intravascular hemolysis beginning as long as 10 days after transfusion when the stimulated antibody titer reaches a critical level. The members of the Rh system (anti-D, -c, -E, -e) follow an immunizing stimulus and destroy cells more slowly by splenic sequestration.

IgM antibodies bind complement. Although they may follow incompatible transfusion, they more often appear spontaneously and, therefore, unpredictably. They include anti-Lewis^a and anti-Lewis^b, anti-P$_1$, and anti-M. Transfusion reactions may vary from intravascular hemolysis to unexplained shortened red cell survival. The most lethal IgM antibodies are anti-A and anti-B, involved in major blood group incompatibility. These antibodies are not detectable by identification techniques since all the test red cells are group O.

Once identified, antibodies must be permanently recorded since they may fade with time only to reappear with incompatible transfusions or be so weak that truly incompatible units appear compatible.

DIRECT ANTIGLOBULIN TEST (DAT)—DIRECT COOMBS TEST

Purpose

The DAT detects antiglobulin coating of circulating red cells, presumably by antibody (1, 2). It does not distinguish alloantibody from autoantibody. After transfusion, in the absence of autoantibody, the red cells coated are donor cells, as confirmed by testing red cell antigens.

Principle

Antihuman globulin manufactured in rabbits agglutinates globulin-coated red cells regardless of the reason for coating. Broad-spectrum reagents react with IgG, IgM, or complement globulins, whereas monospecific serums agglutinate only red cells coated with the specific globulin to which the reagent is directed.

Procedure

Posttransfusion red cells are centrifuged with antiglobulin reagent, and the agglutination is graded 0–4+. The reagent used is usually broad spectrum to detect any possible reaction. All tests whose results are positive require elution of the globulin coat and testing to identify the globulin as red cell antibody.

Specimen

The patient's posttransfusion red cells are used as a specimen. They are collected in EDTA to prevent nonspecific adsorption of globulin in the presence of cold autoagglutinins.

Interpretation

Positive results may vary from ±–4+ depending on the cause. Unlike reactions with autoimmune hemolytic anemia, these tend to be 1+ or weaker. After massive intravascular hemolysis, the DAT may show negative results since all coated cells are now lysed. The donor cells are a minor population in the patient's circulation giving a "mixed-field" appearance that is characteristic. Positive test results may be extremely transient. The antibody specificity of the eluate does not match the patient's red cell antigens, although in patients transfused with many units or in those with a DAT of 4+, the antigens may be difficult to determine. Repeat testing while withholding further transfusions may clarify the picture.

SERUM HAPTOGLOBIN

Purpose

Absent haptoglobin implies recent complexing with free hemoglobin from red cell destruction (2).

Principle

Haptoglobin, an alpha$_2$ globulin, binds free hemoglobin molecule for molecule. The Hp:Hb complex is completely metabolized in the reticuloendothelial system. It requires four days to manufacture new haptoglobin molecules in the liver. Thus complete haptoglobin binding and degradation results in an absent haptoglobin level. The implication is hemolysis, providing liver disease is clinically excluded.

Procedure

Semiquantitative measurement by residual hemoglobin-binding capacity is performed using agar or cellulose electrophoresis.

Specimen

Usually anticoagulated whole blood is drawn atraumatically. Plasma is separated immediately from red cells.

Interpretation

The normal range of haptoglobin is 40–180 mg/dl. Levels less than 25 mg/dl are consistent with hemolysis. Haptoglobin levels may be transiently decreased after massive transfusion as a result of destruction of senescent red cells without hemolysis.

PLASMA HEMOGLOBIN

Purpose

Tests for plasma hemoglobin are performed since hemoglobinemia indicates intravascular hemolysis (2,3).

Principle

IgM antibodies to red cell antigens activate the classic complement pathway resulting in intravascular hemolysis. IgG antibodies of very high titer may also result in intravascular cell destruction.

For sections on *Procedure, Specimen,* and *Interpretation,* see Chapter 5.

URINE HEMOGLOBIN

Purpose

Free plasma hemoglobin at levels above 150 mg/dl appears in the urine (2,3). The test for urine hemoglobin confirms intravascular hemolysis, particularly when venous specimens have been technically difficult to obtain or when obtaining them has been delayed.

Principle

Plasma proteins, haptoglobin, transferrin, and albumin bind free hemoglobin in normal metabolism. When the renal threshold is exceeded, free hemoglobin is detected in the urine. In incompatible transfusion, this is usually a transient occurrence until the incompatible red cells are lysed.

Procedure

Urine is tested with a dip-stick (see Chapter 5).

Specimen

Random urine is collected within two to three hours of the clinical episode.

Normally, no hemoglobin is present in the urine. Significant reactions are 1+ or greater (scale: 0–3+). The urine sediment should be examined for red cells (hematuria) not seen with transfusion reactions but accompanying bladder or prostate surgery and catheters. If red cell destruction has been occurring slowly over several days, urine hemosiderin may be present without overt hemoglobinuria.

NEONATAL ANEMIA WITH ALLOANTIBODIES OF FETOMATERNAL INCOMPATIBILITY

Many of the characteristics of incompatible transfusions are similar in fetomaternal incompatibility (erythroblastosis fetalis). In fetomaternal incompatibility the fetus receives antibody passively from the mother, who has been exposed to foreign antigens by previous transfusion or has received small infusions of red cells across the placenta during the current or some past pregnancy. Serologically in all cases the mother will be negative for the red cell antigen, and her fetus will be positive by virtue of the genetic input of the father. Neonatal hemolytic disease depends on the physicochemical characteristics of the maternal antibody (e.g., only IgG antibodies cross the placenta), and they must be avid to bond strongly with the fetal red cell membrane. Coated red cells are sequestered in the spleen and liver causing enlargement of these organs in the newborn.

The two major types of fetomaternal incompatibility are ABO group incompatibility and Rh incompatibility. The characteristics of each are seen in Table 11-2. ABO group incompatibility is very common but usually not clinically severe. The condition is produced by a mother who is blood group O with a group A or B fetus. It may occur during any pregnancy, even the first, since it is postulated that secreted A or B substance, not just red cells, cross the

Table 11-2. Characteristics of Erythroblastosis Fetalis Caused By ABO and Rh Incompatibility

Clinical and Laboratory Findings	ABO	Rh_o
Clinical		
Number of antigen-positive pregnancy	Any, including the first	After the first pregnancy
Clinical severity	Unpredictable	More severe with each antigen-positive pregnancy
Prenatal evaluation	None needed	Anti-Rh_o titer Amniocentesis
Onset of jaundice[a]	3–4 days postdelivery	Immediate
Treatment[a]	None, bilirubin lights, or rare exchange transfusion	None, early delivery, bilirubin lights, exchange transfusion, or intrauterine transfusion
Laboratory		
Direct Coombs test	±–1+	2–4+
Fetal blood group	A or B	Rh_o positive
Fetal antibody	Anti-A or anti-B	anti-Rh_o
Maternal blood group	O	Rh negative
Maternal antibody screening	Negative	Positive
Peripheral blood (newborn)	Microspherocytes	Not diagnostic

[a]Treatment options are listed by increasing severity of erythroblastosis.

172

placenta to the mother inducing her to produce IgG anti-A, or anti-B antibodies; the antibody recrosses the placenta to attach to the infant cells. Antibody avidity is usually poor so disease is slow to appear, three to four days after delivery.

Rh_o (anti-D) incompatibility appears after the first pregnancy as a result of infusion of red cells across the placenta at the first delivery. It is increasingly severe with each pregnancy but is becoming clinically less common with the use of anti-Rh_o gamma globulin. Given at each abortion or delivery, it prevents immune recognition of D antigen and provides immunity to the mother. Occasionally other antibodies are involved in fetomaternal incompatibility; anti-c, anti-E, and anti-Kell are the commonest. The mechanism is the same as for anti-D, but the antibodies are less efficient at causing jaundice in the newborn. Anti-Kell antibodies in a mother almost always indicate past transfusion, not incompatible previous pregnancy, since 90% of the population is Kell-negative including mother, father, and their infant.

DIAGNOSTIC EVALUATION OF NEONATAL ANEMIA

The type of fetomaternal incompatibility producing hemolytic disease of the newborn can be anticipated by transfusion and gestation history and the following tests:

1. Maternal blood group and antibody screening.
2. Newborn blood group.
3. Direct antiglobulin test of newborn cells and eluate of positive red cells.
4. Peripheral blood smear from cord blood or infant examined for microspherocytes.
5. If serologic evidence is present for erythroblastosis fetalis, serum bilirubins are ordered serially.
6. The father's blood is tested with the mother's if serologic evidence of erythroblastosis is not present, yet the newborn is hemolyzing for undetermined causes and the newborn DAT is positive. This test-

ing is expected to exclude "exotic" incompatibilities between paternal antigens (reflected in the child) and maternal antibody.

7. Although neutralization studies can be performed to classify the maternal antibody as IgG or IgM to estimate likelihood of placental passage, they are rarely necessary or clinically helpful.

LABORATORY STUDIES OF NEONATAL ANEMIA

Hematologic Tests

GENERAL FEATURES

Serologic evidence may exist for erythroblastosis fetalis without clinical evidence of hemolysis, particularly in ABO group incompatibility. Destruction of red cells is primarily caused by reticuloendothelial sequestration, so that fetal liver and spleen are enlarged and variable jaundice is present. In severe Rh erythroblastosis, red cell destruction occurs in utero; the infant may be born severely anemic but is not jaundiced until after birth, when placental transport of bilirubin is lost and the neonatal liver must assume bilirubin metabolism.

PERIPHERAL BLOOD

Blood cell count

Levels of hemoglobin in mild anemia are 14–16 g/dl; in moderate anemia, 10–14 g/dl; and in severe anemia, 8–10 g/dl. The white cell count is 10–20,000 cu mm, and the reticulocyte count is greater than 10%.

Morphology

Morphology shows polychromasia, correlating with the increased reticulocyte count and nucleated red cells greater than 10 per 100 white cells. Microspherocytes usually indicate ABO hemolytic disease.

BONE MARROW

Bone marrow examination is not necessary.

Other Useful Tests

DETERMINATION OF BLOOD GROUP

Purpose

Testing of the blood group of both the mother and the newborn determines if the mother is negative for antigen and the infant is positive (1).

Principle

Maternal red cell antigens and newborn antigens are determined for ABO and Rh_o. Tests can be performed for further antigens if indicated.

Procedure

Standard typing procedures are direct agglutination of red cells by anti-A, anti-B, and anti-D antibodies. All Rh_o (D) negative cells are tested for D^u, the partial or gene-suppressed D antigen.

Specimen

Red cells from clots or anticoagulated specimens are well washed with saline before testing. Specimens are stable for at least seven days. Cord red cells and plasma can be used if the red cells are well washed to remove contaminants. Infant heel-stick specimens can also be used.

Interpretation

In ABO hemolytic disease, the mother's blood is group O (i.e., negative for A or B) and the infant's blood is group A or B. In Rh hemolytic disease, the mother is Rh negative and the infant is positive. Where the serologic possibility of both ABO and Rh disease is possible, that is, an O-negative mother with an A- or B-positive child, hemolytic disease is more likely caused by ABO, since the group incompatibility has usually lysed Rh-incompatible cells throughout pregnancy. Mothers who are Rh positive are not excluded from having infants with hemolytic disease, since they may be c (hr') negative, E negative, and so forth, and their infants positive for these antigens.

MATERNAL ANTIBODY SCREENING AND IDENTIFICATION

Purpose

A positive antibody screening may indicate anti-Rh_o type of hemolytic disease rather than ABO type, where screenings are negative.

Principle

Maternal serum is screened for antibody, usually early in pregnancy and sporadically thereafter to detect IgG and/or IgM antibodies. The antibody is then identified to assess fetal risk and, if necessary, the father's red cell antigens are tested as a predictive measure of fetal involvement.

Procedure

Serum is incubated with test red cells at room temperature in saline suspension to detect IgM antibodies, and by incubation at 37 C with antiglobulin reaction to detect IgG antibodies. All antibodies are identified using the same techniques.

Specimen

Serum less than 48 hours old is obtained at the first obstetric visit. A specimen should also be obtained in the third trimester and more frequently if the early specimen showed positive results or if the obstetric history warrants it.

Interpretation

In ABO hemolytic disease only the expected anti-A and anti-B antibodies are found in the group O mother, so the antibody screen is negative. In all other types of hemolytic disease, the antibody screen is positive. The antibody must be identified to determine its significance to the newborn. Only IgG antibodies cross the placenta and they must coat infant red cells to produce symptoms. A common antibody found in pregnant women is anti-Lewis[a] and/or anti-Lewis[b]. Yet they do not produce neonatal disease because they are IgM and cannot cross the placenta and because all infants are Lewis[a] and Lewis[b] negative. Thus some antibodies are more significant for the mother in a postpartum hemorrhage than for the infant in hemolytic disease of the newborn (HDN).

DIRECT ANTIGLOBULIN (COOMBS) TEST IN THE NEWBORN

Purpose

The DAT detects globulin coating on newborn's red cells (2).

Principle

Fetal red cells are coated with passively transmitted IgG antibody specific for antigen.

Procedure

Broad-spectrum antiglobulin reagent is centrifuged with newborn's red cells that have been washed with saline to free them of all contaminating substances and serum proteins. Agglutination is graded 0–4+. For all tests producing positive results, adsorbed globulin is eluted and tested for antibody specificity.

Specimen

Red cells from specimens of cord blood that is either clotted or anticoagulated can be used. Small capillary specimens from newborn heel-sticks are also adequate. Cord samples are stable for at least one week and can be tested when and if clinical findings appear.

Interpretation

Infant DATs are ±–1+ for ABO hemolytic disease, 2–4+ for Rh hemolytic disease, and 2–4+ for hemolytic disease caused by other antibodies. The antibody eluted from the neonatal red cells should match that found in the maternal serum. Antibody found only in cord plasma, but not on cord red cells, is of doubtful significance, indicating poor avidity and, therefore, less likely clinical disease. Antibodies such as anti-c, anti-E, and anti-Kell, adsorbed to fetal red cells produce a strong DAT but usually minimal jaundice. Improved antiglobulin reagents make false-negative tests less common; additional saline wash of the cells diminishes false-negatives resulting from neutralization of the Coombs reagent. Rarely, elution of an antiglobulin negative red cell yields antibody because of indetectable numbers of molecules concentrated in the elution process.

Positive DAT results on cord specimens without detectable antibody may indicate adsorption of Wharton's jelly, but the cell control is usually positive. The test should be repeated on blood from a heel-stick or venous sample. If results are still positive private antibody limited to this family should be considered, and maternal serum or infant's plasma should be tested against paternal red cells for agglutination.

IMMUNE HEMOLYSIS CAUSED BY DRUGS

Drugs can damage red cells by interaction with intrinsic enzyme systems (see Chapter 5) and by inducing extrinsic antibodies. The latter may be caused by several mechanisms: toxic immune complexes (quinidine, quinine), hapten formation (penicillins), a positive DAT without hemolysis (cephalothin–Keflin), or a true, warm autoimmune hemolytic anemia (AIHA) (alpha methyldopa). Except for the last category, the incriminated drug must be present for hemolysis to occur, although the antibodies persist for life. (See Table 11-3 for a list of drugs commonly involved and their mechanism of action.) Drugs that cause immune hemolysis have a benzene ring often activated by $-OH$, $-NH$, or $-S$ groups. They must have firm binding to a protein carrier, serum proteins, or red

Table 11-3. Drugs Commonly Associated with Immune Hemolysis and the Mechanism of Cell Destruction

Drugs	Route of Administration	Duration of Therapy	Antibody Class	Hemolytic Symptoms
Toxic immune complex of (drug = drug Ab = C') Quinidine, quinine Para-amino salicylate Phenacetin Ethacrynic acid	Oral, variable dose	10–14 days	IgG, IgM, C'	Intravascular hemolysis can occur; single case reports of involved drug; infrequent cause of anemia
Hapten formation Penicillin Methicillin Ampicillin Oxacillin Carbenicillin	i.v. > 20 M U/day	10–14 days	IgG	Splenic sequestration; intravascular hemolysis is rare
				Commonly occurring
Nonspecific protein absorption Cephalothin Cephaloridine	i.m. or oral, >4 g/day	4–6 days	Any protein	Common cause of weakly positive DAT; proven hemolysis rare
True, warm AIHA Alpha methyldopa L-dopa Mefenamic acid Flufenamic acid Chlordiazepoxide hydrochloride (Librium)	Oral	6 weeks– 3 months	IgG	10% of patients have positive DAT, 1% hemolyze; splenic sequestration; drug not present for hemolysis

179

cell membrane in order to produce antibody, and the antibody must have sufficient binding capacity to produce hemolysis. Although by these criteria many drugs are potentially candidates to cause hemolysis, most clinical cases are caused by penicillin or alpha methyldopa.

DIAGNOSTIC EVALUATION OF IMMUNE HEMOLYSIS

Proper diagnostic evaluation requires an awareness of drugs that commonly cause immune hemolysis and a suspicion of their involvement in a patient who is currently receiving or has recently received such drugs and has unexplained anemia. Without that suspicion and without narrowing investigation to a specific drug class, proper testing will probably neither be timely nor diagnostic. Evaluation proceeds with the following:

1. Hematologic findings, which determine normochromic anemia that may be actively hemolytic. Bone marrow aspiration is not usually indicated.
2. Direct antiglobulin test, which must show positive results, although it may be of variable degree depending on the mechanism of drug action. If the DAT results are not positive, immune hemolysis cannot be proven.
3. Serum antibody screening tests, which are usually negative with standard reagent red cells.
4. Special testing of eluates from Coombs-positive red cells in parallel with serum against specific drug-treated red cells.

LABORATORY STUDIES OF IMMUNE HEMOLYSIS

Hematologic Tests

GENERAL FEATURES

The anemia with intravascular hemolysis may be severe or mild to moderate if well compensated, depending on the drug mechanism of action, the dose, and the type of antibody evoked. Drug-immune hemolysis is usually brief, stopping when the drug is withdrawn, so that splenomegaly is not common. Jaundice is not prominent although intravascular hemolysis can occur with hemoglobinuria.

PERIPHERAL BLOOD

Blood cell counts

Hemoglobin can be as low as 2 g/dl in fatal hemolysis. An MCV in the range of 105–110 cu μ reflects reticulocytosis, while the MCHC is usually 30%–34%. The WBC count is 10–20,000 cu mm or may be leukemoid in brisk hemolysis, with a left shift to the myelocyte phase.

Morphology

Nucleated red cells and polychromasia are general findings. Spherocytes may be seen with alpha methyldopa. Target cells are present if jaundice occurs.

BONE MARROW

The bone marrow is hypercellular with normoblastic erythroid hyperplasia and increased marrow iron (4+).

Other Useful Tests

For specimen collection in immune hemolysis, whole blood is obtained fresh and allowed to clot at 37 C before the serum is separated. Freezing sera should be avoided since this frequently disrupts immune complexes. The red cells for testing can be obtained from the clot or from a separately collected EDTA specimen, which prevents nonspecific adsorption of complement.

DIRECT ANTIGLOBULIN TEST (DAT)—DIRECT COOMBS TEST

Purpose

The DAT must show positive results for drug-induced immune hemolysis to be considered seriously. Absorbed globulin may be IgG, IgM, or complement (1,4).

Principle

No matter what the mechanism of antibody production, all types have in common antibody globulin and/or complement attached to the red cell and detectable by the DAT. Without a positive direct antiglobulin test, drug-immune hemolytic anemia is unlikely. The adsorbed globulin, once detected, is eluted and tested in parallel with the patient's serum against drug-treated red cells and untreated red cells. The effects of neutralization of the eluate with the suspected drug are also studied.

Procedure

The DAT uses a broad-spectrum reagent. If results are positive the reaction can be characterized further using monospecific antisera for IgG, IgM, and complement. Eluates are made by organic solvent techniques since these methods precipitate red cell stroma and antibody globulin and, therefore, may detect weak antibody, often critical in drug-immune hemolysis. Tests of the eluate versus drug-treated red cells frequently require supplemental complement to reproduce the effect in vitro.

Interpretation

Findings for each category of drug-immune hemolysis are summarized in Table 11-4.

SERUM ANTIBODY TESTS AND TESTS WITH DRUG-TREATED RED CELLS

Purpose

Agglutination of drug-treated cells is consistent with drug-immune hemolysis but is not as diagnostic as the globulin actually absorbed to the red cell (2,3). For alpha methyldopa, reactions are positive with untreated patient red cells, which defines the antibody as autoantibody.

Table 11-4. Summary of Serologic Findings in Drug-Immune Hemolytic Anemia

Mechanism of Action	DAT	Drug-Treated Red Cell[a]	Untreated Red Cell	Drug Neutralization
Toxic immune complexes (quinine, quinidine)	±–3+ anti-C'			
Red cell eluate	Complement	0	0	0
Serum antibody	IgG, IgM	w+[b] with C'	0	0
Haptens (penicillins)	2–4+ anti-IgG			
Red cell eluate	IgG	4+	0	4+
Serum antibody	IgG	4+	0	4+
		Reacts with and neutralized by related drugs		
Nonspecific protein absorption (cephalothin)	±–2+ all or any protein			
Red cell eluate	No antibody	1–4+	0	0–+
Serum antibody	Rarely	1–4+	0	0–+
		Cross-reactions with penicillins		
True, warm AIHA (alpha methyldopa)	±–4+ anti-IgG			
Red cell eluate	IgG	+–4+[c]	+–4+	0
Serum antibody	IgG	+–4+	+–4+	0

[a]Drug is the specific drug suspected.
[b]w+, weakly positive.
[c]Agglutination is unrelated to drug treatment of red cells and reflects untreated red cells.

183

In general the organic drug binds with a serum protein or the red cell membrane to produce a hapten. Antibody production, strength, and avidity vary with the drug and with the patient, as well as the duration and route of exposure to the drug. Avidity of the drug or its complexes for the red cell membrane appears to be the final common pathway to cell sequestration or hemolysis. Ease of demonstration of the drug antibody varies with the mechanism of action.

Procedure

Tests for the following are available in reference laboratories and most sophisticated hospital blood banks:

1. Toxic immune complexes: Drug pretreated red cells + patient serum + fresh complement, or drug + red cells + patient serum + C'. Concentrations of drugs and sera are varied to achieve optimum antigen-antibody concentration. Drug neutralization is not demonstrable.
2. Haptens: Red cells pretreated with weak dilutions of penicillin drugs can be stored in the refrigerator for two to three weeks for future testing. Treated cells incubated with the patient serum are either positive directly (IgM antibody) or after the indirect antiglobulin reaction (IgG antibody). Antibody can be titered against drug-treated cells or neutralized by the appropriate drug.
3. Nonspecific protein absorption: Red cells can be pretreated with phosphate-buffered cephalothin solutions. Treated cells are incubated with patient serum. Drug neutralization studies are usually not successful. Tests must be performed in parallel with penicillinized red cells to evaluate cross-reactions.
4. True, warm AIHA: Serum agglutinates red cells untreated with the drug. Weak autoantibodies may be demonstrated only against enzyme-treated red cells.

Interpretation

1. Toxic immune complexes (quinine-quinidine): Negative test results do not exclude the diagnosis of hemolysis since many unknown variables exist. However, this is one of the least common causes of

184

hemolytic anemia in general and of drug-associated immune hemolysis in particular. The DAT is usually ±, generally because of C', which can on rare occasions provoke intravascular hemolysis not seen in other types of drug-immune hemolytic anemia. If hemolysis occurs, results of the DAT may be negative. Red cell eluates, since they usually contain insignificant amounts of antibody globulin, may not react with drug-treated red cells.

2. Haptens (penicillins): This type of antibody is common and easily demonstrated, but only IgG antibodies have significance in producing clinical hemolysis. The antibody may react with one or more penicillin cogeners, varying for each patient. Cross-reactions with cephalothin-treated cells occur as a result of similarities in chemical structure. Titer of antibody does not correlate well with clinical hemolysis. The DAT is 2–4+ with anti-IgG reagents. Weakly positive (±) DAT results are not usually associated with clinical hemolysis. The appearance of a positive DAT is dose- and time-related, requiring intravenous administration, 10–20 M units daily, for at least 10 days. Eluates of patients' red cells and the serum react only with penicillinized red cells (or related drugs), and reactivity is neutralized by solutions of the specific drug or any cross-reacting drugs, for example, methicillin, ampicillin, oxacillin, and so forth. Serum antibody alone is not diagnostic since much of the population has IgM antibodies from dietary exposure. Atopic reactions (urticaria, asthma, etc.) are unrelated and are caused by IgE antibody.

3. Nonspecific protein adsorption (cephalothins): Occurring with moderate frequency, cephalothin-induced protein absorption must be separated from the clinically significant hapten type of antibody. Cephalothin most often produces nonspecific protein absorption with no activity with drug-treated red cells. Occasionally an occult antipenicillin antibody reacts with cephalothin-treated cells, which is misleading. To prove true hemolytic anemia for this category, the eluate must react with cephalothin-treated cells after cross-reactions with penicillin have been excluded by prior absorption. The DAT varies from ±–2+. Eluates do not react with drug-treated red cells in most cases since the adsorbed globulin is not antibody but may be anything from fibrinogen to albumin to transferrin.

Only two rather doubtful cases of hemolysis caused by cephalothin have been reported. The process is dose- and time-related; the DAT results become positive within four to six days after oral or intramuscular doses of 6 g/day.

4. True, warm AIHA (alpha methyldopa): This group is very common and, since antibodies may persist after the drug is withdrawn, its presence is unsuspected until blood is cross-matched for transfusion. The DAT results vary from ±–4+, appearing in 10% of patients receiving 1 g/day or more for longer than three months. Direct antiglobulin becomes progressively stronger followed by the appearance of serum antibody. Despite the serologic evidence, only 1% of patients taking alpha methyldopa actually hemolyze. These patients should be monitored with a DAT every three to six months. Withdrawal of the drug reverses the process, with decrease in serum antibody followed by disappearance of the DAT. The presence of antibody and its specificity determines risk with transfusion. Without serum antibody transfusion risk is negligible. With serum antibody in a patient with active hemolysis, red cell survival is decreased as for any warm hemolytic anemia.

REFERENCES

1. Issitt PD, Issitt CH: *Applied Blood Group Serology*, ed 2. Oxnard, CA, Spectra Biologicals, 1975, pp 21–27
2. Dacie JV, Lewis SM: *Practical Haematology*, ed 4. New York, Grune & Stratton, 1968, pp 208–214
3. Davidsohn I, Henry JB: *Todd-Sanford Clinical Diagnosis by Laboratory Methods*, ed 15. Philadelphia, W. B. Saunders Co, 1974, pp 61–66, p 200
4. Bell CA: Serologic evaluation of drug induced immune hematologic disorders. In Nakamura RM (ed): *Immunopathology: Clinical Laboratory Concepts and Methods*. Boston, Little, Brown, 1974, pp 398–417

chapter **12**

Autoimmune Hemolytic Anemias

Autoimmune hemolytic anemia (AIHA) is caused by self-induced antibody to one's own red cell antigens. The pathogenesis of the antibody is unknown although some abnormality of the normal immune pathways is suspected. It can appear at any age including infancy. The mechanism of cell destruction is mediated through red cell coating by IgG or IgM antibodies and complement. In the case of IgG antibodies, monocyte receptors on the molecules are recognized by macrophages in the reticuloendothelial system, predominantly the spleen, and the red cell is gradually ingested over several days. IgM antibodies activate the classic complement pathway, resulting in cell lysis within hours to a few days, and the cell products are usually sequestered in the liver.

Autoimmune hemolytic anemia is divided into two major categories by the laboratory characteristics of the autoantibody: autoantibody that is maximally active at 37 C (warm AIHA) and autoantibody that is maximally active at 4 C (cold AIHA). The clinical and laboratory characteristics of each type are summarized in Tables 12-1 and 12-2. Cold AIHA can be further divided clinically into acute postviral, chronic idiopathic, and cold agglutinin disease (CAD). Table 12-3 indicates pertinent characteristics seen in patients with cold AIHA as compared with healthy persons, in whom cold agglutinins are found in low titer. Serologically all three types of cold AIHA are similar varying in the titer of the cold agglutinin. Clinically chronic idiopathic disease is usually seen in elderly

187

Table 12-1. Characteristics of Autoimmune Hemolytic Anemia (AIHA)

Clinical and Laboratory Findings	Warm AIHA	Cold AIHA
Clinical onset	Abrupt	Insidious
Jaundice	Usually present	Often absent
Splenomegaly	+	0
Age	All ages	All ages
Sex	Slightly increased in females	Increased in females
Associated diseases	SLE, chronic lymphocytic leukemia, lymphoma	Viral pneumonia Histiocytic lymphoma
Laboratory		
Peripheral blood	Spherocytes, nucleated red cells	Red cell agglutinates

Table 12-2. **Serologic Findings in Autoimmune Hemolytic Anemia (AIHA)**

Test	Warm AIHA	Cold AIHA
Direct Coombs test	2–4+	2–4+
Monospecific sera		
Anti-IgG	+	0
Anti-IgG + anti-C'	+	0
Anti-C' only	Rare	+
Serum antibody	IgG	IgM
Specificity	Anti-e, C, c; Rh precursor; LW; U; Wright[b]	Anti-I/i Pr(Sp$_1$), I^T
Technique	Indirect antiglobulin, enzyme	Saline or enzyme
Cold agglutinin titer	Normal	> 256
Serum complement	Normal or decreased	Decreased
Osmotic fragility	Increased	Normal

women while chronic cold agglutinin disease is usually associated with an underlying lymphoproliferative malignancy.

Paroxysmal cold hemoglobinuria (PCH) is closely related clinically to cold AIHA but differs in that the antibody is IgG and has a characteristic biphasic mode of action, first adsorbing to red cells at low temperature and then causing intravascular hemolysis and hemoglobinuria as the temperature rises to 37 C. This biphasic hemolysin is the Donath-Landsteiner hemolysin. It is important to diagnose PCH since it is usually self limited and treated by keeping the patient warm.

As indicated in Table 12-4, cold agglutinins are normally present. They become abnormal as the titer rises above 1:256; the temperature of agglutination rises toward 37 C; and antibody with complement fixes to the patient's red cells as detected by a positive direct Coombs test.

189

Table 12-3. Characteristics of Cold Agglutinins

Clinical Parameter	Physiologic	Postinfection	Chronic Idiopathic AIHA	CAD
Age	Any	Young	Older	Older
Onset	Asymptomatic	Acute, 10–14 d	Insidious	Insidious
Splenomegaly	No	Frequent	No	With lymphoma
Titer	$\leq 1:32$	$\geq 1:64$	$\geq 1:256^a$	$> 1:10,000^a$
Specificity	Anti-I	Anti-I, i	Anti-I, i, Sp$_1$	Anti-I
DAT	0	+ (G,M,C3)	+ (C3)	+ (C3)
Intravascular hemolysis	No	40%	No	Rare
Transfuse?	Yes	Avoid	Avoid	Avoid

^{a}Representative range for titer.

190

Table 12-4. Serologic Characteristics of Cold Agglutinins

Laboratory Finding	Physiologic Cold Agglutinins	Pathologic Cold Agglutinins
Titer	≤ 16	> 256
Thermal range	4 C	Above 16 C
Direct Coombs test	Negative	Positive

Approximately 70% of AIHA is associated with some underlying disease and classified as secondary (Table 12-5). In general warm AIHA is associated with systemic lupus erythematosus (SLE) or other collagen disease, chronic lymphocytic leukemia, or lymphocytic lymphomas. The hemolytic anemia may precede the associated disease by several years, so these conditions should be screened for by physical examination, complete blood count, and testing for antinuclear antibody periodically. The association of warm AIHA with carcinoma is rare and unpredictable. Cold AIHA is frequently associated with *Mycoplasma* pneumonia, so that radiographs of the chest and *Mycoplasma* titers should be obtained. Cytomegalovirus (CMV), Epstein-Barr virus (EBV), measles, and mumps can be associated with AIHA as can infectious mononucleosis. Cold AIHA can also be seen with lymphomas, usually of the histiocytic type. True AIHA secondary to drug is of the warm antibody type, as discussed in Chapter 11.

DIAGNOSTIC EVALUATION

The approach to diagnosis begins with the following:

1. Hematologic evaluation, to establish anemia and study increased erythrocyte turnover (e.g., reticulocyte count, etc.) to determine whether anemia is hemolytic (see Chapter 5).
2. Serologic diagnosis, which tests red cells and serum for antibody. The DAT screens the patient's red cells for adsorbed globulin. The

Table 12-5. Disease Association in Autoimmune Hemolytic Anemia (AIHA)

	Antibody Specificity	
	Warm Ab	Cold Ab
Malignancy		
Lymphocytic leukemia	Anti-Rh, LW, Wright[b]	
Lymphocytic lymphoma	Anti-U, En[a]	
Carcinoma (ovary, thymus, gastrointestinal)		
Histiocytic, lymphoma, Hodgkin's disease		Anti-I, I^T, Pr (Sp$_1$)
Collagen disease		
SLE, rheumatoid arthritis, ulcerative colitis	Anti-Rh, LW, Wright[b] Anti-U, En[a]	
Infection		
Virus, *Mycoplasma*		Anti-I
Infectious mononucleosis		Anti-i
Clostridia, *E. coli*	Anti-T	
Drugs		
Methyldopa (Aldomet)	Anti-Rh	
L-dopa		
Indomethacin		

serum is screened for antibody by indirect antiglobulin test, testing with enzyme-treated red cells, and other techniques as necessary. If the DAT is positive, the adsorbed globulin is eluted and tested in parallel with the serum.

3. Serum antibody is identified for blood group specificity and characterized for temperature of maximum reactivity to classify the type AIHA as cold or warm. Appropriate red cell antigens are tested to determine if the antibody is directed at self antigen (autoantibody) or foreign antigen (incompatible transfusion).

4. Once identified, serum antibody is titered against appropriate red cells to follow therapy. In cold AIHA cold agglutinin titers serve this purpose.

5. The Donath-Landsteiner test for the biphasic hemolysin of PCH.

6. Ham's acid hemolysis test to screen for paroxysmal nocturnal hemoglobinuria (PNH). Positive Ham's tests may be confirmed by the sucrose lysis test.

7. Tests to determine the underlying cause of AIHA include: (a) for cold AIHA, radiography of the chest and tests to determine serum complement levels and specific virus titers; (b) for warm AIHA, peripheral smear for lymphocytosis, antinuclear antibody tests, and evaluation for occult lymphoma.

8. Other tests of limited help are those for red cell osmotic fragility, which increases with spherocytes, and for serum complement.

LABORATORY STUDIES

Hematologic Tests

GENERAL FEATURES

The clinical history often suggests the type of AIHA present. Warm AIHA is of abrupt onset, with jaundice and splenomegaly, and anemia may be severe. Cold AIHA may be postinfectious with a similar abrupt onset, and in children it may be associated with intravascular hemolysis. Classically, however, cold AIHA is more often insidious and well compensated, and, therefore, without jaundice or splenomegaly, despite marked anemia.

PERIPHERAL BLOOD

Anemia may be severe ($\leq$ 3 g/dl Hb) with variable reticulocytosis. Nucleated red cells, marked polychromasia, and anisocytosis are usually seen. In warm AIHA microspherocytes are present, the result of piecemeal ingestion of antibody-coated red cell membrane by macrophage. Cold AIHA may have marked morphologic changes if it is acutely postinfectious. However, clumping of red cells on the smear caused by cold agglutinins is more common. In acute hemolysis granulocytosis with a left shift, a nonspecific stress reaction, may be present. The leukocytosis can reach leukemoid proportions above 50,000/cu mm.

BONE MARROW

The marrow is hypercellular, often approaching 80% cellularity as a result of normoblastic erythroid hyperplasia. Marrow iron is usually markedly increased reflecting the accelerated erythroid turnover. Prolonged severe hemolysis may result in relative deficiencies of folic acid or vitamin B_{12} with a megaloblastic marrow and ultimately hypoplasia.

In idiopathic, cold AIHA, erythroid bone marrow aspiration may not indicate the underlying etiology, but in cold agglutinin disease, it may reveal underlying lymphoma. In warm AIHA, marrow aspiration is most informative when the peripheral blood shows the presence of lymphocytosis or lymphadenopathy is present. In the elderly occult retroperitoneal lymphoma may be present, which will not be diagnosed by marrow aspirate.

Other Useful Tests

The following procedures require 15–20 ml blood, which should be obtained and kept at 37 C until clotted; the serum is promptly removed from the cells and frozen to preserve complement. An EDTA specimen is also obtained. EDTA blocks nonspecific absorption of C', which allows a more accurate assessment of the DAT.

DIRECT ANTIGLOBULIN (DAT)—COOMBS TEST

Purpose

The DAT detects globulin adsorbed to the patient's red cells and identifies immunoglobulin class (1,2).

Principle

Antihuman globulin reagent manufactured in rabbits detects, as the name indicates, human globulin adsorbed to red cells. It does not determine the cause of the globulin coating, which may be autoantibody or not antibody as in myeloma or cephalothin therapy.

Procedure

Patient's red cells are tested for agglutination with broad-spectrum antihuman globulin reagent, which detects globulin coats of IgG, IgM, and complement fragments, particularly C3d. This fragment is believed to be the clinically significant complement fraction in AIHA. Monospecific antiglobulin reagents are also available to detect specifically IgG or complement.

Interpretation

A clinically significant DAT is positive 1–4+ with broad-spectrum reagents. Monospecific reagents are used automatically by sophisticated hospital blood banks and by all reference laboratories to identify the adsorbed globulins in an effort to categorize the AIHA as warm or cold type. In warm AIHA monospecific reagents for IgG or IgG and complement are positive. Monospecific reagents in cold AIHA show only complement since IgM antibody quickly separates from red cells collected at 37 C. Very weak complement reactions (±) are not significant and do not indicate AIHA, whereas such reactions with anti-IgG may be clinically significant occasionally.

Very rarely AIHA is present without a positive DAT. In such

195

cases ultrasensitive methods of Coombs consumption or radioisotopes may reveal antibody molecules on the red cells; however, these tests are not generally available.

SERUM ANTIBODY DETECTION

Purpose

These tests detect serum antibody, identify its blood group specificity, and characterize the temperature of reactivity (1,3,4).

Principle

An indirect Coombs test, which is often ordered, is only one method for screening the serum for antibody. Other techniques used include treating cells with enzymes (ficin, papain, bromelin, or trypsin) to detect very low levels of antibody, and direct agglutination of saline-suspended cells. If screening tests show positive results, the antibody is identified (see also Chapter 11).

Procedure

The patient's serum and red cell mixtures are tested using the previously mentioned techniques at 37 C and at 4 C. In addition to panels of reagent red cells, the patient's own cells are included as well as specimens of cord blood. The presence of agglutination or of hemolysis is significant and is graded 0–4+ (see also Chapter 11).

For information on specimen, see page 194.

Interpretation

Warm autoantibodies are IgG, and, rarely, IgM, which agglutinate test cells by indirect antiglobulin tests and enzyme techniques strongly at 37 C and with no increase at 4 C. Specific antibody is found in 30% of cases and is Rh related (e, C, D, c), although the appearance of narrow specificity may only reflect differences in titers of antibody components. In the remainder, the antibody is directed at some primitive precursor of the Rh system or of the

Wright system, and all cells are agglutinated except very rare test cells used at reference laboratories, for example, Rh null cells.

Since antibodies may be present from previous transfusions concurrent with autoantibodies, specificity should be determined. Although transfusions should be avoided, antibody specificity may help in selection of blood that is least incompatible if life-saving transfusion is needed. With steroids serum antibodies may change specificity or disappear although the positive DAT often persist. The presence of serum antibody correlates more with active AIHA.

Cold autoantibodies are IgM, strongly reactive at 4 C and weaker at 37 C, sometimes seen better with diluted serum. Tests use saline suspensions or enzyme-treated cells. The antibodies may be hemolytic in vitro. Specificity is usually anti-I (reactive with all normal adult cells but not with cord red cells). Anti-i specificity (stronger reactions with cord red cells than adult cells) is seen with the rare AIHA occurring in infectious mononucleosis. Cold autoantibodies should be titered. In order to determine whether antibodies are autoantibodies, the patient's red cell antigens must be determined for the Rh and I systems.

ELUATES OF PATIENT RED CELLS

Purpose

Eluates are prepared to determine if the globulin on red cells detected by the DAT is antibody and, if so, to determine blood group specificity (1,3).

Principle

Red cell antibody-antigen bonds are disrupted by heat or by destroying the red cell membrane.

Procedure

The test is usually performed automatically by the blood bank or reference laboratory. When the DAT is positive, heating the red cells at 56 C or chemically destroying them with cold organic solvents yields (elutes) the adsorbed antibody, which is then tested in parallel with the serum.

Interpretation

In warm AIHA eluate antibody identity duplicates the serum. After recent incompatible transfusion in the absence of AIHA, the DAT may yield positive results because of the presence of coated donor cells, but the serum antibody is alloantibody. Antigen typing of red cells in such cases often indicates a mixed field of donor red cells and patient cells. After incompatible transfusion in the presence of AIHA, specificity of eluate and serum antibody may not be clarified until transfused cells have been cleared, usually several days. If eluate does not react with red cells, nonspecific globulin absorption as in myeloma or recent cephalothin therapy should be suspected. In cold AIHA antibody material is not elutable, and there is no reaction with red cells.

COLD AGGLUTININ TITER

Purpose

The presence of abnormal cold agglutinins usually establishes that the AIHA is of the cold antibody type (3,4). Titer may indicate underlying disease and follows its progress.

Principle

Cold agglutinins usually have anti-I specificity and agglutinate saline suspensions of adult red cells because of the I antigen present on the membrane. Rare cold agglutinins with anti-i specificity should not be expected to agglutinate adult red cells to the same titer and cord blood specimens are needed for accurate titers.

Procedure

The patient's serum is titered in small-volume dilutions of 4, 8, 16, 32, and so forth, and incubated two hours at 4 C with a standard suspension of red cells, usually of the patient or of a group

198

O donor, to avoid ABO blood group incompatibility. Cell-serum suspensions are read for agglutination. Titer is the highest serum dilution producing 1+ agglutination.

Interpretation

As indicated in Table 12-3 cold agglutinins are normally present. They become abnormal as the titer rises above 1:256. With the rise in titer the temperature of agglutination often rises toward 37 C, and antibody with complement fixes to the patient's red cells as detected by a positive direct Coombs test. Physiologic cold agglutinins have titers less than or equal to 16. Titers to 64 are seen after recent respiratory viral infections. Titers are 256 and above in cold AIHA of elderly women or, with viral pneumonia, usually 1000–8000. In chronic cold agglutinin disease titers are often 50,000 or higher but may not always be associated with clinical hemolysis, although vascular occlusion may occur at low temperatures.

Progress of cold AIHA can be followed by repeating titers weekly in viral pneumonia or idiopathic disease and monthly in cold agglutinin disease, particularly in lymphoma for which the patient is receiving chemotherapy.

DONATH-LANDSTEINER TEST (BIPHASIC HEMOLYSIN)

Purpose

The Donath-Landsteiner test diagnoses PCH, which may have a clinical history similar to cold AIHA but is usually a self-limited disease that is treated conservatively by keeping the patient warm (3,4).

Principle

The Donath-Landsteiner test reproduces in vitro a reaction that occurs in vivo. The hemolysin, a complement-dependent IgG antibody, agglutinates cells at 4 C and lyses them at warmer temperatures, usually considered as 37 C. Other hemolysins may react at single temperatures, 4 C or 37 C, but are not biphasic. The

Donath-Landsteiner hemolysin does not lyse cells with reverse incubations, 37 C to 4 C.

Procedure

The patient's serum is incubated with test red cells at 4 C and then at 37 C, and serum-cell suspension is observed for hemolysis, which is usually marked (3–4+). If biphasic hemolysis is present it is tested against panels of reagent red cells to determine blood group specificity, which is often in the P or I system.

Interpretation

A biphasic hemolysin indicates PCH, occasionally seen in patients with a history that suggests cold AIHA. If intravascular hemolysis has recently occurred, the DAT results may be negative. Paroxysmal cold hemoglobinuria is commonly postviral but can be seen with congenital syphilis so that definitive syphilitic serology, that is, the fluorescent treponemal antibody test (FTA), should be performed.

HAM'S TEST FOR ACID HEMOLYSIS

Purpose

Ham's test is performed to exclude PNH, which is not caused by serum antibody but by an acquired clonal defect of the red cell membrane (3,4). Whenever antibody hemolysis is suspected, PNH should be considered and excluded.

Principle

The patient's red cell is supersensitive to human complement lysis activated at a low serum pH. Human complement and its activator, C_3PA, is present in all normal serums including the patient's. The patient's serum is shown to have no antibody against the patient's or any other red cell.

Procedure

Normal sera acidified to pH 6.8 are incubated at 37 C with the patient's red cells and observed for hemolysis, which may be faint to 4+. Controls are established to prove the defect is limited to the patient's red cells.

Interpretation

False-positive hemolysis is seen if the sera acidified contain a cold agglutinin. True positives are positive only with human, not guinea pig, complement. The test can be confirmed by sucrose lysis.

SERUM COMPLEMENT

Purpose

A decrease in serum complement is most often associated with IgM antibody and cold AIHA (4,5). It can, however, be decreased in warm AIHA as well and therefore is not absolute in categorizing AIHA as the warm rather than the cold type.

Principle

Sheep red cells are lysed in the presence of antibody to sheep red cells from rabbits (amboceptor) if complement is present. The source of the complement is the patient's fresh serum. The reaction can be used to quantitate complement.

Procedure

Lytic complement tests are not easily performed and often require reference laboratories. Serum complement is measured by lysis of 50% of a spectrophotometrically determined red cell suspension in one hour. $C'H_{50}$ is 50–100 units in most laboratories but normal ranges must be determined for each.

Specimen

Fresh serum, separated from red cells and immediately frozen, is used as a specimen.

Serum complement is decreased in cold AIHA since the antibodies are complement binding. Levels are also often decreased in warm AIHA, with serum showing anticomplementary activity.

SERUM HAPTOGLOBIN (Hp)

Purpose

The absence of haptoglobin is seen in hemolysis or in liver failure (4). The serum haptoglobin test indicates that hemolysis may be present if liver function is normal.

For sections on *Principle*, *Procedure*, and *Specimen*, see Chapter 5.

Interpretation

As measured by hemoglobin binding, normal values are usually 40–180 mg/dl; with active hemolysis values are less than 10 mg/dl. In cold AIHA when pneumonia is present, haptoglobin as an acute reactant protein may be markedly increased, obscuring expected low levels seen with hemolysis, and the test is no longer helpful (see Chapter 5).

OSMOTIC FRAGILITY

Purpose

This test is of limited usefulness but is positive in the presence of spherocytes (4).

Principle

Spherocytes with increased cell volume have little margin remaining for increased cell water imbibed from hypotonic solutions, and they undergo osmotic lysis.

Procedure

The patient's red cells are suspended in a series of 10 saline solutions that are increasingly hypotonic. The amount of hemolysis is measured by colorimeter or spectrophotometer and converted to a percentage of cells lysed as compared to a totally lysed specimen. Red cells do not normally lyse until saline is .45% or less.

Interpretation

Hemolysis increases with the presence of spherocytosis, usually seen in warm AIHA. It is quicker and clinically satisfactory to review the peripheral smear instead.

VIRAL ANTIBODY TITERS

Purpose

Testing for viral antibody titers identifies, usually in retrospect, the viral etiologic agent in cold AIHA.

Principle

Viral antibodies require acute- and convalescent-phase sera obtained 7–10 days apart to show a rise in titer of antibody-killing specific viruses.

Procedure

The tests are usually performed at county or state reference laboratories, which require both specimens to be submitted. The virus suspected should be specified; most common is *Mycoplasma*, occasionally EBV or cytomegalovirus.

Interpretation

A three-dilution rise in titer is required for the test to be diagnostic since previous exposure to these viruses is fairly common.

ANTINUCLEAR ANTIBODY

Purpose

Antinuclear antibody by indirect immunofluorescence should be ordered when warm AIHA is diagnosed, particularly in young females, to determine if SLE is the underlying disease (3,5). Warm AIHA can precede SLE by months or years.

Principle

The patient's serum contains antibody to nuclear material shared by many species and if present attaches to the material.

Procedure

The patient's serum is incubated with a nuclear antigen source (rat kidney, human granulocytes, etc.). The antigen-antibody combination is detected by antiglobulin reagent that has been tagged with a fluorescent dye. Microscopy with ultraviolet light causes antinuclear antibody combinations to glow. The patient's serum can be titered.

Interpretation

Titers above 1:20 in most laboratories are suspicious and titers of 1:80 or greater are diagnostic of SLE. Positive tests of low titer are seen in 3% of the elderly; high titers in the elderly suggest drug-induced AIHA of the methyldopa (Aldomet) type (see Chapter 11).

EVALUATION OF OCCULT LYMPHOMA

Purpose

Warm AIHA may precede lymphoma by years but AIHA may be the only visible symptom in concomitant unsuspected disease, usually in the elderly patient.

Principle

Physical examination should include evaluation of all lymph node areas and evaluation of hepatosplenomegaly.

Procedure

Noninvasive procedures are utilized. These may include computerized axial tomography of the retroperitoneum and/or pulmonary hilus, radionuclide scans, and intravenous pyelograms for lateral displacement of ureters.

Interpretation

Positive findings should be biopsied to confirm the diagnosis.

TRANSFUSION

Transfusion should generally be avoided if possible since it induces other antibodies, further complicating cross-matching, and may accelerate the autoantibody titer and avidity for red cells. It is a temporizing measure since survival is less than one week in warm AIHA and may be minutes or hours in cold AIHA.

REFERENCES

1. Issitt, PD, Issitt CH: *Applied Blood Group Serology*, ed 2. Oxnard, CA, Spectra Biologicals, 1975, pp 21–30

2. American Association of Blood Banks: *Technical Methods and Procedures*, ed 6. Washington, DC, 1974, pp 38–39

3. Bell CA: Laboratory evaluation of autoimmune hemolytic anemias. In Nakamura RM (ed): *Immunopathology: Clinical Laboratory Concepts and Methods.* Boston, Little, Brown & Co, 1973, pp 367–397

4. Dacie JV, Lewis SM: Practical Haematology, ed 4. New York, Grune & Stratton, 1968, pp 191–202

5. Gewurz H, Suyehira LA: Complement. In Rose NR, Friedman H (eds): *Manual of Clinical Immunology.* Washington, DC, American Society for Microbiology, 1976, pp 38–40

chapter 13

The Polycythemias

Although polycythemia is defined as too many blood cells, without reference to cell type, the word is commonly used in reference to excessive numbers of red cells in particular. Other more precise terms are used to delineate the polycythemic disorders. Erythrocytosis (true erythrocytosis, absolute erythrocytosis) is an absolute increase in red cell volume. Secondary erythrocytosis refers to the increased red cell volume found in disorders other than polycythemia vera. Spurious erythrocytosis is a condition in which red cell measurements such as hematocrit are increased in the peripheral blood but in which red cell volume is normal. Polycythemia vera (PV) is a disorder characterized by a panmyelosis in which elevated red cell volume is characteristically associated with increased numbers of circulating platelets and granulocytes.

Erythropoiesis is regulated by the hormone erythropoietin (EP), which the kidney elaborates. According to one prevailing concept, it is secreted as an inactive form known as renal erythropoietic factor, which reacts with a plasma protein of hepatic origin to form erythropoietin. Erythropoietin regulates the differentiation of the committed erythroid stem cell, and the rate of production of erythropoietin determines the rate of production of red cells. The physiologic stimulus of erythropoietin is tissue hypoxia.

The classification of the polycythemias in Table 13-1 incorporates pathophysiologic mechanisms. Table 13-2 presents the diagnostic differences among spurious erythrocytosis, the secondary erythrocytotic states, and PV. In practice, spurious erythrocytosis is the

Table 13-1. **Classification of the Polycythemias**

Spurious erythrocytosis (relative erythrocytosis, stress erythrocytosis, Gaisböck's syndrome)

Secondary erythrocytosis—increased erythropoietin production

  Physiologically appropriate—tissue hypoxia
    Diminished O_2 transport
      Pulmonary disease
      Congenital heart disease—right-to-left shunt
      High altitude
      Carboxyhemoglobinemia (smokers)
      Hyperventilation syndromes (massive obesity)
    Diminished O_2 release
      High-affinity O_2 hemoglobinopathies
      Congenital decreased 2,3-diphosphoglyceric acid (DPG)

  Physiologically inappropriate—no tissue hypoxia
    Aberrant erythropoietin production from renal lesions: renal carcinoma, cysts, hydronephrosis
    Aberrant erythropoietin from other lesions: cerebellar hemangioma, hepatoma, adrenal adenoma, pheochromocytoma, uterine fibroids
    Familial erythropoietin overproduction—excessive familial erythrocytosis, benign familial erythrocytosis

Polycythemia vera

---

condition most frequently confused clinically with PV. In contrast to the prolonged and at times aggressive therapy of PV, spurious erythrocytosis does not require treatment. Therefore, these conditions must be differentiated. Also, because of therapeutic considerations, it is important to pinpoint the relatively uncommon lesions associated with aberrant production of erythropoietin and with erythrocytosis. When such a lesion is removed, the blood count returns to normal.

The commonest group of disorders causing true erythrocytosis is that caused by tissue hypoxia secondary to decreased oxygen trans-

Table 13-2. Differential Diagnosis of Polycythemias

Findings	Spurious Erythrocytosis	Secondary Erythrocytosis	PV
Clinical findings			
Age at onset	Middle age	All ages	Middle age or elderly
Sex incidence—male:female	9:1	1:1	1.5:1
CNS symptoms[a] with modest increase in hematocrit (< 60%)	Present	Absent	Absent[b]
Splenomegaly	Absent	Absent	Present in 75%–90%
Hematologic findings			
Hematocrit	Modest elevation (PCV > 60%)	Usually modest[c]	Usually marked (PCV > 60%)
White cell count	Normal	Normal	Increased in 80% with left shift

Platelet count	Normal	Normal	Increased in 50%
Nucleated red cells	Absent	Absent	Often present
Bone marrow	Normal	Erythroid hyperplasia	Generalized increase in cellularity; increased megakaryocytes
Other laboratory findings			
Red cell volume	Normal	Increased	Increased
Arterial oxygen saturation	Normal	Low or normal	Normal
Unsaturated serum B_{12} binding capacity	Normal	Normal	Elevated in 75%
LAP[d]	Normal	Normal	Elevated in 80%
Erythropoietin	Not elevated	Frequently elevated	Not elevated

[a] Headaches, dizziness, tinnitus, visual disturbances.
[b] CNS symptoms frequent when erythrocytosis prominent.
[c] May be marked increase with congenital heart disease and high altitude.
[d] *LAP*, leukocyte alkaline phosphatase.

port. Awareness of the association of erythrocytosis with heavy cigarette smoking can obviate unnecessary extensive evaluation. Subjects smoking more than 1.5 packages of cigarettes a day may show mild elevations in hematocrit (approximately 55% for males, 52% for females) that return to normal with cessation of smoking. In patients with chronic pulmonary disease and in those with congenital heart disease associated with right-to-left cardiovascular shunts, the clinical findings of the underlying disorder overshadow those resulting from erythrocytosis.

Occasionally it may be difficult to distinguish PV from another myeloproliferative disorder, such as myelofibrosis with myeloid metaplasia. This occurs when a patient presents with splenomegaly and particularly prominent leukocytosis (greater than $20,000/\mu l$) together with a normal or barely elevated red cell count. Normal red cell count in PV can be caused by occult blood loss, by therapeutic phlebotomy, or by marked splenomegaly with red cell sequestration.

DIAGNOSTIC EVALUATION

Erythrocytic patients with diagnosed disorders known to be associated with secondary erythrocytosis require no special evaluation provided that the degree of erythrocytosis is compatible with the underlying order and there are no unexplained ancillary findings, such as leukocytosis, thrombocytosis, or splenomegaly. A reasonable sequence for a laboratory diagnosis of occult erythrocytosis is as follows (Figure 13-1):

1. Hematologic evaluation with complete blood count including white count and evaluation of red cell morphology and bone marrow study.
2. Measurement of red cell volume to rule out spurious erythrocytosis.
3. Measurement of arterial oxygen saturation to rule out secondary erythrocytosis.

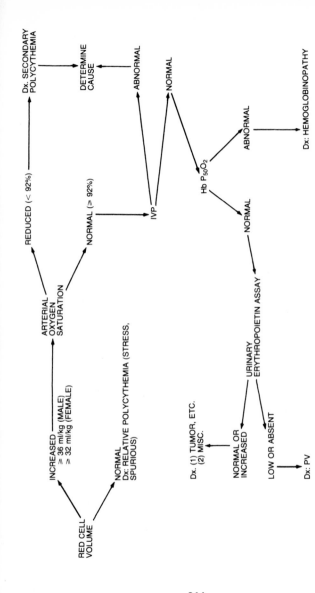

Figure 13-1. Sequence of studies for diagnosis of erythrocytosis. (Modified with permission from Jacob HS: The polychthemias and their relationship to erythropoietin. DM: Disease-a-Month. Chicago, Year Book Medical Publishers, Inc., August, 1974.)

211

4. In a case of true erythrocytosis with normal arterial oxygen saturation for confirmation of the diagnosis of PV, leukocyte alkaline phosphatase, and serum B_{12} and unsaturated B_{12} binding capacity.

5. If diagnosis is still reasonably uncertain after this evaluation, intervenous pyelography should be performed because of the relatively common association of renal lesions with erythrocytosis and, in the presence of a normal intravenous pyelogram, a $P_{50}O_2$ is performed to rule out one of the hemoglobinopathies known to be associated with increase in hemoglobin affinity for oxygen.

6. In one of the uncommon cases of an otherwise inapparent tumor associated with increased erythropoietin and the even more uncommon familial erythrocytosis associated with excessive erythropoietin, measurement of plasma or urine erythropoietin can provide useful information.

LABORATORY STUDIES

Hematologic Tests

GENERAL FEATURES

The initial laboratory finding that characterizes the polycythemias is erythrocytosis as determined by the usual red cell measurements. The minimal values for red cell count, hemoglobin, and hematocrit or packed-cell volume (PCV) compatible with the diagnosis of erythrocytosis are given in Table 13-3. The red cell measurement most often referred to is the PCV. With manual procedures the PCV and hemoglobin are more reproducible than the red cell count. With electronic counters such as the Coulter S, PCV has no apparent advantage. In fact, with such counters, PCV is derived from the MCV and the red cell count. The latter two values, along with the hemoglobin, are direct measurements.

The degree of erythrocytosis with which a patient presents can provide some clue to etiology. Packed-cell volumes less than 60% are seen in patients with spurious erythrocytosis or with some of the more common types of secondary erythrocytosis, such as those occurring in heavy smokers or in chronic pulmonary disease. On

Table 13-3. Blood Cell Values Just Exceeding the Normal Range[a]

Value	Men	Women
Red cell count × 10⁶/μl blood	6.0	5.5
Hemoglobin, g/dl blood	18.0	16.0
Volume packed red cells, ml/100 ml blood	52.0	47.0
Platelet count × 10³/μl blood	400	400
Total leukocytes × 10³/μl blood	11.0	11.0
Total neutrophils × 10³/μl blood	8.0	8.0

[a]More than two standard deviations greater than the normal mean based on automated counts.

the other hand, erythrocytosis in congenital heart disease with right-to-left shunt can be marked, with reported values up to 90%.

The only one of the erythrocytotic states that has a characteristic pattern of findings in the peripheral blood and bone marrow is PV. In the presence of these findings, PV can be diagnosed with a high degree of probability.

PERIPHERAL BLOOD IN POLYCYTHEMIA VERA

Blood cell measurements

Erythrocytosis is present, with MCV usually 56%–80% when first seen. Moderate leukocytosis with the white cell count usually 12,000–25,000/μl with relative and absolute increase in neutrophils is seen. The differential shows a left shift with some increase in nonsegmented neutrophils and occasional metamyelocytes and myelocytes. There is a variable increase in basophils and eosinophils. Platelet count is increased, usually 450,000–1,000,000/μl. The percentage of reticulocytes is normal.

213

Morphology

Morphology is normochromic normocytic. An occasional nucleated red cell may be present. There may be large bizarre platelets with megakaryocytic fragments. In the event of either spontaneous or therapeutic blood loss, red cells may be hypochromic microcytic.

BONE MARROW IN POLYCYTHEMIA VERA

Prominent generalized hyperplasia is best appreciated on bone marrow biopsy because of the presence of panmyelosis with normal M:E ratio. The pronounced increase in megakaryocytes is in keeping with the generalized increased cellularity. Absent iron stores and increased reticulum with special stains are also seen.

Other Useful Tests

RED CELL VOLUME (RCV)

Purpose

Testing for RCV is necessary to establish the diagnosis of erythrocytosis when this finding is not readily apparent by routine red cell measurements, particularly when the underlying diagnosis is clinically obscure (1). Red cell volume is especially useful in distinguishing spurious erythrocytosis from PV. Measurement of RCV is the only definitive way to diagnose spurious erythrocytosis.

Principle

A sample of the patient's red cells is labeled in vitro and reinjected intravenously. The extent of the intravascular dilution of the label is a measure of RCV. The most widely used red cell label is ^{51}Cr-Na chromate, which binds firmly to hemoglobin.

Procedure

Blood is withdrawn into a citrate anticoagulant, red cells are labeled with ^{51}Cr, and the labeled cells are returned to the circulation. A sample of blood is withdrawn 15–30 minutes later, and the extent of the dilution of the injected label is calculated. In patients with splenomegaly, a longer wait before sampling is necessary to assure complete mixing. Red cell volume is obtained from the following formula:

$$RCV = \frac{\text{total radioactivity of injected red cells}}{\text{radioactivity/ml of red cells after mixing}}$$

Specimen

After red cells are labeled, excess label remaining in the plasma is either removed by removing plasma and washing the red cells or, more commonly, a correction is made for ^{51}Cr remaining in the plasma. In the latter event, ascorbic acid is added to the blood specimen before reinfusion to reduce the free ^{51}Cr and thereby prevent labeling of additional cells in vivo.

Interpretation

Red cell volume is reported in relation to either body surface area (ml/M^2), or, more commonly, in relation to body weight (ml/ kg). Representative normal values at sea level are 25 ± 5 ml/kg for women and 30 ± 5 ml/kg for men. Because RCV is related to mean body mass, spuriously low values can be reported with marked obesity. Most patients with PV present with marked elevation of RCV, and values greater than twice normal are commonly seen. Patients with spurious erythrocytosis have normal RCVs with values frequently in the upper normal range.

Notes and precautions

Although the procedure described requires meticulous care, RCV determinations with ^{51}Cr-labeled red cells are highly accurate and reproducible. ^{51}Chromium does not label red cells properly in patients receiving antibiotics or ascorbic acid. These medications act as reducing agents that render chromium incapable of tagging red cells during in vitro labeling, resulting in false lowering of values for RCV.

ARTERIAL OXYGEN SATURATION

Purpose

Arterial oxygen saturation (S_aO_2) is performed to demonstrate the presence of hypoxemia (2).

Principle

More than 98% of oxygen in the blood is bound to hemoglobin as oxyhemoglobin. The remainder is physically dissolved in plasma. The dissolved arterial oxygen is measured as oxygen tension or partial pressure of oxygen (P_aO_2). Arterial oxygen saturation is the ratio of hemoglobin-bound oxygen or oxyhemoglobin to the total amount of hemoglobin, that is, oxyhemoglobin plus reduced hemoglobin. There is a constant relationship between S_aO_2 and P_aO_2 at a given pH as represented by the oxyhemoglobin dissociation curve.

Procedure

In most laboratories S_aO_2 is determined by using a nomogram based on P_aO_2 pH and temperature. pO_2 is measured by the pO_2 (Clark) electrode. S_aO_2 is also determined directly using spectrophotometric methods that measure oxyhemoglobin and reduced hemoglobin in hemolyzed blood specimens at different wave lengths.

Specimen

Arterial blood specimens for blood gas determinations are collected with a minimum amount of heparin, maintained under anaerobic conditions and analyzed promptly.

Interpretation

Erythrocytotic hypoxia requires an S_aO_2 of less than 92%. Careful evaluation for hypoxemia should include blood sampling after exercise, with the patient in the recumbent as well as the upright position. A few patiens with PV do not have associated pulmonary disease or other anoxemic disorders but have unexplained lowering of S_aO_2 in the range of 88%–92%.

Notes and precautions

Use of a nomogram to determine S_aO_2 from P_aO_2 is based on the assumption that all the hemoglobin in the sample is capable of binding oxygen. With liganded hemoglobins such as carboxyhemoglobin or methemoglobin, which are unable to bind O_2, this assumption is incorrect and falsely normal S_aO_2 values are derived. Direct measurements of oxyhemoglobin and total hemoglobin by spectrophotometric methods are required in these instances. This is an especially important consideration in cases of decreased oxygen-carrying capacity associated with increased carboxyhemoglobin in smokers. An instrument that is particularly suited to measuring S_aO_2 in the presence of carboxyhemoglobin is the Co-Oximeter.* This instrument utilizes the principle of reflectance photometry and can monitor the absorbance of hemoglobin, oxyhemoglobin, and carboxyhemoglobin simultaneously at three different wavelengths.

LEUKOCYTE ALKALINE PHOSPHATASE (LAP)

Purpose

Leukocyte alkaline phosphatase can be helpful in differentiating PV from other forms of erythrocytosis (3).

For sections on *Principle*, *Procedure*, and *Specimen*, see Chapter 14.

Interpretation

Normal subjects have scores from 13–130. However, the normal range varies with different coupling dyes and should be determined in each laboratory. An increase in LAP is seen in 80% of cases of PV. Levels tend to remain increased throughout the course of the disease and are not modified by therapy or change of status. Normal

---

*Manufactured by Instrumentation Laboratory, Inc., Lexington, MA.

or high values are usually seen in myelofibrosis whereas low levels are characteristically found in chronic myelogenous leukemia.

Notes and precautions

Before elevated LAP can be used as corroborative evidence for PV, the existence of infectious or inflammatory diseases must be excluded, since elevated values are also found in the latter disease states. Elevated values are also found in pregnant women and in women taking oral contraceptives.

SERUM B_{12} AND UNBOUND B_{12} BINDING CAPACITY (UBBC)

Purpose

Tests of serum B_{12} and UBBC are helpful in differentiating PV from other causes of erythrocytosis (4,5).

Principle

Most of the vitamin B_{12} in plasma is bound to one of two proteins, transcobalamin I (TC I) and transcobalamin II (TC II). Transcobalamin II, the chief B_{12} transport protein, is present largely in the unsaturated state. It is apparently produced by the liver. Transcobalamin I, which is largely saturated with B_{12}, is produced by granulocytes and may function as part of the storage B_{12} pool. Vitamin B_{12} bound to TC I accounts for the major fraction of B_{12} found in normal plasma and is responsible for the elevated B_{12} levels found in conditions associated with granulocytosis. A third B_{12} binder, transcobalamin III (TC III), is a protein of unknown function that is only capable of significant B_{12} binding in vitro; it may also be of leukocyte origin. Transcobalamin III is often increased in PV.

Procedure

The procedure for measuring serum B_{12} is discussed in Chapter 4. UBBC is determined by incubating serum with radioactive labeled B_{12} and removing excess B_{12} that remains unbound to serum protein with hemoglobin-coated charcoal. The supernate in which the serum protein is now saturated with B_{12} is counted to quantitate the uptake of radioactive B_{12}.

Specimen

Vitamin B_{12} and UBBC are measured in serum.

Interpretation

Representative ranges of values for normals, PV, and chronic myelogenous leukemia (CML) are given in Table 13-4. Patients with secondary erythrocytosis show normal values. Patients with myelofibrosis and myeloid metaplasia show values for B_{12} and UBBC in the same range as those with PV. The characteristic finding in PV is an increase in UBBC out of proportion to or in the absence of an increase in B_{12}. This is in contrast to CML, in which UBBC rises concomitantly with B_{12}. This difference is caused by the fact that the major increase in PV is the exogenous binder TC III, whereas the increase in CML is a result of the endogenous binder TC I. Increased B_{12} is seen in 36% of patients with PV, whereas increased UBBC is seen in 70% of such patients. UBBC remains elevated in patients with PV who are treated for phlebotomy or who receive ineffective myelosuppressive therapy.

Notes and precautions

Elevated UBBC and B_{12} levels can be associated with leukemoid reactions secondary to malignancies and chronic infection.

Special Studies

INTRAVENOUS PYELOGRAPHY

More than half the reported tumors associated with inappropriate production of erythropoietin and erythrocytosis have been renal carcinomas. When these cases are considered along with the significant number of nonneoplastic renal lesions, that is, cysts and hydronephrosis associated with this type of erythrocytosis, the

Table 13-4. Serum B_{12} and Unsaturated B_{12} Binding Capacity (UBBC)

Diagnosis	Serum B_{12} (pg/ml)	UBBC (pg/ml)
Normal	300–900	1219–1991
PV	300–2056	1757–4667
CML	2097–8810	7505–17,850

kidney is by far the organ most frequently responsible for cases of aberrant erythropoietin production. Therefore, incidences of absolute erythrocytosis without hypoxemia that do not present as clear-cut PV should be screened for renal disease with an intravenous pyelogram.

$P_{50}O_2$

A growing number of hereditary hemoglobin abnormalities have been reported in which there is an increased affinity of the hemoglobin molecule for more oxygen, decreased oxygen release to tissue, and ensuing erythrocytosis. These hemoglobinopathies have been associated with PCVs in fewer than 60% of patients.

Altered affinity of hemoglobin for oxygen is measured by the $P_{50}O_2$, that is, the PO_2 of arterial blood at which 50% of hemoglobin is saturated with oxygen. P_{50} is derived from the oxyhemoglobin dissociation curve, which in turn is determined by equilibrating aliquots of blood with gases at different oxygen tensions and determining pH, PO_2, and S_aO_2 for each equilibrated sample. Representative normal values for $P_{50}O_2$ range from 25–30 mm. Patients with erythrocytotic hemoglobinopathies have values below 20 mm.

ERYTHROPOIETIN ASSAY

Although attempts are under way to develop an in vitro assay of erythropoietin using such immunologic techniques as hemagglutination inhibition and radioimmunoassay, the only established way of measuring erythropoietin is the bioassay. This assay employs

Table 13-5. Diagnostic Criteria of the Polycythemia Vera Study Group[a]

Category A
1. Increased red cell volume
   (Males $\geq$ 36 ml/kg,
   Females $\geq$ 32 ml/kg)
2. Normal arterial O_2 saturation $\geq$ 92%
3. Splenomegaly

Category B
1. Thrombocytosis
   Platelet count $>$ 400,000/mm³
2. Leukocytosis
   White cell count $>$ 12,000/mm³
3. Elevated LAP score
4. Elevated serum B_{12} ($>$ 900 pg/ml) or UBBC ($>$ 2200 pg/ml)

[a]The diagnosis of PV is accepted in the presence of the following combinations: A1 + A2 + A3 or A1 + A2 + any two from Category B.

mice in which endogenous erythropoietin is first abolished by hypoxia or by transfusion polycythemia. Incorporation of ^{59}Fe into circulating erythrocytes of mice after injection of serum or urine is then used to measure erythropoietic activity. The assay of concentrated 24-hour urine is more sensitive than that of serum. The normal value for urinary excretion of erythropoietin is about 2–3 units.

On theoretic grounds the assay of erythropoietin should be useful in differentiating the various forms of polycythemia. In reality, however, the bioassay is a crude and laborious method that is not widely available and, therefore, is generally impractical. Its greatest usefulness is in occult erythrocytosis in which a suspect lesion is associated with aberrant production of erythropoietin. In such cases, levels of erythropoietin are often markedly elevated.

CRITERIA OF THE POLYCYTHEMIA VERA STUDY GROUP

In 1968 the Polycythemia Vera Study Group developed a set of criteria for the diagnosis of polycythemia vera to ensure uniformity in the patient population studied (Table 13-5). These criteria provide helpful diagnostic guidelines.

REFERENCES

1. International Committee for Standardization: Panel on Diagnostic Applications of Radioisotopes in Haematology: Standard techniques for the measurement of red cell and plasma volume. Br J Haematol 15:801–814, 1973

2. Maas AHJ, Hamelink ML, DeLeeuw RJM: An evaluation of the spectrophotometric determination of oxyhemoglobin, carboxyhemoglobin and hemoglobin in blood with the CO-Oximeter IL 182. Clin Chim Acta 29:303–309, 1970

3. Beutler E: Leukocyte alkaline phosphatase. In Williams WJ, Beutler E, Erslev AJ, et al: *Hematology*, ed 2. New York, McGraw-Hill, 1977, pp 1628–1629

4. Gilbert HS, Krauss S, Pasternack B, et al: Serum vitamin B12 content and unsaturated vitamin B12 binding capacity in myeloproliferative disease. Ann Intern Med 71:719–729, 1969

5. Zittoun J, Zittoun R, Marquet J, et al: The three transcobalamins in myeloproliferative disorders and acute leukemia. Br J Haematol 31:287–298, 1975

PART B/DISORDERS OF THE LEUKOCYTES AND THE RETICULO-ENDOTHELIAL SYSTEM

chapter 14

Reactive Disorders of Myelomonocytic Leukocytes

Granulocytes are derived from a pluripotential stem cell in the bone marrow. The stem cell may also give rise to the monocyte cell line. Granulocytic maturation progresses to immature forms, myeloblasts, progranulocytes, and myelocytes in a series of three or four cell divisions. Metamyelocytes, bands, and segmented forms are intermediate and mature nondividing cells. Granulocyte distribution is divided into three phases: marrow production (four to five days), circulating granulocyte pool (six hours), and tissue phase (four to five days). The total granulocyte pool is approximately evenly distributed between the circulating granulocytes and those temporarily sequestered in the microcirculation, the marginated pool. In normal granulocytic kinetics, neutrophils enter the tissue phase randomly without return to the circulation and die there. The number of circulating or countable granulocytes is determined by marrow production, rate of entry into the peripheral circulating pool, shifts between circulating and marginated fractions, and rate of exit into the tissues. The first two factors are the most important in protracted peripheral granulocytosis, the third in physiologic granulocytosis.

Leukocytosis is an absolute increase in peripheral white cells above 10,000/mm^3. Although the term leukocytosis can include esoinophils and basophils, it is generally interpreted as an increase in neutrophilic granulocytes. Thus granulocytosis is defined by an absolute count greater than 8000/mm^3, or the percentage of segmented neutrophils and band cells exceeds 80%. A list of the commonest causes of neutrophilic granulocytosis is shown in Table 14-1. The most frequent categories are infection, usually from pyogenic bacteria; inflammation caused by tissue or tumor necrosis; hematologic disorders; and physiologic stress of cold, heat, or exercise. Elevation of the granulocyte count above 50,000/mm³ with some immature cells may simulate chronic granulocytic leukemia (CGL) and is therefore categorized as a leukemoid reaction.

Granulocytes act as phagocytic cells mediated in part by their cytoplasmic granules. The immature cells, blasts and progranulocytes, contain primary granules, seen as dense azurophilic masses in progranulocytes. Smaller secondary or specific granules first appear at the myelocyte phase. In the intermediate cells, myelocytes and metamyelocytes, both primary and secondary granules are visible with secondary granules predominating in the mature forms, bands and polymorphonuclear neutrophilic leukocytes (PMNs). The staining characteristics of the secondary granules with Romanovsky dyes (Wright's or Wright-Giemsa) label the leukocytes as neutrophilic, eosinophilic, or basophilic. Both primary and secondary granules contain enzymes; in the secondary granules these enzymes are alkaline phosphatase, lysozyme, and aminopeptidase.

DIAGNOSTIC EVALUATION

The differential diagnosis of leukocytosis is reactive, or leukemoid, versus CGL. Helpful characteristics are summarized in Table 14-2. A clinical history is indispensable.

1. Hematologic findings include total white cell count and differential with repeated determinations to establish persistence and magnitude. These findings also help in evaluating prognosis.

2. Bone marrow aspiration is performed when the granulocytosis does not appear to be physiologic or reactive; for example, when the clinical history is not definitive, the granulocytosis persists or is above 20,000/mm³, increased immature granulocytes are present, or another cell line is also abnormal. An aliquot should be submitted for karyotype analysis.

Table 14-1. Causes of Neutrophilic Granulocytosis

Physiologic stress or physical agents (usual range: 13,000–30,000/mm^3)
    Excessive cold or heat
    Exercise
    Postprandial
    Pregnancy (3rd trimester)
    Newborn
    Emotional states (excitement, depression)
    Nausea, vomiting

Infection
    Bacterial
        Gram positive: *Staphylococcus, Streptococcus,* pneumococcus
        Gram negative: *E. coli, P. aeruginosa, Pasteurella*
    Rickettsiae: typhus
    Parasitic: liver fluke
    Fungal: coccidioidomycosis

Inflammation or tissue necrosis
    Myocardial infarction
    Pneumonia
    Peritonitis
    Collagen disorders (vasculitis, myositis)
    Tumor necrosis

Drugs
    Etiocholanolone
    Epinephrine
    Digitalis
    Steroids
    Heparin
    Histamine
    Endotoxin

Metabolic
    Diabetic acidosis
    Eclampsia
    Gout (with acute inflammation)
    Thyroid storm

Hematologic disorders
    Acute hemorrhage
    Hemolysis (hemolytic anemia, transfusion reaction)
    Myeloproliferative (PV, myeloid metaplasia, or myelofibrosis)
    CGL

Idiopathic (10–15,000/mm^3)

Table 14-2. Laboratory Findings for Leukemoid Reaction and Chronic Granulocytic Leukemia

Test	Leukemoid Reaction	CGL
White cell count/mm^3	< 100,000	May be 30,000–50,000
% PMNs	Up to 95%	May be normal (60%–70%)
Immature granulocytes	To myelocyte phase	May include occasional progranulocytes or blasts
Eosinophils, basophils	Often decreased	Often slightly increased
Nucleated red cells	Rarely seen	Late, may be common
Bone marrow M/E ratio	6–8:1	≥ 15:1
LAP	> 100	< 10

3. Leukocyte alkaline phosphatase is helpful in distinguishing leukemoid reactions from CGL (see Chapter 18).

4. Appropriate bacteriologic studies are performed if the cause of granulocytosis is suspected to be infection.

LABORATORY STUDIES

Hematologic Tests

GENERAL FEATURES

Acute granulocytosis caused by physiologic stimuli is transient, usually resulting from a shift of marginated granulocytes to the circulating pool; no change in bone marrow cellularity is therefore expected. Chronic granulocytosis is reflected in increased marrow granulopoiesis with as much as a tenfold increase in granulocyte turnover, more marked in children than adults. A hypercellular marrow results. As the rate of turnover increases, cells may be released prematurely from the marrow producing a left shift. Increased production of granulocytes in benign conditions has no effect on the size of liver, spleen, or lymph nodes.

PERIPHERAL BLOOD

The magnitude of granulocytosis and the relative proportion of band cells to segmented neutrophils may indicate the etiology and the ultimate prognosis.

White cell count

A total white cell count of 10,000–20,000/mm^3 is consistent with inflammation or physiologic causes. With a count of 20,000–50,000/mm^3 leukemoid reaction versus CGL should be considered. A white cell count greater than 100,000/mm^3 is consistent with CGL. In the elderly, the total count may be less than 10,000/mm^3 but a left shift indicates inflammation.

Differential diagnosis

When more than 80% of cells are PMNs, contained inflammation above the diaphragm (e.g., otitis media, pneumonia, abscess) should be considered. When more than 10% of cells are band forms, perforated viscus, inflammation below the diaphragm (e.g., perforated diverticulum or appendix, ulcer, or carcinoma of the colon with peritonitis) or hemorrhagic pancreatitis should be considered. A left shift to the myelocyte phase is seen in severe infections. The presence of blasts or more than occasional progranulocytes indicates extreme marrow stress or CGL. Increased numbers of bands without granulocytosis, clinical symptoms, or other immature forms suggest Pelger-Huët anomaly. A left shift with nucleated red cells (leukoerythroblastosis) indicates severe marrow stress as in anoxia or myelophthisis from tumor or leukemia. Granulocytosis or left shift with concurrent eosinophilia and/or basophilia suggests CGL.

Platelet counts above 400,000/mm^3 can be seen with inflammation, but counts greater than 600,000/mm^3 suggest that the granulocytosis is myeloproliferative or CGL.

Morphology

Toxic granulations are primary granules seen in granulocytes that either result from abnormal persistence during maturation or are caused by premature marrow release, a characteristic of inflammation or infection. Abnormally large granules are also seen in Chédiak-Higashi syndrome. Döhle bodies are amorphous, cytoplasmic masses seen in severe inflammation, massive burns, or infections. They are also present in May-Hegglin anomaly. Prolonged granulocytosis produces pseudohypersegmented PMNs with four or five lobes.

BONE MARROW

In reactive granulocytosis the marrow is hypercellular (70%–80%), with increased M/E ratio as great as 6:1 or 8:1 associated with a left shift to the myelocyte phase. A shift to myeloblasts or progranulocytes suggests CGL or myeloproliferative disorder. Usually the only cell line that is increased is granulocytic although megakaryocytes may be slightly increased. If megakaryocytes are increased profoundly or the erythroid series appears dysplastic, myeloproliferative disorders should be considered. In prolonged infection or inflammation, plasma cells may be increased. Karyotype analysis that yields Philadelphia chromosome (Ph[1]) is consistent with CGL. Absence of Ph[1] does not exclude CGL, however.

Other Useful Tests

LEUKOCYTE ALKALINE PHOSPHATASE (LAP)

Purpose

The LAP test is useful in differentiating CGL from leukemoid reactions (see also Chapter 18).

Principle

Leukocyte alkaline phosphatase is an enzyme present only in the secondary granules of maturing neutrophils from the myelocyte phase onward. It is not present in lymphocytes, monocytes, or abnormal and immature neutrophils. Stimulated neutrophils contain increased amounts of LAP. Therefore, the test is useful in distinguishing leukemoid reactions (increased LAP) from the abnormally maturing granulocytes of CGL (decreased LAP).

Procedure

The LAP test is routinely available in most hospital laboratories. Although LAP can be determined quantitatively by enzymatic release from freshly lysed granulocytes, it is usually determined semiquantitatively by specific cytochemical staining of peripheral blood smears. The LAP present in the neutrophils hydrolyzes a substrate of naphthol AS-BI phosphate substrate at pH 8.6, and the hydrolyzed product couples to a soluble diazonium dye, Fast Blue RR, forming insoluble brown-to-black azo dye particles in the cytoplasm of the cells at the enzyme sites. The smears are then counterstained with hematoxylin, examined microscopically, and 100 segmented or band neutrophils are counted and graded 0–4+. The LAP score is calculated by addition of the number of cells times the grade, as shown in the following example. The range of normal scores is 13–130.

No. cells × grade	=	Score
20 × 0		0
30 × 1+		30
30 × 2+		60
40 × 3+		120
10 × 4+		40
		250 = LAP Score

Specimen

Freshly prepared patient and control blood smears, obtained from a finger stick, capillary blood, or heparinized venous blood, and less than four hours old are fixed for 30 seconds in 10% formalin in absolute methanol. Edetate (EDTA) anticoagulant inhibits the reaction and must not be used. If not stained immediately, the fixed slides may be stored up to six months in a freezer without significant loss of enzyme activity.

Interpretation

Normal peripheral smears show 0–1+ staining PMNs, band cells, metamyelocytes, and myelocytes yielding scores of 13–130 (Table 14-3). Leukemoid reactions have granulocytes with increased LAP (3–4+) so that scores are above 100. Intermediate degrees of elevation are seen in pregnancy, in women taking oral contraceptives, in myocardial infarction, and with steroid therapy. Pathologic granulocytes (as in CGL) lack normal enzymatic activity and produce scores less than 10. Other causes of low scores are paroxysmal nocturnal hemoglobinuria (PNH) and congenital hypophosphatasia, an inborn error of metabolism.

Table 14-3. **Leukocyte Alkaline Phosphatase Scores**

< 10	10–100	> 100
CGL	Pregnancy	Leukemoid reaction
PNH	Contraceptives	Pyogenic infection
Idiopathic thrombocytopenic purpura (ITP)	ACTH therapy	
Infectious mononucleosis	Myocardial infarction	
Pernicious anemia		
Congenital hypo-phosphatasia		

Notes and precautions

Lymphocytes or blasts of any cell line do not stain and peripheral smears with marked increases in either cannot be interpreted. Improperly stored smears lose enzymatic activity and give falsely low LAP scores.

EOSINOPHILIA

Eosinophils spend 3–6 days in production in the marrow, have a very short circulation time (less than one hour), and survive for 8–12 days in tissue, where they apparently function in sequestering immune complexes and in limiting chronic inflammatory reactions. They do not have bacteriocidal activity; the specific eosinophilic granules contain peroxidase and acid phosphatase but no alkaline phosphatase or lysozyme. They have limited phagocytic activity. Eosinophils are chemotactically attracted to tissue sites of foreign antigen, antigen-antibody complexes, and vasoactive amines. They limit inflammation by counteracting vasoactive amines and kinins.

Response of eosinophils to inflammation involves an immediate transient accumulation in tissues and prolonged tissue accumulation for days, weeks, or months associated with peripheral eosinophilia and increased bone marrow production of eosinophils. Tissue eosinophils are ingested by macrophages, and Charcot-Leyden crystals are found in secretions or tissue in association with disintegration of eosinophils.

Eosinophilia is defined as an increase in peripheral eosinophils above 3% or an absolute increase above $250/mm^3$. Conditions associated with eosinophilia are summarized in Table 14-4. The commonest causes are drug association, allergy, or parasites. Parasitic infestations that cause eosinophilia are characterized by a prominent tissue infestation either during migration or encysting of the parasite and often have pulmonary involvement. Allergic reactions associated with eosinophilia are often IgE dependent reactions and immune complex disease.

DIAGNOSTIC EVALUATION OF EOSINOPHILIA

Eosinophilia is usually a benign process; its evaluation depends heavily on clinical history. Persistent eosinophilia with levels above 10% should be evaluated by:

1. Hematologic findings to determine persistence. Bone marrow aspiration is rarely helpful except to exclude CGL when the peripheral blood is suggestive of that disease. Absolute eosinophil count is useful to evaluate therapy.
2. Examination of stool and urine sediment for ova or parasites. Infestation by *Strongyloides*, *Ascaris*, *Taenia*, or *Schistosoma* parasites frequently causes eosinophilia.
3. Determination of serum IgE, which is frequently elevated in allergic eosinophilia.
4. Radiography of the chest to exclude sarcoid, Löffler's syndrome or infiltrates secondary to parasites.
5. Muscle biopsy if trichinosis is suspected. In fatal trichinosis eosinophilia may be absent.
6. Biopsy of lymph nodes if persistent lymphadenopathy is associated to exclude Hodgkin's disease or sarcoid.

Table 14-4. Conditions Associated with Eosinophilia

Drug therapy
- Allopurinol
- Phenothiazine
- Heparin
- Streptomycin, penicillins, cephalothin
- Digitalis, quinidine, procainamide, propranolol

Parasitic infestation
- Trichinosis
- Visceral larva migrans (*Ascaris*)
- Filariasis
- Echinococcus
- *Clonorchis sinensis* (liver fluke)

Chronic infections
- Brucellosis
- Fungal infections
- Leprosy
- Tuberculosis

Malignancies
- Carcinoma of the lung, ovary, stomach

Hematologic disorders
- Pernicious anemia
- CGL
- Hodgkin's disease

Collagen disease
- Periarteritis nodosa
- Rheumatoid arthritis

Dermatitis
- Dermatitis herpetiformis
- Exfoliative dermatitis caused by drug

Pulmonary disease
- Löffler's syndrome (eosinophilic pneumonia)
- Farmer's lung (moldy grain)
- Bagassosis (cane fiber, insulation material)

Allergy
- Asthma
- Hay fever
- Urticaria
- Angioneurotic edema

Miscellaneous
- Sarcoidosis

7. Serologic tests for parasites. The available serologic techniques vary with the parasite (Table 14-5). Skin test antigens are not generally available and are not reliable.

LABORATORY STUDIES OF EOSINOPHILIA

Hematologic Tests

GENERAL FEATURES

The cause of eosinophilia is either clinically obvious or obscure. For this reason, when levels of eosinophils are less than 10%, the disease is often ignored in the absence of clinical signs or symptoms or other hematologic abnormality. With significant eosinophilia, the liver, spleen, and lymph nodes may be enlarged; the skin or lungs may be involved; and fever may be present depending on the cause.

PERIPHERAL BLOOD

Eosinophilia is present when levels of eosinophils are greater than 3% (the normal range is 1%–3%), or when an absolute increase in eosinophils above 250/mm^3 is present (the normal range is 50–250/mm^3). The highest elevations are seen in trichinosis, in *Clonorchis sinensis* infections, and in dermatitis herpetiformis.

BONE MARROW

Variable eosinophilia is present that is unrelated to the degree of tissue or blood eosinophilia. Immaturity of the granulocytic series or M/E ratio greater than 10:1 suggests CGL. Granulomas may be seen in sarcoidosis or tuberculosis.

Table 14-5. Serologic Test Methods for Parasitic Diseases

Parasite	CF[a]	BF[a]	LA[a]	IHA[a]	Ind. IF[a] P[a]	Skin[b]	Comment
Ancylostoma							No reproducible satisfactory tests
Ascaris	+	+		+	+		All methods unreliable and little used
Clonorchis	+			+			
Echinococcus	+	+		+	+	+	90% correlation with active disease if titer above 256, low titer has poor correlation; some cross reactions with other parasites
Filaria		+		+	+		60% correlation; false positive at low titer; cross-reactive
Schistosoma	+			+	+		No tests available
Taenia							
Trichina	+	+		+	+	+	CF correlates with active disease cross reaction with *Schistosoma*
Toxocaris (visceral larva migrans)		+		+			False negatives are a problem; less than 60% are positive

[a]Abbreviations: *BF*, bentonite flocculation; *CF*, complement fixation; *IHA*, indirect hemagglutination; *Ind. IF*, indirect immunofluorescence; *LA*, latex agglutination; *P*, precipitin.
[b]Skin antigens are not regularly available but parasites for which they are used are listed.

Other Useful Tests

STOOL EXAMINATION FOR OVA AND PARASITES

Purpose

Examination of stool identifies *Strongyloides*, *Ascaris*, and *Taenia*, which may cause eosinophilia (4). Urine sediment should be examined for *Schistosoma mansoni*.

Principle

Parasites with strong tissue phases are those associated most commonly with eosinophilia.

Procedure

Preparation of slides for examination is a standard procedure for most hospital laboratories.

Specimen

Fresh stool specimens are examined on at least three occasions.

Interpretation

Significant parasites for diagnosis of eosinophilia are *Strongyloides*, *Ascaris*, *Taenia*, or *Schistosoma*. Parasites such as *Amoeba*, *Giardia*, *Trichuris*, and *Enterobius vermicularis* (pinworm) are not associated with eosinophilia.

SEROLOGIC TESTS FOR PARASITES

Purpose

Serologic tests confirm exposure to antigens of parasites that encapsulate in tissue and are not readily detected in stool.

Principle

Serologic tests detect rising antibody titer to parasitic antigens. Antibodies may vary with each patient's immune response, the antigenicity of the organism, and the stage of the disease. Not all antibodies react by the same method since some fix complement, some are flocculins or precipitins, and others are agglutinins. In general a battery of tests is needed to confirm the diagnosis.

Procedure

Tests are not generally available except in county, state, or Center for Disease Control laboratories. Methods of testing vary with each parasite but usually include complement fixation (CF), indirect hemagglutination (IHA), indirect immunofluorescence (IFA), or bentonite flocculation. Latex agglutination tests lack sensitivity as a general class. Skin test antigens are not generally available. Commonly used tests are listed in Table 14-5.

Specimen

Acute and convalescent serum specimens should be obtained at least 10 days apart. Sera can be stored frozen.

Interpretation

Rises in titer are clinically significant for active disease although in many cases titers are already maximal at the time of serologic diagnosis. They usually require three weeks to develop although eosinophilia may precede the antibodies. In chronic disease or in inactive disease, titers fade after one to two years. Significant titers vary with each disease and technique and are reported by the testing agency.

SERUM IMMUNOGLOBULIN E (IgE)

Purpose

Levels of IgE are elevated in eosinophilia caused by parasitism or atopic disease, for example, dermatitis, hay fever, or asthma (5).

Principle

IgE (reaginic) antibodies result from skin-sensitizing antigens, which may be introduced through the skin or through broncho-pulmonary or gastrointestinal systems. IgE is present in minute amounts that can be measured only in nanograms and requires sensitive radioimmunoassays for quantitation.

Procedure

Several radioimmune assay (RIA) variations are available commercially as test kits. Radioimmunoassay by competitive protein binding is sensitive to 5 ng/ml. Although serum inhibitors can interfere with the test, it is reasonably accurate for elevated levels. Noncompetitive protein-binding RIA uses a double antibody sensitive to picogram levels and unaffected by serum inhibitors. The most widely available method is radioimmune precipitation assay, which also uses a double-antibody technique. Antibody to IgE plus I^{125}-labeled IgE is incubated with the patient's serum. The antibody becomes complexed with radiolabeled IgE and IgE of the patient. The complexes are precipitated with a second IgG antibody and the insoluble immune complexes are counted.

Specimen

Heparinized plasma or serum, which may be stored frozen, is used as a specimen. Specimens should be shipped frozen.

Interpretation

The normal range for serum IgE is 0.4–4000 IU/ml. Values are age dependent; they are very low in cord blood and approach adult levels by the time the patient is 12. Serum IgE levels fluctuate with exposure to the inciting allergen but may rise several times their original levels. T-lymphocytes influence IgE levels so that T cell malignancies and Hodgkin's disease may be associated with increased IgE.

Low levels of IgE do not rule out parasitic or allergic disease.

OTHER USEFUL TESTS

1. Nasal smears or sputum cytology for eosinophils. Sputum eosinophils suggest Löffler's pneumonia. Nasal eosinophilia is common in allergic rhinitis. Charcot-Leyden crystals may be present.

2. A chest radiograph is useful to exclude Löffler's pneumonia or sarcoid.
3. Biopsy of enlarged lymph nodes to exclude Hodgkin's disease or filariasis in endemic areas.
4. Biopsy of the gastrocnemius muscle, diagnostic in most cases of trichinosis, is used only in severely ill patients in whom the diagnosis is in doubt.

BASOPHILIA

The precursor cell is a marrow, pluripotent stem cell for the granulocytic series. The basophil circulates briefly before ending in tissue, usually at the site of antigen-induced injury. Circulating basophils appear in levels of less than 1%, and, therefore, little is known of disease entities with basophilia. Basophils are known to be increased in some hypersensitivity reactions, myeloproliferative disorders including polycythemia vera and myeloid metaplasia, and CGL. Basophilia is defined as a peripheral proportion greater than 1%.

DIAGNOSTIC EVALUATION OF BASOPHILIA

Because of the association with granulocytic proliferative disorders, evaluation is dependent on the degree of associated abnormality of the granulocytic series. Bone marrow aspiration may be helpful. Tissue basophils or mast cells are a nonspecific, nondiagnostic reaction to many stimuli including metastatic tumor, marrow hyperplasia, and urticaria pigmentosa.

MONOCYTOSIS

The marrow precursor cell, while not identified, is suspected to be a stem cell leading to both monocytic and granulocytic cell lines and, therefore, many similarities in metabolism and function are seen. Monocyte cytoplasm contains many hydrolytic enzymes including lysosomes. Monocytes function, as does the neutrophil, in bacterial phagocytosis and may be the processor of many antigens. The peripheral blood monocyte is an intermediate step that leads to the tissue macrophage. In animals, circulating monocytes have a half-life of approximately one to three days with a tissue phase of months to years. Tissue macrophages may be seen as histiocytes, giant cells, and epithelioid cells in granulomas.

Monocytosis is often transient and correlates poorly with disease states. Of the diseases listed in Table 14-6, monocytosis is associated most commonly with neutropenia of all types (familial, cyclic, and drug induced), the recovery phase of infection or inflammation, and Hodgkin's disease. Before 1965, infectious disease with tissue destruction was considered the most important cause, but changes in therapy have altered this. Tissue destruction in chronic infection, for example, subacute bacterial endocarditis (SBE) and disseminated candidiasis, is an important factor in monocytosis. Recent studies no longer show the diagnostic correlation with tuberculosis.

DIAGNOSTIC EVALUATION OF MONOCYTOSIS

The proportion of monocytes in the peripheral blood is correlated with clinical history. Since destruction of tissue is associated with monocytosis, radiographs of the chest and appropriate cultures of blood or tissue may be helpful.

LABORATORY STUDIES OF MONOCYTOSIS

Hematologic Tests

GENERAL FEATURES

In a healthy person monocytes comprise 0%–9% of total white cells with an absolute count of 300–500/mm^3, somewhat higher in

Table 14-6. Diseases Associated with Monocytosis

Physiologic
    Normal newborn

Infections
    Bacteria
        Brucellosis
        M. tuberculosis
        M. leprae
        Subacute bacterial endocarditis
        Recovery phase of acute infections
    Rickettsiae
        Rocky Mountain spotted fever
        Typhus
    Protozoa or parasites
        Malaria

Hematologic disorders
    Myeloproliferative disorders
    Myelogenous and monocytic leukemias
    Hodgkin's disease
    Agranulocytosis
    Cyclic neutropenias

Collagen disorders
    SLE
    RA
    Polyarteritis

Gastrointestinal
    Sprue
    Ulcerative colitis
    Regional enteritis

Miscellaneous
    Postsplenectomy
    Lipidoses (Gaucher's, Niemann-Pick, Hand-Schüller-Christian diseases)

children. Monocytosis is normal in the first two weeks of life. Physical findings depend on the underlying cause; hepatosplenomegaly is associated with myeloproliferative disorders and lipidoses. In some of the infectious diseases, fever may be present. Monocytes are phagocytic and in reticuloendothelial hyperplasia (e.g., SBE), monocytes may be seen in peripheral blood or tissue with ingested red cells, or, rarely, white cells and platelets. Stasis encourages this phenomenon so that specimens from the ear lobe are more helpful than finger sticks or venous specimens.

PERIPHERAL BLOOD

White cell count

A proportion of greater than 10% monocytes in the peripheral blood defines monocytosis. Absolute values are greater than 500–800/mm^3 for adults, greater than 750/mm^3 for children, and greater than 1000–1200/mm^3 for newborns.

An absolute value on white cell counts of less than 1000/mm^3 is compatible with the compensatory monocytosis of neutropenia. When absolute values of white cells are greater than 10,000/mm^3, the increase in monocytes parallels increase in granulopoiesis.

Morphology

Ingestion of red cells seen in monocytes on specimens from the ear lobe often indicates SBE.

BONE MARROW

Bone marrow studies are helpful only if hematologic disorders are suspected. Clot sections may show granulomas in miliary tuberculosis. Cellularity varies from aplastic to myeloproliferative. Bone marrow cultures are not helpful since the specimen is too limited; blood cultures should be performed.

Other Laboratory Tests

CULTURES

Blood cultures may be considered negative after three have yielded no organism if anaerobic techniques have been included.

RICKETTSIAL SEROLOGY

Rickettsial serology is usually tested using febrile agglutination titers. Results are significant only if one titer is elevated. Anamnestic elevations of all titers increase with fever of any origin.

GRANULOCYTOPENIA

Granulocytopenia, defined as a decrease in neutrophilic granulocytes to less than $2500/mm^3$, is often associated with a relative lymphocytosis. Thus the peripheral white cell differential may be misinterpreted as a lymphocytic disorder unless the low total white cell count is noted and absolute granulocyte count is calculated. Granulocytopenia may be caused by decreased production of marrow, increased utilization (i.e., loss to the tissues), or shifts from the circulating to the marginated pool (Table 14-7). The commonest causes are related to drugs, collagen disease, viral infection, and hypersplenism, usually secondary to hepatic cirrhosis.

Granulocytopenia becomes clinically significant in terms of infection when the total neutrophil count is less than $1000/mm^3$. Since granulopoiesis in the marrow requires four to five days, a time lag may follow toxic insult to the marrow before granulocytopenia is evident, and, similarly, before recovery is noted.

Drug-associated neutropenia may be caused by direct chemical suppression of marrow production or may be secondary to toxic immune complexes formed by the drug, its antibody, and complement, destroying cells peripherally. These complexes adhere to the surface of the target cell (platelet, leukocyte, or red cell) resulting in cell lysis. Drugs frequently responsible for neutropenia are listed in Table 14-8.

Table 14-7. Causes of Granulocytopenia[a]

Decreased marrow production
    Toxicity caused by drugs, chemicals, or irradiation
        Chemotherapeutic (cytotoxic)
        Noncytotoxic drugs (see Table 14-8)
        X-ray, gamma irradiation
        Chemicals (benzene, CCl_4, DDT)
    Bone marrow replacement (myelophthisis)
        Cancer
        Leukemia or lymphoma
        Myelofibrosis
    Abnormal granulopoiesis, congenital
        Fanconi's anemia (neonatal aplasia)
        Familial cyclic neutropenia—exaggerated oscillation
        Familial benign neutropenia
    Abnormal granulopoiesis, acquired
        PNH
        Immune injury
        Collagen disease
          SLE
          RA with splenomegaly (Felty's syndrome)
    Aplastic anemia
    Nutritional
        Vitamin B_{12}
        Folic acid

Increased destruction or utilization in peripheral blood or tissue
    Hypersplenism
        Splenomegaly with RA (Felty's syndrome)
    Virus
    Immune
        Leukocyte antibody
        Drug antibody—innocent bystander cell
    Surface injury
        Hemodialysis
        Pump-oxygenator in open heart surgery
    Prolonged inflammation

Shift from circulating to marginated pool
    Peritoneal dialysis

[a]May be part of pancytopenia in some categories.

Table 14-8. **Noncytotoxic Drugs Associated with Neutropenia**

Antimicrobial drugs
 Chloramphenicol
 Sulfonamides
 Nitrofurantoin
 Tranquilizers or psychotropic drugs

Antithyroid drugs
 Thiouracils

Antiinflammatory drugs
 Phenylbutazone
 Indomethacin

Diuretics
 Thiazides
 Ethacrynic acid

Hypoglycemic agents
 Sulfonamide derivatives

Miscellaneous
 Quinidine
 Procainamide
 Allopurinol

Granulocytopenia seen in SLE is of moderate degree and unknown etiology, possibly antibody. It may be associated with thrombocytopenia and is most often seen in young females. Rarely, rheumatoid arthritis is associated with splenomegaly and hypersplenism (Felty's syndrome), which produces sequestration granulocytopenia.

Cyclic neutropenia is a diagnosis made by excluding all other likely causes. It is frequently familial with slightly increased frequency in black females. The mechanism of disease may be exaggerated oscillation in granulopoiesis and distribution between circulating and marginated pools.

Viral infections appear to have a direct inhibiting effect on maturation of granulocytes resulting in transient neutropenia with lymphocytosis.

DIAGNOSTIC EVALUATION OF GRANULOCYTOPENIA

Diagnostic evaluation should include extensive history of current and recent (six weeks) drug therapy and physical examination to estimate size of the spleen.

1. Hematologic evaluation. The total white count and differential determine granulocytopenia with or without relative lymphocytosis.
2. Bone marrow aspiration is usually necessary when the white cell count is persistently below $3000/mm^3$ or when another cell line is also abnormal to determine marrow cellularity or arrest in cell maturation. Arrest of normal maturation usually suggests drug or other toxic etiology and a thorough investigation of drug history is necessary.
3. Screening tests for antinuclear antibodies in SLE or RA.
4. Testing for rheumatoid factor to exclude the rare Felty's syndrome (rheumatoid arthritis with hypersplenism).
5. ^{51}Chromium survival studies of red cells to evaluate size of the spleen and sequestration, since hypersplenism may be associated with leukopenia as well. Studies of leukocyte kinetics are not generally available.

LABORATORY STUDIES OF GRANULOCYTOPENIA

Hematologic Tests

GENERAL FEATURES

In granulocytopenia total granulocyte counts are below $1500/mm^3$. Hematologic tests should define whether the disease is caused by lack of production, as in aplasia, myelofibrosis, or granulocytic arrest, or is caused by peripheral destruction by toxic immune complexes, virus, leukocyte antibody, chemicals, or splenic sequestration. Splenomegaly and/or hepatomegaly support splenic sequestration as the cause.

Relative lymphocytosis usually indicates peripheral, specific destruction of granulocytes by drug, virus, or arrest of the granulocyte series in the marrow. Decrease in more than one cell line suggests generalized marrow suppression or peripheral splenic sequestration. Major damage to the marrow generally maintains the relative distribution of granulocytes and lymphocytes.

PERIPHERAL BLOOD

Morphology of granulocytes is normal but the total number is decreased. Neutrophil counts below $1000/mm^3$ indicate significant risk from infection so that toxic granulations or Döhle bodies may be present. A left shift with neutropenia indicates severe infection or inflammation, with increased tissue utilization and destruction of granulocytes. Monocytosis may be seen and is partly compensatory. Associated thrombocytopenia indicates severe insult to the marrow or peripheral sequestration.

BONE MARROW

Bone marrow biopsy supplements the aspirate in evaluating cellularity. Neutropenia and hypocellular marrow ($< 20\%$) or aplasia are seen with drug or chemical toxicity and are associated with decreases in megakaryocytes or erythroid precursors resulting in peripheral pancytopenia. Neutropenia and hypercellular marrow ($> 80\%$) with a normal maturation sequence suggest splenic sequestration. Normal cellular or hypercellular marrow with partial or complete arrest in granulocytic maturation may be seen with drug insults. The effects of marrow arrest on peripheral blood are delayed for four days. Partial arrests are difficult to appreciate unless a careful marrow differential is made; less than 6% stab cells and PMNs is consistent with arrest.

Other Useful Tests

ANTINUCLEAR ANTIBODIES

Purpose

The presence of antinuclear antibodies suggests that the cause of granulocytopenia is collagen disease, probably SLE, and, less frequently, rheumatoid arthritis (4–6).

Principle

Patient serum containing antinuclear antibodies may react with a variety of nuclear constituents. The antibodies are not species specific so that nuclear material may include rat kidney, human granulocytes, or tumor cells taken from tissue culture. Various indicator systems can be used, but indirect immunofluorescence has 98% sensitivity.

Procedure

The patient's serum is incubated with a source of nuclear antigen. The antibody globulin attaches to the antigen and is detected by antihuman globulin reagent tagged with fluorescein dye. Microscopic evaluation under ultraviolet light causes all positive attachments to glow. Serums can be titered; the normal value is a titer of less than 10.

Specimen

Serum is stored in a refrigerator or frozen.

Interpretation

A titer greater than 80 is consistent with SLE, while a titer of 10–80 may indicate either SLE or rheumatoid arthritis, so that this test result should be followed by testing to detect rheumatoid factor. Tests for antinuclear antibody are more sensitive and specific than LE cell preparations. Screening for anti-DNA antibodies can be performed to assess the disease further.

RHEUMATOID FACTOR (RF)

Purpose

The presence of RF suggests that rheumatoid arthritis is the cause of granulocytopenia (5).

Principle

Rheumatoid factor is IgM antibody against IgG. All tests are based on incubating an indicator particle coated with IgG with the patient's serum. If IgM RF is present, it will agglutinate or clump the indicator. The serum can be titered.

Procedure

Tests for RF include latex particles coated with IgG from rabbits or humans, and the Rose-Waaler test, which uses enzyme-treated sheep red cells tested in parallel with untreated sheep red cells.

Specimen

Serum is used as a specimen.

Interpretation

Significant titers for the latex test for RF are 1:80 or above, while significant titers for the Rose-Waaler test are 1:640. Nonspecific sheep-cell antibodies can be detected and excluded by the parallel testing. False-positive tests correlate with increased fibrinogen levels, and false-negative tests are common in inactive disease.

LEUKOAGGLUTININS

Purpose

Detection of leukoagglutinins implies a direct immune cause for leukopenia (7,8). Positive test results only in the presence of specific drugs imply drug-induced immune neutropenia. The test has low sensitivity and poor correlation, and is available on a research basis only.

Suspensions of test granulocytes are incubated with the patient's serum. Evidence of cytotoxicity or leukoagglutination is determined by a variety of indicator systems including leukoagglutination, complement fixation, indirect immunofluorescence, and vital dye exclusion. No single technique is satisfactory since the antibodies involved may be direct-reacting IgM or indirect IgG and not all are complement binding. The tests can be performed in the presence or absence of specific drugs to attempt to correlate neutropenia with drug-dependent antibody.

Procedure

Fresh granulocytes are separated from whole blood collected in EDTA using Ficoll-isopaque gradient centrifugation. For a wider antigen pool three to five donors should be tested. Cell suspensions are incubated briefly with the patient's serum at room temperature, and reactions are evaluated by agglutination under phase microscopy, indirect immunofluorescence, or trypan blue dye exclusion. In drug studies dilutions of drug (1:10, 1:40, 1:100) and of patient serum are necessary to strike the optimum antigen-antibody concentrations. Supplemental complement may be necessary.

Specimen

Fresh serum is stored frozen to preserve complement. The patient's granulocytes are usually not used since collection of adequate numbers is difficult with neutropenia. For drug studies the patient must be free of all suspect drugs for five days to allow clearing of plasma proteins in order to obtain a baseline.

Interpretation

All results must be 3–4+ since cell damage resulting from the test is a major technical difficulty. Nonspecific aggregation yields false-positive interpretations. Alloantibodies in previously pregnant or previously transfused patients may give agglutination but are not necessarily significant. False-negative reactions are a major problem, and these tests cannot be used to exclude antibody-induced leukopenia.

OTHER USEFUL TESTS

Other tests to study phases of granulocyte production, circulation, and pool sizes are research tools that are not generally available, and their interpretation is not well established. Such tests include measurement of total granulocyte pool by serum vitamin B_{12} binding capacity, granulocyte survival time measured by ^{51}Cr half-life as for red cells, and granulopoiesis measured indirectly by serum lysozyme. In the latter test low levels of lysozyme are difficult to measure, and significantly low levels are not established. The normal fragility of granulocytes further limits all three tests.

FUNCTIONAL DEFECTS OF GRANULOCYTES

Neutrophil function involves chemotaxis, phagocytosis, and bacterial killing. Chemotaxis and phagocytosis are dependent on external factors involving immune (antibody) globulin and complement opsonins, C_{3a}, C_{5a}, and C_{567}. Bacterial killing requires production of hydrogen peroxide intracellularly by anaerobic glycolysis and the hexose monophosphate shunt and utilizes myeloperoxidase of granulocytic primary granules.

Diseases associated with functional defects of granulocytes are summarized in Table 14-9. These diseases are characterized by repeated bacterial or fungal infection beginning early in life or infections with otherwise low-virulence organisms in patients with normal granulocyte counts. Most of these involve inherited disorders of immune globulins, complement, or the hexose monophosphate shunt. Acquired transient defects secondary to drugs are poorly understood. One of the most severe is a heritable defect at multiple functional levels seen in chronic granulomatous disease.

Chronic granulomatous disease (CGD) is generally a sex-linked disorder of granulocyte function in males, and, rarely, an autosomal

Table 14-9. **Summary of Conditions Associated with Functional Defects of Granulocytes**

Extrinsic defects
    Immune globulin opsonin defects
        Agammaglobulinemia, congenital or acquired
        Immune suppression
        Pathologic immunoglobulins (myeloma)
    Complement deficiencies
        C_3
        C_5
    Drugs, toxins
        Adrenocorticoids—inhibit chemotaxis
        Alcohol—inhibits chemotaxis
        Cytotoxic drugs
        Diabetes mellitus—inhibits phagocytosis

Intrinsic defects
    Defective hydrogen peroxide generation
        Chronic granulomatous disease
        Complete G-6-PD deficiency (whites)
    Myeloperoxidase deficiency
    Unknown mechanism
        Chèdiak-Higashi syndrome

recessive disease of females that leads to early death from infection. The PMNs are defective in their bacteriocidal activity for *Staphylococcus aureus*, in activity of the hexose monophosphate shunt, and in production of peroxide after phagocytosis. In some cases CGD has been associated with absence of red cell antigens in the Kell system and with bizarre red cell morphology. With repeated infections granulomas appear in the liver, spleen, lymph nodes, and lungs. Macrophages in these involved organs and in bone marrow contain gold-brown pigment, lipochrome.

Myeloperoxidase deficiency is a rare autosomal recessive disorder of primary granules that results in defective production of myeloperoxidase. Some patients show repeated infections particularly with

Staphylococcus aureus; however, other patients show no increased incidence of infection.

DIAGNOSTIC EVALUATION OF FUNCTIONAL GRANULOCYTIC DEFECTS

Neutrophils function as phagocytes by a complex interaction of immunoglobulins, complement, and neutrophil enzymes. Total evaluation of patients who show an inability to handle infections screens for defects of all phases.

The specific tests of defective granulocyte function as seen in CGD and myeloperoxidase deficiency measure the contribution of peroxidase to phagocytosis by the following tests:

1. The nitroblue tetrazolium (NBT) dye is a test of nonimmune phagocytosis and measures the contribution of peroxidase qualitatively.

2. Myeloperoxidase stain, which identifies the presence of the enzyme in neutrophil cytoplasm, also provides qualitative measurement.

3. Additional tests for CGD include Kell red cell antigen typings, absent in some types of CGD, and G-6-PD screening tests since the hexose monophosphate shunt works poorly in CGD and myeloperoxidase deficiency, as well as in primary enzyme deficiency.

4. Tests of extrinsic factors indirectly involved in granulocyte function are quantitation of immunoglobulins to diagnose agammaglobulinemia and total lytic complement (CH_{50}) as a screening test of complement function. If CH_{50} is decreased specific assays for C_3 and C_5, the chemotactic complement, can be performed.

LABORATORY STUDIES OF FUNCTIONAL GRANULOCYTIC DEFECTS

Hematologic Tests

GENERAL FEATURES

Associated findings in patients with diseases of granulocyte dysfunction are secondary to infection and can include regional lymphadenopathy, fevers, hepatosplenomegaly, and eczematoid or lupuslike skin eruptions.

PERIPHERAL BLOOD

White cell count

The presence of granulocytosis reflects infection. Granulocytopenia is seen in the Chédiak-Higashi syndrome.

Morphology

In some types of CGD marked red cell poikilocytosis is seen, even in asymptomatic patients.

Red cell antigens

Kell blood group antigens (Kell, Cellano, Js^a, Js^b, Kp^a, Kp^b) are absent producing Kell null cells in CGD. The serum may contain antibodies to all Kell antigens, agglutinating all red cells except the patient's own or those of other patients with CGD and defective Kell antigens.

BONE MARROW

Granulocytic hyperplasia in a hypercellular marrow with a left shift reflects infection. Granulomas are seen in marrow clot sections in CGD, and histiocytes with lipochrome pigment may also be seen.

Other Useful Tests

NITROBLUE TETRAZOLIUM (NBT) DYE TEST

Purpose

The NBT test is used to evaluate granulocyte phagocytic function. Results are negative in CGD (6). Originally devised to differentiate bacterial from nonbacterial infections, it is now used most often to measure opsonin ability.

Principle

Unstimulated PMNs do not ingest the dye NBT, but PMNs stimulated in vivo by bacterial infection or in vitro by latex particles or endotoxin do ingest the dye. Once ingested, cell peroxidases reduce the dye to blue crystals (formazan) which can be seen microscopically. This does not occur in CGD.

Procedure

Heparinized blood samples from patients incubated with and without endotoxin for a brief period are added to NBT dye solutions and incubated further. The colorless dye is reduced by peroxidase to blue-black formazan granules in neutrophils and monocytes. Blood smears are prepared from each reaction mixture and stained with Wright's stain. A control sample is treated similarly. One hundred PMNs are counted and the percentage with formazan granules is reported. If untreated smears are negative, the results of the endotoxin-stimulated smear are reported.

Specimen

Fresh heparinized whole blood is used as a specimen. Edetate specimens are not satisfactory since EDTA inactivates C1q, reducing the results of this complement-dependent reaction.

Interpretation

A positive range for the NBT test is 29%–47%, while negative results are less than 10%. The normal unstimulated PMN contains less than 10% formazan crystals. Stimulated PMNs can contain up to 90% formazan granules but usually contain less. Each laboratory determines its own normal range. Negative results on NBT tests are seen in CGD, complement deficiencies, and agammaglobulinemia; stimulation by endotoxin is of no help in these instances. Patients with normal responses may have a negative test even during infection if antibiotic therapy is being given; however, in this case the endotoxin-stimulated NBT test gives positive results. True negatives remain negative. NBT dye reduction is low in patients receiving aspirin, steroids, or phenylbutazone. Negative results should be confirmed by demonstrating leukocyte bactericidal defects.

MYELOPEROXIDASE STAIN

Purpose

Cytochemical staining detects absence of myeloperoxidase in granulocytes (1,3). Active myeloperoxidase implies that opsonin function is intact. Myeloperoxidase deficiency produces a clinical picture similar to that of CGD.

Principle

Peroxidase of granulocytic secondary granules reduces azo dyes producing insoluble complexes at the site of enzyme action.

Procedure

Hydrogen peroxide (H_2O_2) and colorless dye are layered over the peripheral smear. Peroxidase converts H_2O_2 to O_2 and H_2O, which oxidizes the colorless dye such as benzidine to blue-black. A methyl-green or safranin counterstain allows easier identification of granulocytic cell series and monocytes.

Specimen

Freshly prepared blood films are used as a specimen. They should be stained within a few hours since peroxidase is unstable in light. Smears stored in the dark are usable for two to three weeks.

Interpretation

Normally maturing granulocytes are strongly positive. Absent staining is seen in some acute leukemias and in cells with deficient peroxidase. Myeloperoxidase deficiency is a rare defect of bactericidal activity against *Staphylococcus aureus* and *Candida*.

OTHER USEFUL TESTS

Other tests that may be useful include biopsy of lymph nodes for granulomas and lipochrome-pigmented histiocytes in CGD and detection of quantitative immunoglobulins G, A, and M by radial immunodiffusion or antigen-antibody nephelometry to document agammaglobulinemia.

LEUKOCYTIC DISORDERS OF ABNORMAL MORPHOLOGY

A varied class of hereditary disorders of granulocytic morphology is summarized in Table 14-10. In general, the disorders are of nuclear morphology or are characterized by persistence of primary type granules or by abnormal granules. Except for Pelger-Huët anomaly, all are associated with major clinical abnormalities, such as albinism, gargoylism, and, with thrombocytopenic hemorrhage, repeated severe infections and early death.

DIAGNOSTIC EVALUATION OF LEUKOCYTIC DISORDERS

Except in Pelger-Huët anomaly it is unlikely that the hematologic findings will call attention to the disease. Instead, clinical findings of thrombocytopenic hemorrhage and severe or repeated infection in early life warrant close examination of:

1. Peripheral smear for morphologic abnormalities in both the patient and close relatives, for example, siblings, parents, and children.
2. Leukocyte count.
3. Platelet count.

LABORATORY STUDIES OF LEUKOCYTIC DISORDERS

Hematologic Tests

GENERAL FEATURES

Clinical findings vary with the anomaly (see Table 14-10). However, patients with Pelger-Huët anomaly and the majority of those

Table 14-10. Granulocytic Disorders of Abnormal Morphology

Disorder	Morphology	Inheritance	Frequency	Associated Clinical Findings
Pelger-Huët anomaly	Bilobed nuclei in mature PMN	Autosomal dominant	1:6000	None
May-Hegglin anomaly	Leukopenia, Döhle bodies, bizarre platelets	Autosomal dominant?	Rare	Thrombocytopenic bleeding, infection, lymphomas, death in childhood
Alder-Reilly anomaly	Giant granules			Associated with gargoylism
Chédiak-Higashi syndrome	Giant granules in PMNs, red cells, and platelets; leukopenia; occasionally granules in lymphocytes, monocytes	Autosomal recessive		Thrombocytopenic hemorrhage, repeated infection, histiocytes in hepatosplenomegaly, lymph nodes, brain; albinism

with May-Hegglin anomaly are asymptomatic. Thrombocytopenia or functional platelet disorder is common to two anomalies, May-Hegglin and Chédiak-Higashi. The latter may be related to the lipidoses and, as such, may have hepatosplenomegaly with infiltration of these organs by lipoid histiocytes. The Chédiak-Higashi syndrome may show decreased granulopoiesis and shortened survival of granulocytes.

PERIPHERAL BLOOD

White cell count

Values for granulocytes are less than 2500/mm^3 for the Chédiak-Higashi or May-Hegglin anomaly. Giant granules are seen in the Chédiak-Higashi or Alder-Reilly anomaly, Döhle bodies are found with the May-Hegglin anomaly or severe infection, and large azurophilic inclusions in lymphocytes accompany the Chédiak-Higashi anomaly.

Platelet morphology

Platelets are large in the May-Hegglin and Bernard-Soulier anomalies.

BONE MARROW

There are no diagnostic morphologic findings. Lipoid histiocytes may be seen in sections of marrow clot in lipidoses.

REFERENCES

1. Beutler E: Leukocyte alkaline phosphatase. In Williams WJ, Beutler E, Erslev AJ, et al (eds): *Hematology*, ed 2. New York, McGraw-Hill, 1977, pp 1628–1629
2. Bauer JD: Numerical evaluation of red blood cells, white blood cells and platelets. In Frankel S, Reitman S, Sonnenwirth AC (eds): *Gradwohl's Clinical Laboratory Methods and Diagnosis: A Textbook on Laboratory Procedures and Their Interpretation*, ed 7. St. Louis, C. V. Mosby Co, 1970, pp 499–504

261

3. Bauer JD: Staining technics and cytochemistry. In Frankel S, Reitman S, Sonnenwirth AC (eds): *Gradwohl's Clinical Laboratory Methods and Diagnosis: A Textbook on Laboratory Procedures and Their Interpretation*, ed 7. St. Louis, C. V. Mosby Co, 1970, pp 508–509

4. Davidsohn I, Henry JB: *Todd-Sanford Clinical Diagnosis by Laboratory Methods*, ed 15. Philadelphia, W. B. Saunders Co, 1974, pp 1020–1036

5. Adkinson JF Jr: Measurement of total serum immunoglobulin E and allergen-specific immunoglobulin E antibody. In Rose NR, Friedman H (eds): *Manual of Clinical Immunology*. Washington, DC, American Society of Microbiology, 1976, pp 590–599

6. Nakamura RM: Approach to the diagnosis of immune deficiency diseases. In *Immunopathology: Clinical Laboratory Concepts and Methods*. Boston, Little, Brown, 1974, pp 71–74

7. Verheugt FWA, von dem Borne AEG Kr, Prins HD, et al: The detection of granulocyte antibodies in relation to granulocyte transfusion. Exp Hematol 5[suppl]: 151–155, 1977

8. Payne R, Perkins HA, Najarian JS: Compatibility for seven leucocyte antigens in renal homografts: Utilization of a microagglutination test. In *Histocompatibility Testing*. Copenhagen, Munksgaard, 1967, pp 237–245

Reactive Disorders of Lymphocytes and Lymph Nodes

Lymphocytes are derived from stem cells of thymic origin (T cells) or from bone marrow (B cells). T cells are located in the interfollicular and subcapsular areas of lymphoid tissue in lymph nodes, spleen, and gastrointestinal tract. In a complex interdependent relationship with monocytes, they recognize and process foreign antigens. B cells are found in follicles of lymphoid tissues. When processed antigen is presented to B cells in soluble form, they enlarge (blast transformation), with cell division and production of clones of daughter lymphocytes or plasma cells. The latter produce specific antibody to the antigen. Antibody either destroys the antigen by cell or particle lysis or coats it so that phagocytic cells, neutrophils and monocytes, can ingest and destroy the particle. Thus, T cells are the primary agents in cellular immunity, as in skin rashes and skin tests. B cells are involved in humoral, or antibody, immunity since they are directly involved in antibody production. Lymphocytes participating in the recognition process, antibody production, and killing process are permanently committed to respond to the particular antigen on every subsequent exposure but to no other and are therefore said to have "memory." When the antigenic stimulus is removed, the lymphocytes return to a waiting state. These lymphocyte subpopulations are identifiable

263

by markers on the cell membrane, including receptors for complement, Fc fragment, and surface immunoglobulins.

T cells comprise 80%–90% of circulating lymphocytes, B cells only 10%–15%. T cells may survive up to 30 years, B cells for shorter periods of time. Lymphocytosis may be neoplastic and therefore monoclonal in origin with one subpopulation type or reactive with a heterogeneous population of lymphocytes. The spectrum of antigens that may incite the immune sequence of cell division and antibody production are legion. Antigen reactivity may be reflected in peripheral lymphocytosis and antibody production or may be reflected in hyperplasia and enlargement of lymphoid tissue, most often in lymph nodes but occasionally in the spleen.

Lymphocytosis is defined by an absolute increase in lymphocytes above 3000/mm^3; its causes are listed in Table 15-1. Leukocytosis, which is secondary to an absolute lymphocytosis, is seen in pertussis, infectious mononucleosis (IM), infectious lymphocytosis, and lymphocytic leukemia. A relative lymphocytosis without leukocytosis is seen in acute viral exanthems, measles, roseola infantum, and the like. The lymphocytosis seen in postperfusion syndrome is believed to result from acute infection by cytomegalovirus (CMV) transmitted by the lymphocytes of whole blood transfusion. Lymphocyte leukemoid reactions are associated most often with infectious lymphocytosis (40,000–100,000/mm^3) or pertussis (15,000–50,000/mm^3). Infectious lymphocytosis may be caused by adenovirus, enterovirus, or Coxsackie A virus.

The significance of lymphocytosis, and, therefore, the aggressiveness with which it is evaluated, differs with age. Newborns and children less than four years are considered to be "lymphoid organs" and tend to respond to all antigenic stimuli with lymphocytosis. This characteristic fades as the child reaches puberty, at which time reactive lymphocytosis is stimulated by a narrower range of antigens: infectious mononucleosis, respiratory viruses, hepatitis virus, cytomegalovirus, or toxoplasma. Beyond age 30, the range narrows as infectious mononucleosis, respiratory viruses, and toxoplasmosis are less likely to be primary infections, although they still may be suspected.

Table 15-1. Causes of Lymphocytosis

Physiologic—4 months to 4 years

Acute infections
   Infectious mononucleosis
   Infectious lymphocytosis
   Cytomegalovirus infection (including postperfusion syndrome)
   Pertussis
   Brucellosis
   Typhoid—paratyphoid
   Viral exanthems—measles, rubella, varicella, mumps, roseola infantum
   Toxoplasmosis
   Infectious hepatitis
   Mycoplasma pneumoniae

Chronic infection
   Congenital syphilis
   Tertiary syphilis

Endocrine
   Thyrotoxicosis
   Adrenal insufficiency

Neoplasm
   Acute lymphoblastic leukemia
   Chronic lymphocytic leukemia
   Circulating lymphosarcoma cells

Drug sensitivity
   Diphenylhydantoin (Dilantin)
   Para-aminosalicylic acid

DIAGNOSTIC EVALUATION

The urgency of testing and its sequence depends on clinical history, symptoms, and age of the patient. The differential diagnosis of reactive versus pathologic lymphocytosis begins with:

1. Hematologic findings. Examination of the peripheral blood determines the magnitude and duration of the lymphocytosis as well as lymphocyte morphology. Bone marrow aspirate is rarely helpful in reactive processes, but the pattern and extent of infiltration on marrow clot sections or biopsy are helpful in persistent, and therefore possibly pathologic, lymphocytosis.

2. Serologic tests are performed to document the underlying cause if hematologic and clinical findings are of short duration suggesting a reactive process. These tests include screening for heterophile and differential absorption tests for infectious mononucleosis, screening for hepatitis B surface antigen (HB_sAg) if lymphocytosis is associated with elevated liver enzymes, tests for cytomegalovirus, toxoplasma titers, or Epstein-Barr virus (EBV) titer.

3. Biopsy of enlarged lymph nodes is performed if serologic testing is not diagnostic, if lymphadenopathy persists or progresses, and if clinical symptoms such as fever or malaise persist beyond three to six weeks. Lymph nodes are cultured for virus or bacteria and are also examined microscopically.

4. T and B cell classification may be performed in the few cases where the differential diagnosis of reactive versus pathologic lymphocytosis cannot be made. Changes in the normal proportion may indicate an emerging monoclonal process; this aids in prognosis, if not in diagnosis.

LABORATORY STUDIES

Hematologic Tests

GENERAL FEATURES

The significance of lymphocytosis varies with age; in children under four years mature lymphocytosis is more likely to be a physiologic process. Reactive lymphocytosis caused by infection is usually of short duration, three to six weeks, and associated with systemic symptoms, fever, exanthems, pharyngitis, or malaise. Lymphadenopathy is variable but usually involves at least cervical nodes; generalized lymphadenopathy is rare. Splenomegaly is seen more often than hepatomegaly although both may be found in infectious mononucleosis or CMV infection. Reactive lymphocytosis is not associated with anemia but can be associated rarely with thrombocytopenia. Calculation of the absolute lymphocyte count will avoid misinterpreting relative lymphocytosis associated with neutropenia as absolute lymphocytosis.

PERIPHERAL BLOOD

Red cell count

No anemia is present.

White cell count

Normal values are 5000–30,000/mm^3.

Lymphocytes

Greater than 30%, or greater than 3000/mm^3, lymphocytes are present. Normal levels vary with age; at birth, 30% lymphocytes are present; at six months, 60%; at four years, 50%; at six years, 40%; and in adults, 30%.

Platelet count

Platelet count is normal. Rarely, it is less than 100,000/mm^3 with acute viral exanthems.

Morphology

Both T- and B-lymphocytes appear as small, uniform cells with scanty cytoplasm. Antigenically stimulated, B cells are seen on the peripheral smear as large ameboid cells, termed reactive or atypical lymphocytes (Figure 15-1). Atypical lymphocytes comprise more than 20% of the total, most often in infectious mononucleosis, CMV infection, and infectious hepatitis. Lymphocytes in infec-

267

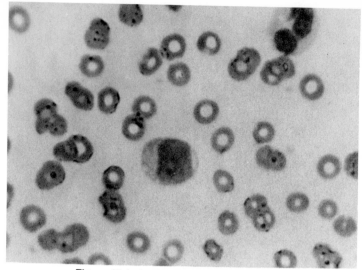

Figure 15-1. Atypical, or reactive, lymphocyte.

tious lymphocytosis generally remain small. Lymphocytes of varied size and shape usually indicate a reactive process, while morphologic monotony suggests pathologic lymphocytosis. Azurophilic granules may be prominent as may cytoplasmic vacuoles, the site of lysosomes dissolved in the staining process.

BONE MARROW

Both aspirated particles and sections of the marrow clot should be examined for distribution of lymphocytes. Bone marrow *biopsy* may be of further help. Lymphocytosis may be diffuse, in small aggregates of 3–10 cells, or in nodules. Lymphoid nodules, which are small and discrete, are usually a reactive phenomenon and are often seen in elderly patients. Rarely, reactive lymphoid nodules may show actual follicle development. Confluence of nodules or many nodules with ill-defined borders suggest a pathologic lymphocytosis. Lymphocytes comprise less than 20% of cells in normal marrows but may appear as sheets if a nodule in a particle has been smeared. Therefore, to avoid distribution errors, more than one slide must be examined.

In hypoplastic marrows, lymphocytes and lymphoid nodules become more prominent, since they and the stromal support cells are the last to disappear. Lymphocytosis is frequently associated with some degree of plasmacytosis. If both lymphocytes and plasma cells are mature, they are considered reactive.

Other Useful Tests

INFECTIOUS SEROLOGY

Purpose

Serologic tests for infectious agents may determine the specific etiology for reactive lymphocytosis, often retrospectively (1).

Principle

After individuals have been exposed to infectious agents, specific antibody titer rises. Antibodies may be IgG, IgM, complement fixing, or precipitating, and they vary with each patient. Rise in antibody titers usually occurs slightly after the onset of lymphocytosis.

Specimen

Acute and convalescent serum is taken 10–14 days apart during the period of lymphocytosis. Specimens can be stored frozen.

Procedure

Testing is usually available at county or state health department laboratories. Complement fixation, hemagglutination inhibition, direct or indirect immunofluorescence, or radioimmunoassay (RIA) are helpful techniques (Table 15-2). Serum is serially diluted for all except RIA procedures.

Interpretation

Many patients have been exposed to specific agents early in life. Therefore, a single titer is not diagnostic. A threefold or fourfold

Table 15-2. Serologic Tests in the Differential Diagnosis of Lymphocytosis

Disease	Diagnostic Test[a]	Significant Result
Infectious mononucleosis	Heterophile by kit or Davidsohn differential	Positive
		Titer ≥ 224 resistant to guinea pig kidney absorption
	Anti-EBV CF	Positive in 20% cases
Hepatitis A (infectious)	RIA test for antibody to Hep. A	
Hepatitis B (serum)	Hb$_s$Ag by RIA	Reactive
CMV	CF	Titer > 256 for acute infection, > 8 for past infection
Toxoplasmosis	IF	Titer > 64
	CF	Titer > 128
Rubella	HI	Titer > 10 for past infection, > 80 for acute infection
Mycoplasma pneumoniae	CF	Titer > 256
	Cold agglutinin titer	> 64

[a]Abbreviations: CF, complement fixation; HI, hemagglutination inhibition; IF, immunofluorescence; RIA, radioimmunoassay.

rise in titer in a 10–14-day span is considered significant, since laboratory dilution carry-over could not account for the change. Low-antibody titers may persist for years in toxoplasmosis, EBV or CMV infection, or in rubella.

For CMV and *Mycoplasma* infection, titers of 256 or higher suggest acute infection. For toxoplasmosis, a titer of 1:8 is seen in most adults; titers above 64 are suspicious for acute infection. Positive immunofluorescence using IgG conjugates may represent maternal antibody until the newborn reaches three months of age. Therefore, positive test results with IgM conjugates are considered more significant but must be correlated with maternal titers.

Hepatitis B is reported as reactive or nonreactive. The presence of Hb_sAg, its core antigen (Hb_cAg), or the DNA polymerase antigen (Hb_cAg) are consistent with current infection, the latter two with high infectivity. Tests for core antigen and DNA polymerase are not available. Tests for *antibody* to core antigen are available. Of the many techniques for Hb_sAg, RIA is the most sensitive. The presence of Hb_s antibody is not clinically significant unless a baseline nonreactive test result is known, since antibody is found in 10% of healthy blood donors and may remain detectable for months or years. Core antibody is consistent with current virus replication in liver cells, as seen in acute or chronic active hepatitis.

Antibodies to EBV are directed at a spectrum of antigens, so that a diagnostic fourfold rise in titer is seen in only 20% of patients with infectious mononucleosis. Anti-EBV is also present in nasopharyngeal cancer and in Burkitt's lymphoma.

T AND B CELL MARKERS OF LYMPHOCYTES

Purpose

Tests for T and B cell markers determine monoclonal populations of lymphocytes, which, therefore, may be neoplastic, not reactive (2).

Table 15-3. Markers for Human Lymphocytes and Monocytes

	B-Lympho-cytes	T-Lympho-cytes	Monocytes
Surface Membrane immunoglobulin (SmIg)	+	−	±
E rosette	−	+	−
EAC[a] (C₃ receptor)	+	−	+
Aggregated-IgG (Fc receptor)	+	−	+

[a]EAC, erythrocyte :: antigen :: complement.

Principle

Each subpopulation of lymphocytes has membrane markers as defined by laboratory techniques (Table 15-3). T-lymphocytes have membrane attachment sites for sheep red cells and will form a rosette with them. B-lymphocytes, which are related to antibody production, have surface immunoglobulins. In addition they have receptors for the Fc fragment of IgG, the basis of rosette formation with antibody-coated sheep cells, and for C_3. In each population of lymphocytes some do not show markers as presently defined and are termed null lymphocytes.

Procedure

Tests for T and B cell markers are not generally available, but some large hospital laboratories and universities have the capability to perform the test.

Specimen

On the day of the test lymphocytes are collected by centrifuge gradient through Ficoll-isopaque from 10–20 ml of the patient's heparinized whole blood. Red cells layer to the bottom and are discarded. The buffy layer is 90% lymphocytes but the interface zone with red cells is contaminated with unwanted granulocytes.

Interpretation

Monoclonal populations of a lymphocyte type may be neoplastic rather than reactive. Some reactive diseases are apparently associated with transient decreases in one subpopulation. Interpretation is still in the early stages.

Notes and precautions

Since all potential membrane receptors have not been defined, the significance of large populations of null cells cannot be assessed.

INFECTIOUS MONONUCLEOSIS

Infectious mononucleosis (IM), a highly specific cause of lymphocytosis, is a febrile illness of low infectious risk that occurs in all age groups but most often in individuals between the ages of 15 and 25 years. It is probably caused by EBV. The disease has an unknown prodromal period of possibly two to three weeks, followed by clinical symptoms of fever, malaise, and pharyngitis. The virus causes proliferation of B cells in lymphoid tissue that leads to lymphadenopathy and lymphocytosis. There is an associated decrease in T cell activity. Thirty percent of patients have splenomegaly and 10% have hepatomegaly. Although hepatomegaly is not common, nearly all patients have hepatitis with elevated liver enzymes. Hematologic findings appear three or four days after symptoms begin but may be delayed for two or three weeks. Serologic findings, which appear with the onset of peripheral atypical lymphocytosis, include (a) antibody to the causative virus, (b) coincidental antibody-agglutinating sheep red cells (the heterophile antibody), (c) antibody to human red cell antigens (anti-i), (d) hemolysins of ox cells, and (e) an increase in IgM (Table 15-4). Documentation of the presence of heterophile antibody is necessary to establish the diagnosis. Serologic findings persist into and beyond the convalescent phase, which may be four to six weeks. The disease may be epidemic, usually in the spring, or cases may be episodic and

Table 15-4. Antibodies in Infectious Mononucleosis

Antibody	Stage of Disease	Diagnostic Test
Heterophile	With lymphocytosis persists 2–3 months	Sheep-cell agglutinins (Davidsohn differential); horse-cell agglutinins (commercial kit tests)
Anti-EBV	Persists for years	Immunofluorescence titer 1:80 or 3-dilution rise; complement fixation
Anti-i	Rare, during acute phase	Direct antiglobulin test, serum antibody screening; cold agglutinin titer
Ox-cell hemolysin	Convalescent phase	Ox-cell hemolysin test > 480; not generally available
IgM	Mid-disease and 2–3 months after	Quantitative immunoglobulins

isolated. Diagnosis may be difficult when the course is primarily febrile (old terminology, typhoidal) unless the diagnostic tests are repeated over several weeks.

DIAGNOSTIC EVALUATION OF INFECTIOUS MONONUCLEOSIS

Evaluation of lymphocytosis should also include evaluation for infectious mononucleosis, particularly when the patient is under 30 years.

1. Hematologic evaluation with attention to blood lymphocytosis and lymphocyte morphology. Bone marrow examination is rarely needed unless serologic tests remain nondiagnostic.
2. A positive test for heterophile antibody is required to diagnose infectious mononucleosis as the cause of the lymphocytosis. This is

usually accomplished by a screening test. If the test is negative in young patients or is positive in a clinical setting inconsistent with infectious mononucleosis, it should be followed by a Davidsohn differential absorption test.

3. The Davidsohn differential absorption test excludes serum sickness or Forssman antibodies from true heterophile and detects low-titer heterophile seen in young children.

4. Specific viral serology for EBV is rarely needed for the diagnosis and does not influence treatment. It is positive in only 10%–20% of patients.

5. Ancillary procedures that indicate the expected rate of recovery include liver function tests.

6. Serologic tests for autoimmune hemolytic anemia are performed if anemia is present. They include a direct antiglobulin test, serum antibody screening, and a test for cold agglutinin titer.

LABORATORY STUDIES OF INFECTIOUS MONONUCLEOSIS

Hematologic Tests

GENERAL FEATURES

At the peak of the disease marked lymphocytosis with hyperplasia of all lymphoid tissue is present. The lymphocytosis may have a delayed appearance of two to three weeks. Nearly all patients have cervical lymphadenopathy with less involvement of other groups, and 30%–50% have splenomegaly. Although splenic rupture occurs it is rarely a cause of death. Anemia is uncommon but autoimmune hemolytic anemia, cold antibody type, appears in 1% of cases. Antibody specificity is often anti-i but anti-I or anti-Pr have also been reported. The anemia appears two to three weeks after onset of the disease and is self-limited. Thrombocytopenia is rare, less than 0.1%, and usually moderate with hemorrhage a very rare event. The cause of the thrombocytopenia may be direct effects of virus, splenomegaly, or specific antibody. Thrombocytopenia responds quickly to steroid therapy.

Blood cell measurements

No anemia is usually present; rarely, hemolytic anemia may occur with hemoglobin level of 9–11 g/dl. Mean corpuscular volume is greater than 105 μ^3 if hemolysis is present, as a result of the increased reticulocyte count.

White cell count is 10,000–20,000/mm^3 with greater than 60% lymphocytes; 10%–20% lymphocytes is atypical. Platelet count is usually normal, although, rarely, it may be 80,000–100,000 mm^3.

Morphology

Lymphocytes have large nuclei that appear folded with copious ameboid dark-blue cytoplasm rich in RNA. Cytoplasm is often vacuolated. Variants of typical Downey cells are plasmacytoid forms; classification as Downey type I, II, or III is of historic interest only. If hemolytic anemia is present spherocytes and nucleated red cells may be seen.

Bone marrow

Bone marrow aspiration is usually unnecessary. Mild hypercellularity may be present due to reactive granulocytic hyperplasia or to mild diffuse lymphocytosis.

Spleen

The spleen is occasionally removed because of rupture. Histology shows lymphoctye infiltration of vascular trabeculae.

Other Useful Tests

HETEROPHILE SCREENING TESTS

Purpose

Results of the heterophile test must be positive and associated with lymphocytosis to make the diagnosis of infectious mononucleosis (3,4).

Table 15-5. Tissues with Heterophile and Forssman Antigens

	IM Heterophile Antigen	Forssman Antigen
Sheep red cell	+	+
Horse red cell	++	0
Ox or beef red cell	+	0
Guinea pig kidney	0	+

Principle

Subsequent to EBV infection and lymphoid hyperplasia, IgM antibodies are produced in the human that cross react with antigens found in tissues of other animal species, and are, therefore, heterophilic. Rise in heterophile antibody parallels atypical lymphocytosis and declines with decrease in lymphocytes. Animal tissues that have heterophile antigen are listed in Table 15-5. Heterophile must be distinguished from other cross-reacting, Forssman-type antibodies by absorption tests using animal tissue rich in Forssman antigens that remove Forssman antibodies and leave heterophile. Sheep red cells are the classic source of heterophile, but it is more strongly represented on horse red cells. Both cell types are used in screening test kits, usually stabilized by tanning to allow longer storage (Table 15-6). Sheep red cell suspensions are available commercially for the more classic Paul-Bunnell test.

Procedure

Commercial test kits for infectious mononucleosis screening are widely available. The Paul-Bunnell test requires refrigeration of sheep red cell suspension and is usually available in most reference laboratories and large hospitals.

Screening tests with commercial kits mix a drop of stabilized cell suspension with the patient's serum or serum dilutions on a slide or card. Agglutination indicates a positive test result. Positive and negative serum controls are provided and are run simultaneously.

Table 15-6. Summary of Serologic Specificity in Tests Used to Diagnose Infectious Mononucleosis

Test	Test Antigen	Differential Absorption	Antibody Specificity[a]
Paul-Bunnell presumptive	2% sheep red cells in saline		IM, FA, SS
Differential absorption	2% sheep red cells in saline	Guinea pig kidney and beef red cell	IM
Monosticon[a]	Sheep red cell extract		IM, FA, SS
Diagluto[b]	Horse red cells	Guinea pig kidney and beef red cells	IM
Hetrol[c]	Stabilized horse red cells		IM
Monospot[d]	Fresh citrated horse red cells	Guinea pig kidney and beef red cells	IM, FA
Mono-Chek[e]	Aldehyde-treated horse red cells	None	IM
Mono-Test[f]	Stabilized horse red cells	None	IM

[a]Abbreviations: *IM,* infectious mononucleosis; *FA,* Forssman antibody; *SS,* serum sickness.
[b]Manufactured by Organon Diagnostic Products, West Orange, NJ.
[c]Manufactured by Beckman Instruments, Inc., Fullerton, CA.
[d]Manufactured by DifCo Laboratories, Detroit, MI.
[e]Manufactured by Ortho Pharmaceutical Corp., Diagnostic Division, Raritan, NJ.
[f]Manufactured by Wampole Laboratories, Cranbury, NJ.

278

The classic Paul-Bunnell anti-sheep cell titer incubates equal volumes of sheep cell suspension and dilutions of the patient's serum for 30 minutes. The test is read for the highest serum dilution showing agglutination.

Specimen

Kit tests use serum or plasma. For the Paul-Bunnell test serum must be complement inactivated at 56 C for 30 minutes since heterophile antibodies are hemolytic.

Interpretation

In Paul-Bunnell tests titers above 224 are presumptive of infectious mononucleosis. Titers of 56–224 indicate probable infectious mononucleosis but should be confirmed by differential absorption. Diagnosis of IM is not supported by titers less than 28.

Positive agglutination using commercial screening kits suggests infectious mononucleosis. Negative agglutination may indicate that the titer is less than 56. The test should be repeated using differential absorption.

Titers for positive agglutination in kit tests are adjusted by formalinization to detect titers of 56 or 112 and above. Fresh horse red cells may detect lower titers. Titers below 56 are frequently found in infectious mononucleosis in children under 12 years, and kit tests may give false-negative results. False-positive results occur in serum sickness, and approximately 5% of sera contain high-titer horse agglutinins unrelated to infectious mononucleosis. False positives are usually excluded by differential absorption tests, since only in infectious mononucleosis are Forssman antigens unable to remove the sheep cell agglutination. Low levels of heterophile persist for months and may be recalled anamnestically with other diseases; therefore, all positive results should be correlated with the characteristic lymphocytosis. Seronegative infectious mononucleosis is uncommon, usually appearing in young children. The diagnosis of seronegative infectious mononucleosis can be substantiated only if EBV antibody titers show a diagnostic rise. If both heterophile and EBV titers are negative, another cause for the lymphocytosis should be found.

DIFFERENTIAL ABSORPTION TESTS

Purpose

Absorption tests differentiate heterophile from Forssman antibody (3).

Principle

Infectious mononucleosis results in the production of many antibodies directed at antigens shared by humans and other species. The classic diagnosis of infectious mononucleosis is defined by the sheep red cell antibody discovered by Paul and Bunnell. The heterophile antigen found on sheep red cells and beef red cells is not found on guinea pig kidney which has Forssman. Absorption with guinea pig kidney of serum that agglutinates sheep cells and beef cells defines the pattern of heterophile.

Procedure

In the Davidsohn differential absorption test, serial dilutions of the patient's serum are incubated with sheep red cells to determine the presumptive titer. Serum aliquots are then absorbed individually with guinea pig kidney or beef cells and retitered against sheep red cells. A three-tube decrease in titer is considered positive absorption. Some kit tests include suspensions of guinea pig kidney or beef cells so that drops of serum can be absorbed with appropriate drops of suspension, and the drop mixtures can then be mixed with stabilized sheep or horse cells to determine patterns of absorption.

Specimen

For the Davidsohn differential absorption test, serum is complement inactivated immediately before testing. For the kit tests serum or plasma may be used without inactivation.

Table 15-7. **Representative Patterns in the Davidsohn Differential Absorption Test**

Type of Antibody	Absorption with Guinea Pig Kidney Antigen	Absorption with Beef Red Cell Antigen
Heterophile antibody in infectious mononucleosis	Not removed or less than 3-tube change in titer	Antibody removed
Forssman antibody (normal serum)	Antibody removed	Antibody not removed or incompletely removed
Forssman antibody (serum sickness)	Antibody removed	Antibody removed

Interpretation

Table 15-7 summarizes the diagnostic patterns. Antibody resistant to absorption by guinea pig kidney is characteristic of heterophile. Negative findings for heterophile suggest that the disease is not infectious mononucleosis. Titers are a technical means to determine three-tube decrease and do not correspond to activity or severity of disease.

ANTI-EBV SEROLOGY

Purpose

Anti-EBV serology is a confirmatory test of infectious mononucleosis to identify recent infection with the causative virus (1).

Principle

Epstein-Barr virus is the presumed cause of infectious mononucleosis. Its presence early in the disease causes an increase in antibody in two to three weeks. Unfortunately, at the time serologic testing is performed, the diagnostic rise in titer has often been missed.

Procedure

The test is usually available at state viral laboratories. Acute and convalescent sera should produce a threefold increase in titer for diagnosis. Serologic techniques used include immunofluorescence and complement fixation.

Specimen

Acute and convalescent sera obtained during the period of lymphocytosis 10 days apart are used as specimens. They should be stored frozen.

Interpretation

A fourfold rise in titer is suggestive of EBV infection and is found in only 10%–20% of patients. Elevated titers may persist for years so that single determinations are not diagnostic. Elevated titers are also seen in viral hepatitis, Burkitt's lymphoma, and paranasal sinus carcinoma. Titers in these diseases may be greater than in infectious mononucleosis.

LIVER FUNCTION TESTS

Purpose

Magnitude of liver enzyme elevation is associated with severity of clinical symptoms, and duration of enzyme elevation correlates with rate of recovery (3) (see also Chapter 16).

Principle

Mild hepatocellular damage presumably secondary to portal triad lymphocytosis is present. Appropriate tests for liver cell dysfunction are serum glutamic-pyruvic transaminase (SGPT), serum glutamic-oxaloacetic transaminase (SGOT), and alkaline phosphatase. Most cases of infectious mononucleosis produce anicteric hepatitis, but bilirubin can be quantitated if jaundice appears.

Procedure

Baseline determinations of SGOT, SGPT, and alkaline phosphatase are made when clinical symptoms suggest infectious mononucleosis since the differential diagnosis is often hepatitis.

Specimen

Serum that is free of hemolysis is used as a specimen since red cells contain glutamic-oxaloacetic transaminase.

Interpretation

Levels of SGOT and SGPT are elevated in 80%–100% of patients and remain so for three to five weeks. Fatigue usually correlates with elevation of enzymes.

LYMPHOPENIA

Lymphopenia may be secondary to abnormalities of lymphocyte production seen in neoplastic disease or immunodeficiency or secondary to lymphocyte mechanical loss or destruction by drugs or radiation (Table 15-8). Lymphopenia can also occur relative to marked granulocytosis. Since 80% of circulating lymphocytes are T cells, disease processes that affect this subpopulation are usually associated with lymphopenia. Similarly, since T cells are mediators of cellular immunity, lymphopenia is often associated with clinical symptoms of a cellular immune deficit, such as skin rashes or eczema, and mucocutaneous candidiasis. Acquired lymphopenia can result from mechanical interference with lymphocyte kinetics and includes disorders of small intestinal lymphatics and the thoracic duct that are often associated with the malabsorption syndrome.

DIAGNOSTIC EVALUATION OF LYMPHOPENIA

Recognition of the most common disorders causing lymphopenia is based on clinical history followed by:

Table 15-8. Causes of Lymphopenia and Diagnostic Methods

Disease	Diagnostic Method
Immunodeficiency syndromes	Quantitative immunoglobulins
Swiss-type agammaglobulinemia	IgG, IgA, and IgM decrease
Agammaglobulinemia with thymoma	IgG, IgA, and IgM decrease
Lymphopenic dysglobulinemia	IgG, IgA decrease; IgM increase
Wiskott-Aldrich syndrome	Platelet count decrease; IgM decrease
Ataxia telangiectasia	IgA decrease; IgE ? decrease
Lymphocyte destruction	
Corticosteroids—Cushings syndrome, iatrogenic	Plasma cortisol
Radiation	History
Alkylating chemotherapy	History
Intestinal lymphocyte loss	
Intestinal lymphangiectasia	Small bowel biopsy; IgA decrease
Whipple's disease	Small bowel biopsy with PAS stain
Right heart failure	EKG, chest x-ray, physical examination
Occlusion of the thoracic duct or intestinal lymphatics	Chest x-ray
Neoplasm	
Hodgkin's disease	Biopsy
Terminal carcinoma	Biopsy
Miscellaneous	
Sarcoid	Angiotensin-converting enzyme; lymph node biopsy
Renal failure	Serum creatinine
Miliary tuberculosis	Chest film; sputum culture
SLE	Antinuclear antibody
Aplastic anemia	Bone marrow biopsy

284

1. Hematologic findings, with attention to leukocyte differential. Bone marrow aspirate differential may lend supportive evidence.
2. Quantitative immunoglobulin determinations, which are needed to classify immunodeficiency syndromes.
3. Ancillary tests that may determine the underlying cause and are easy to perform are those for antinuclear antibodies (in SLE), angiotensin-converting enzyme (in sarcoidosis), and serum creatinine (in renal failure).
4. If cellular immunodeficiency is suspected, skin tests, including mumps antigen, are applied. Biopsy of lymphoid tissue may be necessary.
5. T- and B-lymphocyte studies are less definitive in the previously mentioned syndromes than in malignancy and are not widely available.

LABORATORY STUDIES OF LYMPHOPENIA

Hematologic Tests

GENERAL FEATURES

Lymphocytopenia may be associated with thrombocytopenia or anemia in some immunodeficiency syndromes, in aplastic anemia, after irradiation, or with some drugs. Significant lymphopenia occurs at a higher level in children. Depending on the underlying cause, there may be a paucity of palpable lymphoid tissue, nodes, or spleen. Alternatively, enlargement may occur as in Hodgkin's disease or sarcoid. In the latter hepatomegaly may also be present.

PERIPHERAL BLOOD

Blood cell measurements

The lymphocyte count for adults is less than $1500/mm^3$, or less than 10%, and for children it is less than $3000/mm^3$. Thrombocytopenia in immune deficiency is moderate—$30-50,000/mm^3$. Anemia is mild, normochromic, or absent.

Morphology

No distinguishing morphologic features are present.

BONE MARROW

Cellularity varies with underlying disease. It is hypocellular in aplasia, hypercellular in Hodgkin's disease, and normocellular in most cases of lymphopenia. Normally, 5%–20% of cells are lymphocytes or plasma cells. Under five months of age, lymphocytes may comprise as much as 40% of cells but are normally absent. Persistent absence of both cell lines after six months suggests immunodeficiency. Clot sections or biopsy may be necessary to detect sarcoid granulomas.

Other Useful Tests

QUANTITATION OF IMMUNOGLOBULINS

Purpose

Acquired and hereditary immune deficiency syndromes associated with lymphopenia are often combined with deficient production of immunoglobulins (5,6).

Principle

Lymphopenia is usually caused by T cell deficiency. When a combined deficiency with B-lymphocytes occurs, production of immunoglobulins is altered. This may result in decreases of one or more immunoglobulins and elevations of others. Combined deficiencies occur in hereditary disorders but also in mechanical loss or toxic destruction of the entire lymphocyte pool. Immunoglobulins that are deficient are usually IgG, IgA, and IgM. Immunoglobulin E is rarely involved and the significance of decreased IgD is unknown.

For sections on *Procedure*, *Specimen*, and *Interpretation*, see Chapter 18.

LYMPHADENOPATHY WITHOUT LYMPHOCYTOSIS

Lymphadenopathy results from either neoplastic proliferation of a clone of lymphocytes or reactive hyperplasia of lymphocytes. Metastatic tumors commonly enlarge lymph nodes. The common causes of reactive lymphadenopathy are toxoplasmosis, viral infections (particularly cytomegalovirus), venereal infection (syphilis, chancroid, and lymphogranuloma inguinale), and, less commonly, granulomatous disease (sarcoid, tuberculosis) (Table 15-9). Lymphoid hyperplasia not only involves regional lymph nodes but in some cases involves spleen and liver as well. Metastatic carcinoma usually enlarges a localized group of lymph nodes that drain the primary site.

DIAGNOSTIC EVALUATION OF LYMPHADENOPATHY

The logical sequence of diagnostic evaluation involves noninvasive techniques to document the underlying disease before tissue biopsy is performed. Physical examination determines the extent of lymphadenopathy and includes:

1. Radiography of the chest to document hilar adenopathy of sarcoid, tuberculosis, other fungal infections, or tumor.
2. Serologic tests for infectious agents including RPR, VDRL, or the fluorescent treponemal antibody absorption test (FTA-Abs) to exclude syphilis. Complement fixation tests for toxoplasma and cytomegalovirus are also performed.
3. Skin tests for tuberculosis, coccidioidomycosis, or histoplasmosis are applied, especially if radiographs of the chest are positive.
4. Biopsy of lymph nodes is often necessary to establish lymph node morphology and to document granulomas or tumors. If facilities are available some material should be submitted for electron microscopy, which can often detect occult organisms including viral particles. Persistent, significantly enlarged lymph nodes (≥ 2 cm) in the absence of obvious infection should be biopsied.

Table 15-9. Summary of Causes of Lymphadenopathy without Lymphocytosis

Infections
    Parasitic
        Toxoplasmosis
        Chancroid
        Lymphogranuloma venereum
        Filaria
    Bacterial
        Plague, tularemia
        Mycobacterium tuberculosis, atypical *Mycobacterium*
        Syphilis, congenital or tertiary
    Fungal
        Coccidioidomycosis
        Histoplasmosis
    Viral
        CMV
        IM

Collagen disease
    RA
    SLE

Drugs
    Diphenylhydantoin (Dilantin)
    Para-aminosalicylic acid

Neoplastic
    Lymphoma or leukemia
    Metastatic carcinoma

Other
    Sarcoidosis
    Reactive follicular hyperplasia
    Cat-scratch hyperplasia

5. Bone marrow biopsy and liver biopsy are less helpful in the diagnosis of benign lymphadenopathy.

6. All biopsied material should be cultured for routine bacteria, fungus, and *Mycobacterium tuberculosis*. Cultures of bone marrow are less successful than those of lymph nodes because of the more limited volume of specimen.

7. Ancillary tests include those for angiotensin-converting enzyme in sarcoid and for antinuclear antibodies in collagen disease.

LABORATORY STUDIES FOR LYMPHADENOPATHY

Hematologic Tests

GENERAL FEATURES

Lymphocytosis may be transient in many diseases that cause lymphadenopathy and absent at the time of diagnosis. Therefore hematologic findings may be minimal. Anemia and thrombocytopenia suggest lymphoproliferative malignancy but may be seen in collagen disease. Regional lymphadenopathy may suggest the cause or port of entry of infection: cervical lymphadenopathy—respiratory disease; inguinal—venereal disease; axillary or inguinal—plague or tularemia; or pulmonary hilus—sarcoid. Regional lymphadenopathy draining tumors may suggest the primary site: cervical—nasopharynx, lung, or thyroid; axillary—upper extremity, breast, or rarely, lung; inguinal—lower extremity, anal or perineal area; or pulmonary hilus—lung, or, rarely, upper gastrointestinal tract.

PERIPHERAL BLOOD

Findings are nonspecific. Variable lymphocytosis may be seen in some infectious diseases, neutrophilia in others.

BONE MARROW BIOPSY OR CLOT SECTION

Bone marrow biopsy or clot section occasionally reveals granulomas in sarcoid, disseminated fungal disease, or miliary tuberculosis. Because of limitations of the specimen, culture is rarely rewarding.

Other Useful Tests

SEROLOGIC TESTS FOR INFECTIOUS AGENTS

Purpose

High titers for ubiquitous organisms (e.g., *Toxoplasma*) or titers of unusual organisms (as in coccidioidomycosis) are consistent with the causative agent (1,7).

Principle

Infection with various organisms produces specific antibody, as in toxoplasmosis, or nonspecific yet consistent antibody, such as the reaginic antibodies of syphilis. The presence of antibody may be documented by direct methods using the organism or indirect methods such as complement fixation (Table 15-10).

Specimen

Serum is used as a specimen. In complement fixation tests, specimens from the acute and convalescent phases of disease are required to detect rises in titer.

Procedure

Indirect immunofluorescence techniques are commonly available. They are performed by incubation of serum dilutions with organisms fixed to prepared glass slides. Specific antibody adheres to the organism. Excess serum is rinsed away and anibody is detected by fluorescein-conjugated antiglobulin reagent. Positive reactions fluoresce on a microscope with ultraviolet light source. Complement fixation techniques are available at state or county health laboratories and other regional reference laboratories. These tests rely upon specific antibody (Ab) attaching to antigen (Ag) (*Coccidioides, Histoplasma,* and so forth) with complement binding (Reaction 1). The presence of complement is then determined by lysis of an indicator system, usually a sheep red cell (SRBC) with anti-sheep cell antibody (anti-SRBC) (amboceptor). If complement

Table 15-10. Diagnostic Methods in Reactive Lymphadenopathy

Disease	Serologic Test Technique[a, b]					Skin Tests	Comments
	CF	IF	HA	LA	FLOC		
Infections							
CMV	> 256						
Toxoplasmosis	128						
Tuberculosis						X	
Histoplasmosis	8–16 (yeast)					X	
Coccidioidomycosis	4 recent, > 16 disseminating					X	
Lymphogranuloma venereum						Frei skin test not available	
Syphilis		FTA-Abs reactive			VDRL, RPR reactive		
Plague			256				
Tularemia	40–80						
Collagen disease							
RA				≥ 80			
SLE		≥ 80					
Nonspecific							
Cat-scratch hyperplasia						Cat-scratch antigen unavailable	
Sarcoidosis						Kveim skin test not available	Angiotensin-converting enzyme

[a] Abbreviations: CF, complement fixation; IF, immunofluorescence; LA, latex fixation; HA, hemagglutination; FLOC, flocculation.
[b] Significant titers are recorded under appropriate serologic technique.

291

was not fixed the indicator system hemolyzes (Reaction 2b). If complement fixation has occurred, the indicator system does not hemolyze (Reaction 2a). The amount of sheep-cell antibody and standardization of the initial amount of complement present in the system must be determined on the day of the test. The test itself is an overnight incubation of 4 C for complement fixation, with addition of the indicator system the following morning. The test is read for hemolysis. Serial dilutions of test serum yield titers.

Reaction 1:
Antigen + patient serum Ab + standardized $C' \rightarrow Ag = Ab = C'$
$\searrow C' + Ag + Ab$

Reaction 2a:
$SRBC + \text{anti-SRBC} + (Ag = Ab = C') \rightarrow \text{no hemolysis}$

Reaction 2b:
$SRBC = \text{anti-SRBC} + (C' + Ag + Ab) \rightarrow \text{hemolysis}$

Excess of antigen or antibody may be anticomplementary, invalidating the test. Microtiter techniques are available.

Interpretation

Reaginic tests for syphilis serology such as RPR or VDRL are sensitive screening tests but should be confirmed by the more specific anti-treponemal test, the fluorescent treponemal antibody absorbed test (FTA-Abs). Lymphadenopathy appears in congenital and tertiary syphilis. The FTA-Abs IgM test on newborn infants of seropositive mothers cannot exclude congenital syphilis until the infant is three to six months old, since some babies with congenital infection do not produce IgM antibody until later than normal. In long latency and tertiary syphilis, lipoidal antibodies may fade but FTA-Abs usually persists weakly for 30 or 40 years. Three percent of elderly adults have biologic false-positive serology with these tests, including FTA-Abs.

Direct immunofluorescence or complement fixation tests are of equal sensitivity and specificity and have replaced the Sabin-

Feldman dye test for toxoplasma. The latter test used live and potentially infectious organisms and is not generally available.

Complement fixation titers above 256 are consistent with recent infection by cytomegalovirus. Complement fixation tests are greater than 90% reliable for fungal titers (coccidioidomycosis and histoplasmosis) since they are very sensitive. However specificity is somewhat less since *Histoplasma* yeast antigen may cross react with coccidioidomycosis or other fungal infections. High titers may indicate disseminated disease. Latex agglutination tests are less sensitive and may give false-positive and negative results.

SKIN TESTS

Purpose

Skin tests show strongly positive results in certain fungal diseases with lymphadenopathy, including tuberculosis, histoplasmosis, and coccidioidomycosis (1,6) (Table 15-10). Frei test antigen (lymphogranuloma venereum), Kveim antigen (sarcoidosis), and cat-scratch antigen are no longer available.

Principle

Prolonged stimulation with fungal or tuberculosis organisms provokes a cellular immune response that is recalled when capsular lipid or killed organisms are injected intradermally. T-lymphocytes aggregate at the site of injection, releasing chemotactic factors for monocytes that then release vasoactive amines, producing redness and induration, and, in some cases, necrosis at the injection site. Skin tests become positive 4–12 weeks after infection.

Procedure

Dilute antigen solutions of tuberculin, coccidioidin, and histoplasmin are injected intracutaneously on the forearm. The sites are observed for 48 hours for redness and induration.

Interpretation

Transient redness is not diagnostic. Induration at 48 hours with or without redness is interpreted as positive. Negative tests occur with anergy. Anergy can be excluded if the mumps skin test (to which most adults are sensitive) is positive.

CULTURES

Purpose

Cultures document the specific organism in infectious lymphadenopathy. They are most applicable for bacterial causes.

Principle

Blood cultures are usually not helpful unless obvious systemic symptoms of high fever and leukocytosis are present. Cultures of specific lymph nodes or, if pulmonary infection is visible on x-ray, of sputum is helpful. Bone marrow culture is not usually diagnostic because limited numbers of organisms are expected to be present.

Procedure

Blood or tissue is inoculated on specific media for bacteria, including *Yersinia-Pasteurella*, Sabourauds's agar for fungus, and Löwenstein-Jensen or Middlebrook 7H10 culture medium or the equivalent for tuberculosis.

Interpretation

If the lymph node contains organisms known to cause lymphadenopathy, the culture is diagnostic. Pyogenic organisms such as *Staphylococcus* and *Streptococcus* are probably contaminants from skin in systemic lymphadenopathy.

RADIOGRAPHY OF THE CHEST

Purpose

Radiography of the chest helps to detect pulmonary hilar lymph nodes.

Procedure

An anteroposterior and lateral chest x-ray are taken.

Interpretation

With sarcoid, a butterfly hilus is seen. With fungal infections, diffuse fibrosis to cavitary single lesions is found.

BIOPSY OF THE LYMPH NODE

Purpose

Biopsy of the lymph node provides specific diagnosis and tissue for culture.

Principle

Easily accessible enlarged lymph nodes, preferably not from inguinal areas, are biopsied. In venereal disease, however, inguinal lymph nodes may be the only enlarged group.

Procedure

Biopsy and culture are taken.

Interpretation

The presence of follicles, acute inflammatory cells, or follicular necrosis suggests a reactive origin. Granulomas, if present, may be epithelioid (in sarcoid and other diseases) or caseating (in tuberculosis, fungus). Eosinophils suggest cat-scratch hyperplasia or toxoplasmosis. Geographic necrosis of previous hyperplastic follicles is seen in toxoplasmosis, fungi, and chancroid. Increased plasma cells as a component of lymphadenitis suggest venereal origin, especially syphilis. Silver stains may reveal spirochetes. Tumors metastatic to lymph nodes from previously unsuspected malignancy may suggest the primary tumor by their histology (i.e., adenocarcinoma versus squamous carcinoma versus melanoma).

295

ANGIOTENSIN-CONVERTING ENZYME (ACE)

Purpose

Angiotensin-converting enzyme test is often positive with pulmonary sarcoidosis, correlating with severity of disease and steroid response (8).

Principle

Angiotensin-converting enzyme is a glycoprotein present at the surface of capillary endothelial cells. It cleaves peptide substrates, including the decapeptide angiotensin I, converting it to angiotensin II.

$$\text{Angiotensin I} \xrightarrow{\text{angiotensin-converting enzyme}} \text{angiotensin II} + \text{L-histidyl-L-leucine}$$

Angiotensin-converting enzyme is important in the renin-angiotensin system. The enzyme is elevated in many sera and particularly in granulomatous lymph nodes of sarcoidosis. It is also elevated in serum and spleen in Gaucher's disease and in neonatal idiopathic respiratory distress syndrome. It is believed that the sarcoid granulomas secrete the enzyme increasing its serum as well as tissue levels.

Procedure

Assay techniques include biologic, spectrophotometric, and spectrofluorometric assays so that an artificial substrate must be substituted. The ultraviolet spectrophotometric method of Cushman and Cheung[9] uses hippuryl-L-histadyl-L-leucine (HHL) as substrate, measuring free hippuric acid released by the enzyme ACE. Hippuric acid is extracted with ethyl acetate from the reaction mixture and quantitated as a measure of enzyme activity. One unit ACE is defined as nanomoles (nmole) hippuric acid released per minute at 37 C under standard assay conditions. Normal values may vary by age and sex but in active sarcoidosis these differences are no longer significant.

Specimen

Serum is used as a specimen. The enzyme is metallodependent so that plasma obtained from EDTA-anticoagulated specimens cannot be used since calcium would be chelated.

Interpretation

Up to 30 units of ACE are considered normal, 30–35 units are suspicious for sarcoidosis, and 35 units or higher are positive. In active sarcoidosis sex and age variables are not critical. Values are increased in 60% of cases of active sarcoidosis. They decrease to normal in chronic disease and after steroid therapy.

REFERENCES

1. Kaufman, L: Serodiagnosis of Fungal Diseases. In Rose NR, Friedman H (eds): *Manual of Clinical Immunology.* Washington, DC, American Society of Microbiology, 1976, p 363–382

2. Hong R: Immunodeficiency. In Rose NR, Friedman H (eds): *Manual of Clinical Immunology.* Washington, DC, American Society of Microbiology, 1976, pp 620–637

3. Davidsohn I, Henry JB: *Todd-Sanford Clinical Diagnosis by Laboratory Methods* ed 15. Philadelphia, W. B. Saunders Co, 1974, pp 261–265

4. Bauer JD: White blood cell pathology. In Frankel S, Reitman S, Sonnenwirth AC (eds): *Gradwohl's Clinical Laboratory Methods and Diagnosis: A Textbook on Laboratory Procedures and Their Interpretation,* ed 7. St. Louis, C. V. Mosby Co, 1970, pp 646–647.

5. Davis NC, Ho M: Quantitation of immunoglobulins. In Rose NR, Friedman H (eds): *Manual of Clinical Immunology.* Washington, DC, American Society of Microbiology, 1976, pp 4–17

6. Nakamura RM: Approach to the diagnosis of immune deficiency diseases. In *Immunopathology: Clinical Laboratory Concepts and Methods.* Boston, Little, Brown, 1974, pp 63–71

7. *Manual of Tests for Syphilis 1969,* Public Health Service Publication no. 411. Washington, DC, US Government Printing Office, 1969

8. Lieberman J: Elevation of serum angiotensin-converting enzyme (ACE) level in sarcoidosis. Am J Med 59:365–372, 1975

9. Cushman DW, Cheung HS: Spectrophotometric assay and properties of the angiotensin-converting enzyme of the rabbit lung. Biochem Pharmacol 20:1637–1698, 1971

chapter 16

Disorders Involving the Spleen: Hypersplenism

Hypersplenism is defined as a reduction in one or more' cellular elements in the peripheral blood associated with splenomegaly and corrected by splenectomy. The spleen is a 150-g vascular organ composed of red pulp and lymphoid tissue or white pulp. The red pulp is a system of sinusoidal blood spaces lined by a fenestrated basement membrane separated by cords of reticuloendothelial cells and monocytes. The lymphoid tissue is found as perivascular sheaths and lymphoid follicles. Blood percolates through the sinusoids into the splenic cords to return through splenic veins to the peripheral circulation. The major functions of the spleen are phagocytosis of damaged red cells, releasing and recycling hemoglobin-bound iron, and reticuloendothelial macrophage ingestion and lymphocyte recognition of antigen, with subsequent production of antibodies. The normally sluggish flow through the 3-μ sinusoid fenestrations to the splenic cords requires red and white cells that are properly deformable if they are to make the transit through the spleen. Thus, abnormal red cells such as spherocytes or target cells become trapped in splenic sinusoids. Increase in the size of the spleen slows the transit time for hematopoietic elements effectively decreasing their presence peripherally. Even without splenic enlargement, increased activity of phagocytic cells decreases the survival of blood elements. The mechanism for the increase in splenic size varies with the disease (Table 16-1).

Table 16-1. **Mechanisms of Splenic Enlargement and Hypersplenism**

Etiology	Mechanism	Disease
Functional	RE hyperplasia or hyperfunction	Hemolytic anemias 　Immune 　Thalassemia major 　Enzyme defects 　Hereditary sphero- 　　cytosis 　PA Infection 　Bacterial endo- 　　carditis 　Malaria 　IM 　Infectious hepa- 　　titis 　Miliary tuberculosis Collagen disease 　Felty's syndrome (RA)
Vascular	Portal hypertension	Cirrhosis, liver 　Portal vein thrombosis
Hematopoietic	Extramedullary hematopoiesis	Myelofibrosis
Metabolic	Macrophage storage of abnormal meta-bolite	Gaucher's disease Niemann-Pick disease Hemochromatosis
Neoplasm	Malignant prolif-erations	Chronic leukemias Lymphomas

DIAGNOSTIC EVALUATION

The diagnosis of hypersplenism is based on "full marrow, empty blood," so that

1. Hematologic findings should show a decrease in one or more cell lines in peripheral blood associated with normal or increased production in bone marrow.
2. Splenomegaly is usually determined by physical examination, but in the obese patient it may be confirmed by radioactive scans of spleen and/or liver using ^{99m}technetium (Tc).
3. Radioactive studies with ^{51}chromium determine sites of red cell sequestration and are used if the diagnosis of hypersplenism is in doubt or splenectomy is being considered.
4. Diagnosis of the underlying cause may require liver function tests or splenic portography in cirrhosis, blood cultures to diagnose SBE, or heterophile tests for infectious mononucleosis. Splenic puncture is discouraged because its risk is high and its diagnostic yield low.

LABORATORY STUDIES

Hematologic Tests

GENERAL FEATURES

In most patients splenomegaly of varying degree is present, although hypersplenism can result from an overactive reticuloendothelial system with minimal enlargement of the spleen. Early in the course of liver disease, hepatomegaly may be present but with advancing cirrhosis the liver may decrease in size. Lymphadenopathy may be present in lymphocytic neoplasms. Jaundice may be secondary to hereditary spherocytosis, malaria, pernicious anemia, or advanced cirrhosis, but it is not a primary symptom of hypersplenism. In the syndrome of "full marrow, empty blood," cellular elements are generally sequestered in the following order: red cells, then platelets, then white cells.

PERIPHERAL BLOOD

Blood cell count

Modest decreases in platelet count ($100,000/mm^3$) to moderately severe decreases ($30,000/mm^3$) are seen. Normochromic anemia may be present, with levels of hemoglobin at 9.0–11.0 g/dl. Leukocytes are decreased with a normal differential, $4500/mm^3$.

Morphology

Smear morphology varies with the following underlying causes:

1. Spherocytes seen in hereditary spherocytosis.
2. Target cells in liver disease (congestive splenomegaly).
3. Tear drop and hand mirror cells—myelofibrosis.
4. Leukoerythroblastosis—nucleated red cells and immature granulocytes, seen in extramedullary hematopoiesis of myelofibrosis.
5. Atypical lymphocytes in chronic infections or infectious mononucleosis.

BONE MARROW

Bone marrow aspiration shows normal to moderate hypercellularity (80%) with all cell lines increased and maturing normally.

Other Useful Tests

TESTS WITH [51]CHROMIUM LABELED RED CELLS

Purpose

Tests with ^{51}Cr-labeled red cells measure red cell survival and splenic uptake of radioactive label (1,2).

Principle

[51]Chromium, a gamma-emitting nuclide with a half-life of 21–26 days, can be used to label red cells or platelets. Increased splenic size leads to increased blood flow and to increased sequestration of red cells. As labeled red cells are trapped or break down, ^{51}Cr is

released at the site of cell sequestration, as detected by external monitoring. Increased splenic sequestration of labeled red cells in the absence of antibody implies hypersplenism. Frequent sampling and gamma counting of the peripheral blood determines the half-life of red cells, which is decreased in hemolysis and in hypersplenism. Radioactive uptake by the spleen is compared to a baseline (precordium) and to the liver to establish ratios of ^{51}Cr uptake. Splenic size can be estimated by radio scan using 1–2 mCi ^{99m}Tc, a nuclear medicine procedure requiring only one or two minutes.

Procedure

Performed in a nuclear medicine facility, tests with ^{51}Cr labeled red cells require three weeks for the complete study. If hemolysis is present, the study may be completed sooner. A sample of the patient's own red cells is withdrawn, labeled with 100 mCi ^{51}Cr, and reinjected. Serial 3-ml aliquots of blood are drawn over a period of 21–26 days to determine the cell half-life. Precordium, spleen, and liver are counted for one to three minutes every two days for three weeks to determine sites and rate of uptake. Radioactive counts are plotted against time. Ratios of radioactivity between liver and spleen are calculated for selected points during the three-week period. Suspensions of donor platelets can be labeled similarly and platelet half-life studied. Leukocyte sequestration studies have not been established and are not commonly available.

Specimen

Small, equal volume (3 ml) aliquots of heparinized blood should be refrigerated and counted simultaneously to minimize specimen variability. Specimens can be counted as whole blood or as red cells, excluding counts leaching into plasma as the result of mechanical hemolysis.

Interpretation

Normal red cell half-life is 26 days. Normal spleen/liver ratio is 1.0. Hypersplenism spleen/liver ratio is 1.5–2.0 and hemolysis spleen/liver ratio is above 3.0.

Normal splenic uptake shows a steady decrease in precordium and peripheral blood radioactivity, with steady, slow increase in speen and liver (reticuloendothelial) counts. In splenic enlargement caused by hypersplenism, peripheral blood radioactivity declines linearly paralleled by decreasing counts in the heart and liver. Since splenic blood flow is increased, counts increase rapidly proportionate to its size and remain constant thereafter, reflecting circulating intact red cells, rather than accumulations seen with red cell degradation as in hemolysis. If radiolabeled donor red cells rather than autologous red cells are used, they must be compatible, since antibody will lead to splenic sequestration and a false interpretation of hypersplenism.

Notes and precautions

The patient's blood volume must remain constant without blood loss or transfusion during the 21–26 days of the test. Other gamma-emitting radioisotopes as used in lung, liver, or spleen scans must be avoided during the three weeks of the test. If platelet concentrates are labeled, they should be relatively free of erythrocytes, which are preferentially labeled.

MYELOFIBROSIS

Myelofibrosis, one of the myeloproliferative disorders, is caused by proliferation of reticulum fibers that efface the marrow gradually obliterating cell production. The fibrosis is associated with extramedullary hematopoiesis in liver and spleen (myeloid metaplasia), which enlarges both. Massive splenomegaly is common; hepatomegaly is seen in 75% of patients. The extramedullary hematopoiesis may be compensatory to the profound pancytopenia but is more likely neoplastic itself. Lymphadenopathy is uncommon. Myelofibrosis is frequently associated with focal osteosclerosis particularly of pelvic bones. The differential diagnosis is most often to distinguish it from CGL. Myelofibrosis may be the terminal event in polycythemia vera or may itself end in acute myelogenous leukemia.

LABORATORY STUDIES OF MYELOFIBROSIS

Hematologic Tests

PERIPHERAL BLOOD

Pancytopenia, leukoerythroblastosis, and poikilocytosis are present.

Blood cell count

Range for hemoglobin is 3–10 g/dl. Anemia is often severe and normocytic but may be mildly macrocytic because of reticulocytosis.

In early stages of disease white cells are 10,000–20,000/mm³ up to 50,000/mm³. In late stages the white cell count is less than 2000/mm³, with marked shift left including progranulocytes and occasional blasts. The platelet count is less than 60,000/mm³ and giant platelets or megakaryocyte fragments are present. Thrombocytosis is present in early stages in some patients. The reticulocyte count is usually elevated, 2%–6% from extramedullary sources.

Morphology

Red cell poikilocytosis is marked. Hand mirror or tear drop forms are said to be diagnostic. Polychromasia is marked, with many nucleated red cells and immature granulocytes (leukoerythroblastosis). Macrocytosis may be present probably representing the reticulocytes.

BONE MARROW

Dry aspirates are common. Biopsy shows variable fibrosis beginning in peritrabecular areas, with prominent clusters of megakaryocytes and residual islands of erythroid hyperplasia. More than one area should be biopsied to avoid sampling error if the diagnosis is in doubt. If particles can be aspirated they are hypercellular. Silver stains show increase in interlacing bands of reticulum fibers.

SPLENIC PUNCTURE

Splenic puncture is discouraged.

Other Useful Tests

Liver biopsy, less hazardous than splenic puncture, may also show extramedullary hematopoiesis. ^{59}Iron uptake studies may provide little additional information but measure marrow uptake of administered dose of ^{59}Fe and identify other sites of red cell production over a three- to four-week period. In myelofibrosis this study is frequently performed before splenectomy is considered as a remedy for hypersplenism.

Other tests for increased leukocyte breakdown or turnover support the diagnosis of CGL or myeloproliferative syndrome. If normal, they support the diagnosis of myelofibrosis. Tests include those for serum uric acid (increased in leukemia and myelofibrosis), leukocyte alkaline phospatase (low in CGL), and Ph^1 chromosome, in marrow karyotype (not seen in myelofibrosis).

LIVER DISEASE WITH PORTAL HYPERTENSION

Hepatic cirrhosis, whatever the etiology, has intrahepatic fibrosis with narrowing of the portal vasculature. It is one of the commonest causes of splenomegaly. The increased portal pressure is transmitted via the portal and splenic veins to the spleen, which gradually enlarges. Ultimately, fibrosis of the splenic red pulp results. Sequestration of red cells, leukocytes, and platelets occurs in the enlarged spleen. Increased pressure in the portal system is also transmitted to gastric and esophageal veins, which may bleed chronically or produce a major hemorrhage.

LABORATORY STUDIES OF LIVER DISEASE WITH PORTAL HYPERTENSION

Hematologic Tests

PERIPHERAL BLOOD

Blood cell counts

Anemia is variable; it is macrocytic if associated with B_{12}-folate deficiency and hypochromic if associated with repeated bleeding. White cell count is mildly decreased with hypersplenism (less than or equal to 3000/mm^3). Platelets are moderately decreased (50–60,000/mm^3).

Morphology

Morphology is variable with target cells seen in hyperbilirubinemia or cirrhosis, burr cells in upper gastrointestinal bleeding, microspherocytes and acanthocytes in abnormal cholesterol exchange with red cell membrane, and cell fragments in hemolysis or severe iron deficiency. Nucleated red cells are very uncommon in splenomegaly resulting from portal hypertension, and therefore some other etiology should be considered.

BONE MARROW

Bone marrow is hypercellular, with normoblastic erythroid hyperplasia of regenerative anemia. Decreased iron results from chronic blood loss.

Other Useful Tests

LIVER FUNCTION TESTS

Purpose

Abnormal liver function supports the diagnosis of cirrhosis as an underlying cause of splenomegaly (3) (see also Chapter 15).

Principle

The most useful tests, listed in Table 16-2, are serum alkaline phosphatase, which is excreted via the intrahepatic biliary tracts; SGPT, in high concentration in liver cells; and bilirubin conjugated by liver cells and excreted via intrahepatic ducts to the major extrahepatic ducts. Intermittent cell destruction by fatty change releases hepatic cell transaminases and causes transient mild hyperbilirubinemia. Cirrhosis causes fibrosis of intrahepatic ducts leading to alkaline phosphatase elevation. Bromsulphalein (BSP) retention tests using an allergenic dye have been supplanted by more modern enzyme tests.

Procedure

Most tests for liver enzymes use kinetic techniques that measure two or three changes in oxidative color development of molybdenum dyes during the following prototype reactions:

1. $A + B \xrightarrow{\text{patient serum enzyme}} P + Q + (H^+)$
   (A, B, P, Q, R = substrates)

2. $NADH + Q \xrightarrow{(H+)\ \text{enzyme Z}} NAD + R$
   (NAD, NADH, enzyme Z = added reagents)

3. $\text{molybdenum} \xrightarrow{\quad NADH \quad} \text{molybdenum}$
   (blue)   (colorless)

Because the substrates vary with each test and each test modification, they are converted to international units (IU) for uniformity.

Specimen

Serum should be separated from red cells promptly since red cells contain transaminases. Sera are stable and can be refrigerated or frozen.

Interpretation

Interpretation is summarized in Table 16-2.

Table 16-2. **Liver Function Tests in Portal Hypertension**

Test	Normal Range	Etiology of Change	Comment
Alkaline phosphatase	24–70 IU/l	Intrahepatic fibrosis	Increased in 40% of Laennec's cirrhosis and 100% of biliary cirrhosis; only abnormality in asymptomatic cirrhosis
SGPT	M:1–21 IU/l F:0–16 IU/l	Focal recurring cell destruction	Episodic elevation
Bilirubin	0.5–1.5 mg/dl	Intrahepatic fibrosis	Episodic elevation

LIVER BIOPSY

Liver biopsy is used to document cirrhosis, an indirect diagnosis of hypersplenism, or to detect extramedullary hematopoiesis. It is a somewhat safer procedure than splenic puncture, but postbiopsy hospital observation for hemorrhage is mandatory.

SPLENIC PORTOGRAPHY

Purpose

Splenic portography is a highly specialized procedure performed in radiology departments to evaluate abnormal hemodynamics in portal hypertension and demonstrate esophageal varices (4). The test is useful in childhood splenomegaly to demonstrate occult cirrhosis.

Principle

The splenoportal venous system can be evaluated by injections of dye percutaneously into the liver or spleen or under direct vision at laparotomy. The pressure of dye injection is then dissipated throughout the system. In some cases, this pressure is sufficient to disrupt the system leading to negative results on studies despite the presence of disease. Percutaneous splenic portography is the benchmark procedure; direct angiography is used less often. The needle is introduced into the splenic pulp for injection of dye. The spleen cushions the transmitted pressure, permitting reasonably accurate determinations of pressure and visualization of intra- and extrahepatic obstruction of the splenic-portal system; retrograde flow of blood away from the liver via collaterals is consistent with portal hypertension. The splenic portagram is helpful in determining surgical procedure for shunt.

Procedure

With the patient flat on his or her back, the position of the splenic hilum is marked in midexpiration in the midaxillary line using x-ray visualization or image intensification. This position is usually at the ninth intercostal space. The needle is inserted percutaneously using local anesthesia. Portal pressure is measured with a water manometer or strain gauge. A 10-cm, 18-gauge spinal needle is used for the puncture and dye injection while the patient is cautioned to hold his or her breath. No more than three punctures should be attempted and repeat studies should not be performed on the same day. Diatrizoate meglumine (Hypaque), 40–45ml, is injected and serial x-ray exposures are obtained. Vital signs and serial hematocrit determinations are monitored at frequent intervals for the remainder of the day.

Interpretation

Normal visualization reveals the splenic pulp, splenic hilar veins, splenic vein, and the portal vein with its intrahepatic branches. Venous radicles that drain to the splenic and portal systems (i.e., inferior and superior mesenteric veins, short gastric veins, and pancreatic and hepatic coronary veins and their collaterals) should not be seen under normal pressure. Errors in interpretation result from (a) extravasation of dye through the splenic capsule, (b) a larger collateral system than the dye bolus can demonstrate such that only some of the collaterals will be demonstrated and not the portal system, or (c) too few films so that collaterals are not seen as they fill. Normal results on splenoportography do not rule out cirrhosis.

REFERENCES

1. Kniseley RM, Korst DR, Nelp WB, et al: The blood. In Wagner NH Jr (ed): *Principles of Nuclear Medicine*. Philadelphia, W.B. Saunders Co, 1969, pp 439–442

2. International Committee for Standardization in Hematology: Recommended methods for radioisotopic erythrocyte survival studies. Am J Clin Pathol 58:71–80, 1972

3. Zimmerman HJ: Tests of Hepatic Function. In Davidsohn I, Henry JB (eds): *Todd-Sanford Clinical Laboratory Diagnosis by Laboratory Methods*, ed 15. Philadelphia, W.B. Saunders Co, 1974, pp 804–805

4. Rousselot LM, Burchell AR: Splenic and arterial portography and hemodynamics in portal hypertension. In Schiff L (ed): *Diseases of the Liver*, ed 4. Philadelphia, J.B. Lippincott Co, 1975, pp 370–373

chapter 17

Acute Leukemia

Acute Leukemia Leukemia is a neoplastic disorder of the hematopoietic system, characterized by an unregulated accumulation or proliferation in the bone marrow of a member(s) of the leukocyte series. The leukemic cells eventually replace the normal marrow elements. In addition to being involved in the bone marrow, the leukemic cells also proliferate in the lymph nodes, spleen, and liver and may be found in many other organs, including meninges, ovaries, testes, skin, gastrointestinal tract, and kidneys.

Acute leukemia is defined as a leukemia that if left untreated runs a rapidly fatal course with an expected life span of less than six months. The leukemic infiltrate consists predominantly of very immature cells, blasts, and closely related cells such as promyelocytes and prolymphocytes. In most patients, the peripheral blood and bone marrow have more than 30% blasts.

Subleukemic leukemia refers to a leukemia in which the total number of white cells in the blood is not elevated but in which immature cells (blasts) are present. The term aleukemic leukemia is used when no abnormal cells are found in the blood. The diagnosis of leukemia, in both instances, is made by examination of the bone marrow. More than 30% blasts usually indicate leukemia.

Classification of acute leukemia is based mainly on morphologic observation of the leukemic cells as seen in Romanovsky-stained smears of blood and bone marrow (Table 17-1). Since treatment is different, every effort, including consultation, should be made to differentiate lymphoid from nonlymphoid leukemia. A variety of

Table 17-1. **Clinical Features of Acute Leukemia**

Clinical Features	Laboratory Abnormalities
Weakness and pallor	Anemia
Bleeding or bruising	Thrombocytopenia, occasionally DIC
Fever, infections	Granulocytopenia, immunosuppression
Bone or joint pain	Leukemic infiltrates
Neurologic symptoms (headache, vomiting, etc.)	Leukemic cells in CSF
Lymphadenopathy	Leukemic infiltrates
Hepatosplenomegaly	Leukemic infiltrates

cytochemical stains may be necessary for subclassification, and, more recently, cell surface markers have been shown to be useful in acute lymphoblastic leukemia.

The etiology of human leukemias is still unknown, and it is evident that multiple pathogenetic factors may be responsible. Some of these factors are viruses, radiation, chemical agents, chromosomal and genetic factors, and abnormal immunologic function. In addition, certain acquired hematologic disorders are associated with increased frequency of acute leukemia. These include myeloproliferative disorders, PNH, sideroblastic anemia, and aplastic anemia.

The overall incidence of acute leukemia in the United States averages 3.5 per 100,000 inhabitants. It is the most common malignant disease of childhood. In children, acute leukemia is usually of the lymphoblastic type, while in adults, acute myeloblastic leukemia is the most common type of acute leukemia.

All forms of acute leukemia are associated with abnormal and usually decreased production of normal granulocytes, erythrocytes, and platelets. The mechanism that leads to failure of normal hematopoiesis is uncertain, but ineffective hematopoiesis is usually present before the number of blast cells in the bone marrow is increased significantly. The deficiency of normal hematopoiesis gives rise to the most serious complications of acute leukemia such as anemia, hemorrhage, and infections.

The presenting clinical features of acute leukemia as related to pathophysiology are summarized in Table 17-1. These clinical manifestations arise mainly from anemia, granulocytopenia, and thrombocytopenia, and to a lesser extent from the proliferation and infiltration of leukemic cells in bone marrow, lymph nodes, spleen, meninges, and other organs.

DIAGNOSTIC EVALUATION

After a clinical history and physical examination have been completed, the laboratory diagnosis of acute leukemia proceeds in the following sequence:

1. Hematologic evaluation.
    a. Complete blood count (CBC) including white cell count and platelet count and review of peripheral blood smear. It is essential to have a technically well-prepared smear. The slide should be reviewed by the patient's physician. The smear should be reviewed for abnormal cells, number of immature and mature cells, and red cell morphology, and an estimate of platelet count should be made. The latter is important as a control measure of the platelet count.
    b. Bone marrow study. The site from which bone marrow is obtained is not usually important since leukemia is a diffuse disease. It may be easier to obtain marrow particles from the sternum, but for safety and the advantage of being able to take a biopsy, the posterior iliac crest is recommended. Multiple smears should be made. One is stained with a Romanovsky-type stain and the rest should be left unstained for special cytochemical procedures. If uncertain about type of fixation to use for special stains, it is best to leave slides unfixed. Not infrequently, the bone marrow aspirate results in a dry tap in patients with leukemia. A bone marrow biopsy should then be performed. This specimen is very useful for evaluation of cellularity, but cytologic detail is not as clear as with smears of aspirated marrow. It is, therefore, essential that imprints be made of the

Table 17-2. Methods for Characterizing Leukemic Cells

Morphology
Cytochemistry
Surface markers
Biochemistry—terminal transferase, lysozyme
Electron microscopy
Cytogenetics

biopsy by touching the biopsy specimen gently on several glass slides. The latter should then be stained with a Romanovsky-type stain and other stains as necessary. Ideally, bone marrow aspirate smears, histologic preparation of aspirate (clot section), and a biopsy with imprints should be available for the initial evaluation of a patient suspected of having leukemia. Repeat bone marrow examination is performed during treatment to evaluate the efficacy of chemotherapy.

2. Studies to delineate the type of acute leukemia to gauge prognosis and therapy include cytochemical stains, tests for serum and urine lysozyme, and the more recently available test for leukocyte terminal deoxynucleotidyl transferase. Other special procedures generally available at some centers include immunologic characterization of leukemic cells, cytogenetic studies, and electron microscopy (Table 17-2).

3. Examination of cerebrospinal fluid for the presence of leukemic cells.

4. Ancillary studies to determine the extent of leukemia and to disclose the presence of complications. These include microbiologic evaluation for fever, chest x-ray and other radiologic studies, blood chemistries, coagulation tests, and, when indicated, tissue biopsy.

LABORATORY STUDIES

Hematologic Tests

GENERAL FEATURES

The initial laboratory findings that suggest acute leukemia are anemia, thrombocytopenia, neutropenia, and immature white cells

314

in the peripheral blood (Table 17-3). The anemia is usually normo-chromic normocytic and sometimes macrocytic. It is progressive and may become severe. The platelet count is usually decreased at clinical onset, and associated skin and mucous membrane hemor-rhages (petechiae) are common. The thrombocytopenia usually be-comes progressively severe. The white cell count may be normal, decreased, or increased, and the number of immature cells varies from an occasional blast cell to 100% blast cells.

PERIPHERAL BLOOD

Review of blood smear usually reveals neutropenia. The white cell count may be normal, low, or high. When high, the differen-tial count reveals a preponderance of blasts—myeloblasts in acute myeloblastic leukemia (AML) and lymphoblasts in acute lympho-blastic leukemia (ALL). When only blasts are present, it is difficult to differentiate AML from ALL without additional studies. In ap-proximately 50% of patients with AML, red or purple rod-shaped structures called Auer rods may be found in the cytoplasm of neu-trophil precursors. The presence of Auer rods is a very useful marker in distinguishing AML from ALL. Auer rods do not occur in ALL. When the white cell count is low, the peripheral blood resembles that found with aplastic anemia. In these instances it may be difficult to find blast cells, and a smear made of a buffy coat preparation may be helpful in locating the immature cells.

In addition to immature cells, abnormalities of neutrophils, such as pseudo-Pelger-Huët anomaly (failure of normal nuclear lobe development) and lack of cytoplasmic granules, may be noted. Nucleated red cells may also be observed.

BONE MARROW

The marrow is usually markedly hypercellular; the normal he-matopoietic elements are replaced by a diffuse proliferation of im-mature cells, with little evidence of cell maturation. Blast cells are increased in number even when none are found in the blood. This

Table 17-3. Acute Leukemia: Summary of Clinical Features, Morphology, and Cytochemistry

Factor	Lymphocytic (ALL)	Granulocytic (AML)	Monocytic (AMOL)[a]
Age	Common in children, rare in adults	Common in adults, rare in children	Common in young adults
Blood	Anemia, neutropenia, thrombocytopenia; lymphoblasts and prolymphocytes	Anemia, neutropenia, thrombocytopenia; myeloblasts and promyelocytes	Anemia, neutropenia, thrombocytopenia; monoblasts and promonocytes
Morphology	Small or medium-sized blasts, scarce cytoplasm, usually no granules; nuclear chromatin and nucleoli indistinct	Medium to large blasts, more cytoplasm than lymphoblasts, cytoplasmic granules and occasional Auer rods; distinct nucleoli	Large blasts, abundant cytoplasm, a few granules; distinct nucleoli; promonocytes have folded nuclei, more mature chromatin
Cytochemistry	Negative for peroxidase and Sudan black; periodic acid-Schiff reaction usually positive in granules or blocks	Positive for peroxidase and Sudan black; periodic acid-Schiff reaction negative or diffusely positive	Positive for non-specific esterase inhibited by NaF; periodic acid-Schiff reaction often positive in blocks; peroxidase and Sudan black negative or weakly positive
Extramedullary and focal disease	Common in lymph nodes, spleen, liver, and CNS; gonads	Common in spleen and liver; less common in lymph nodes and CNS; granulocytic sarcoma (chloroma)	Common in gums and skin; less common in lymph nodes, spleen, and liver

[a]AMOL, acute monocytic leukemia.

finding is useful in differentiating leukemia from other causes of pancytopenia. Not infrequently, megaloblastic changes may be present in normoblasts. Rarely, the marrow is hypocellular with only clusters of blast cells present.

Other Useful Tests

CYTOCHEMISTRY

Purpose

The addition of cytochemistry is helpful in identifying various types of acute leukemias and may also be useful in predicting the prognosis (1–3). It is particularly helpful when no identifiable features such as granules or Auer rods are seen in the leukemic cells.

Principle

Cytochemistry is the application of special cytochemical stains to cells from blood and bone marrow to help in identifying the type of cells present. Enzymatic activity in the cytoplasm is demonstrated by means of specific substrates and appropriate couplers to provide a color localized in the area of enzyme activity. The color is produced by union of one of the products of the enzyme action with the coupler.

Procedure

A variety of cytochemical stains are available and a certain cytochemical profile exists for each hematopoietic cell line. Peroxidase stain, Sudan black B (SBB), and specific esterase stains (naphthol AS-D chloroacetate esterase) show positive results in the granulocytic cell series but negative results in the lymphocytic cell line. Therefore, these stains are useful in differentiating acute granulocytic leukemia (AML) from ALL. The specific esterase stain is less sensitive than the SBB and the peroxidase reactions but is particularly useful in paraffin-embedded tissue sections to separate granulocytic from lymphocytic cell proliferations.

The nonspecific esterase (alpha-naphthyl acetate or alpha-naphthyl butyrate) stains monocytes and histiocytes diffusely and is used to identify monocytic leukemias. Leukemic monocytes appear to stain more strongly than normal monocytes (Table 17-5). The nonspecific esterase stain using naphthol AS-D acetate (NASDA) as substrate together with sodium fluoride inhibition, is also useful for positive identification of monocytes. The same inhibitor can be used with the other two substrates described previously for the nonspecific esterase stain.

The periodic acid-Schiff reaction is not very reliable in the differentiation of acute leukemias. The typical block staining of lymphoblasts in ALL may also be seen in AML and is frequently observed in acute monocytic leukemia. The acid phosphatase stain and the nonspecific esterase (alpha-naphthyl acetate or alpha-naphthyl butyrate acetate) stain may prove to be useful as a T cell marker in ALL, where it has been reported to stain in a localized, dotlike fashion.

Specimen

Blood smears of good quality are made from blood and/or bone marrow. Capillary blood from a finger stick or anticoagulated venous blood may be used. Special fixatives are recommended with many of the previously described stains. Satisfactory preparations can, however, be made from smears that have been air dried only. Ideally, all cytochemical stains should be made on fresh specimens. Since this is often not practical, unstained smears can be stored, covered and away from light in a refrigerator. For the peroxidase stain, however, a fresh smear is necessary.

Interpretation

The interpretation and usefulness of the special stains described are indicated in Tables 17-4 and 17-5. The nonspecific esterase stain, using alpha-naphthyl acetate or alpha-naphthyl butyrate as substrates, produce a dot of dense, localized positivity in the

318

Table 17-4. Practical Value of Cytochemistry in Acute Leukemia

Stain	Diagnostic Utility
Peroxidase or Sudan black	AML vs. ALL
Nonspecific esterase with and without NaF[a]	AMOL vs. AML and ALL
Periodic acid-Schiff reaction	Not very reliable in distinguishing AML, AMOL, or ALL

[a]A number of substrates may be used: alpha-naphthyl acetate esterase, alpha-naphthyl butyrate esterase, and NASDA.

Table 17-5. Cytochemical Profile—Acute Leukemia

Stains	AML	AMML[a]	AMOL	ERL[a]	ALL
Peroxidase	0–3+	1–2+	0–2+	0	0
Sudan black B	1–3+	1–2+	0–2+	0	0
Nonspecific esterase[b]	0–1+	1–3+	3+	0–2+	0–1+
Nonspecific esterase—NaF	1–2+	1–2+	0–1+	0–2+	
Periodic acid-Schiff reaction (PAS)	0–2+	0–2+	0–3+	1–3+	0–3+
Acid phosphate	0–1+	1–2+	1–2+	1–2+	0–1+

[a]Abbreviations: *AMML*, acute myelomonocytic leukemia; *ERL*, erythroleukemia (Di Guglielmo syndrome).
[b]Nonspecific esterase: alpha-naphthyl acetate esterase or alpha-naphthyl butyrate.

cytoplasm of most T-lymphocytes. Similarly, blast cells of T cell ALL show strong localized acid phosphatase activity more frequently than do the cells of non-T ALL. Since non-T ALL have a better prognosis than T ALL, these stains may prove to be of some value in planning therapy. T cell ALL is frequently associated with a mediastinal mass and early involvement of the central nervous system. In general, the addition of cytochemistry reduces the subjectivity and increases the reproducibility in the classification of acute leukemia.

Notes and precautions

Although it may appear that the performance and interpretation of the special stains are relatively easy, this is, unfortunately, not true. Many of the stains require considerable technical expertise to be performed well, and experience with interpretation of acute leukemia is necessary. Leukemic cells may not stain the same way as their normal counterparts. Thus, one may observe neutrophils from patients with AML that stain negatively with peroxidase and SBB. Occasionally, the immature cells in AML are negative with peroxidase stains, but SBB stains produce positive results.

Unless the physician sees patients with leukemia at regular intervals, all of the cytochemical procedures should not be introduced. The peroxidase stain and the nonspecific esterase stain are probably the most useful. The specific esterase stain is very valuable in histologic sections.

CEREBROSPINAL FLUID IN ACUTE LEUKEMIA

Purpose

Cerebrospinal fluid (CSF) is examined for the presence of leukemic cells (4).

Principle

Infiltration of meninges is the most important extramedullary manifestation of acute leukemia. Without treatment directed against the central nervous system (CNS), the incidence of meningeal involvement may be as high as 80% in ALL and 30%–40% in AML. The central nervous system is one of the most common sites of relapse in children with leukemia. A combination of radiotherapy to the cranium and intrathecal chemotherapy is used in ALL as part of the treatment maintenance program.

Procedure

Cerebrospinal fluid is obtained with a lumbar puncture. A variety of methods are available for concentrating CSF leukocytes, including centrifugation, filter techniques, sedimentation methods, and the cytocentrifuge. The cytocentrifuge method has proven to be very effective in providing satisfactory smears of CSF fluid in patients with leukemia. The smears are stained with a Romanovsky-type stain and a differential count is taken.

Specimen

Cerebrospinal fluid is used as a specimen.

Interpretation

Leukemic cell counts vary from a rare blast to numerous blast cells. When only an occasional cell is found, it may be extremely difficult to be certain whether the cell in question represents a leukemic cell and not an atypical mononuclear cell. The appearance of the leukemic cell is similar to that observed in the blood and bone marrow.

Notes and precautions

The specimen must be examined immediately since cytolysis occurs rapidly. After intrathecal chemotherapy, considerable atypia may be seen in nonmalignant mononuclear cells and these may be mistaken for leukemic cells.

LYSOZYME (MURAMIDASE)

Purpose

Lysozyme is a hydrolytic enzyme that is present in many tissues of the body. Among the elements of the blood and bone marrow, lysozyme activity has been demonstrated in neutrophilic granulo-cytes, monocytes, and monoblasts. No activity is seen in erythro-cytes, lymphocytes, eosinophils, basophils, myeloblasts, platelets, or megakaryocytes. Levels of serum and urine lysozyme activity may be useful in the classification of leukemia.

Principle

Micrococcus lysodeikticus bacteria show marked sensitivity to the hydrolytic activity of lysozyme.

Procedure

Serum or urine is added to a suspension of *Micrococcus lysodeik-ticus* bacteria. The rate of clearing of this cloudy suspension, as measured in a spectrophotometer, is proportional to the amount of lysozyme present. This is the turbidimetric method; a lysoplate method is also available. Serum or urine is added to a well in an agar plate containing a suspension of the bacteria. After a period of incubation, lysozyme levels are determined by relating the log of the concentration to the cleared zone-ring diameter of lysis in the agar plate.

Specimen

Serum or aliquot of 24-hour urine is used as a specimen. If specimen cannot be assayed the same day, it should be stored at −20 C.

Interpretation

Normal serum levels range from 4–15 μg/ml and urine levels are normally less than 2 μg/ml. No clear-cut correlation between the white cell count and the lysozyme levels is seen. Lysozyme levels are increased in most myeloproliferative disorders. They are moderately elevated in acute myelomonocytic leukemia and CGL. In acute and chronic monocytic leukemia, the lysozyme levels are markedly increased. The levels in AML may be moderately in-creased, normal, or low depending on the percentage of myeloblasts present. Acute and chronic lymphocytic leukemia and hairy cell leukemia (leukemic reticuloendotheliosis) are associated with decreased levels. Thus, if serum or urine lysozyme levels are increased in a patient with acute leukemia, the diagnosis is unlikely to be acute lymphoblastic leukemia. In malignant histiocytosis (histiocytic medullary reticulosis), the lysozyme levels have been reported to be high.

Notes and precautions

Increased levels of urine lysozyme may be seen in renal disease, even in the absence of a hematologic disorder.

Special Procedures

TERMINAL DEOXYNUCLEOTIDYL TRANSFERASE (TDT)

TDT is a DNA polymerase enzyme that adds deoxyribonucleoside monophosphatase to preformed DNA without a template. Normally, only immature, cortical thymic lymphocytes and bone marrow lymphocytes have TDT activity. The finding of TDT in malignant cells suggests that such cells are derived from normal cells that also have TDT activity.

TDT can be used as a biochemical marker of lymphoid tissue, probably of early T-lymphocytes or null cell lymphocytes. Determination of TDT may be useful in classification of several lymphocytic malignancies.

TDT can be identified in leukocytes from blood, bone marrow, or tumor tissue. Both biochemical assays and immunofluorescent techniques have been used in specialized laboratories. A sensitive assay, which shows promise as a practical test, is based on the use of a radiolabeled (^{3}H) dATP and a cold oligodeoxynucleotide receptor, dA_{10}. The determination of TDT activity is based on measuring the rate at which the deoxynucleotide is transferred to the receptor (5,6).

TDT is found in 95% of patients with untreated acute lymphoblastic leukemia and is present in T cell and null cell types. In addition, TDT activity is present in 30% of patients with CML in blast crisis. Of the latter group of patients, some respond to the chemotherapy normally used for ALL. TDT may also be helpful in the classification of malignant lymphoma, since it appears to be present only in patients with lymphoblastic lymphoma. Unfortunately, TDT is probably not a specific marker for leukemic lymphoblasts or prothymocytes. It has also been identified in a small number (5%–10%) of patients with AML. It is possible, however, that these patients may benefit from treatment similar to that used in ALL.

IMMUNOLOGIC CHARACTERIZATION OF LEUKEMIC CELLS

Immunologic characterization of lymphoid malignancies is based on identification of cell surface markers (7,8) (Tables 17-6–17-8). The latter are characteristic membrane constituents of normal thymus-derived (T) and bone marrow-derived (B) lymphocytes. Lymphocytes that cannot be classified as either B or T cells have been termed null cells. The B-lymphocyte is a lymphoid cell that produces immunoglobulin bound to the plasma membrane (SIg) and is detectable by immunofluorescence. The T-lymphocyte is a lymphoid cell that possesses receptors for sheep erythrocytes (E rosettes). Surface markers are evaluated by examining suspensions of viable cells from blood, bone marrow, or lymph node.

Immunologic characterization of ALL is of considerable prognostic importance and may affect the treatment (Table 17-9). Thus, T cell ALL has a considerably worse prognosis than null cell ALL.

CYTOGENETIC STUDIES

A wide variety of chromosome abnormalities may be found in 50%–60% of patients with acute leukemia (9-11). In general, ALL shows a hyperdiploid pattern whereas AML shows hypodiploid, hyperdiploid, or pseudodiploid patterns. Acute promyelocytis (M3) frequently shows a 15 to 17 translocation.

Chromosome studies in acute leukemia appear to have important prognostic implications; the medium-length survival for pa-

Table 17-6. Characteristics of Human B and T Cells

Characteristic	B Cells	T Cells
Origin	Bone marrow	Bone marrow
Site of differentiation	Bursa equivalent (?)	Thymus
Peripheral localization	Follicles Medullary cords	Paracortex (lymph node); periarteriolar lymphatic sheath (spleen)
Function	Antibody production	Cell-mediated immunity, regulation of antibody production, helper T cells, suppressor T cells
Blood	20%–30%	60%–80%

Table 17-7. Identification of Mononuclear Cells by Surface Markers

Marker	T Cell	B Cell	Monocyte
Sheep red cell rosettes			
E	+	−	−
C_3-EAC (IgM)[a]	−	+	+
Fc-EA (IgG)[b]	−	±	+
Surface Ig	−	+	−

[a]C_3-EAC: Erythrocyte antibody (IgM) and complement (C_3).
[b]Fc-EA: Fc receptor for immunoglobulin (IgG).

tients with normal karyotypes has been reported to be twice as long as that for patients with abnormal karyotypes. The presence of the Philadelphia chromosome (Ph[1]), which was considered fairly specific for CML, has also been described in some patients with adult acute leukemia (AML and ALL).

Distinguishing patients with Ph[1] positive acute leukemia from those with Ph[1] negative acute leukemia appears to have important therapeutic and prognostic significance. Adults with Ph[1] negative ALL survive significantly longer than adults with Ph[1] positive ALL.

Table 17-8. **Immunologic Classification of Lymphoproliferative Neoplasms**

B cell origins
    Chronic lymphocytic leukemia
    Most adult lymphomas
    Waldenström's maroglobulinemia
    Multiple myeloma
    Burkitt's lymphoma

T cell origins
    Acute lymphoblastic leukemia (25%)
    Lymphoblastic lymphoma
    Sézary syndrome
    Mycosis fungoides
    Rare chronic lymphocytic leukemia
    Rare large cell lymphomas

However, no known clinical or morphologic characteristics have been discovered to allow identification of which acute leukemia will be Ph^1 positive. For a discussion of methodology, see Chapter 18.

ELECTRON MICROSCOPIC EXAMINATION

Electron microscopic examination of leukemic cells may be useful in the identification of cell lines involved when other methods have failed (12). Cells from bone marrow aspirate or bloody buffy coat preparations are fixed in glutaraldehyde and submitted to the electron microscopy laboratory. Ultrastructural analysis using enzymes such as peroxidase and nonspecific esterase may be of additional assistance in arriving at a correct diagnosis.

Ancillary Tests

RADIOLOGY

A chest x-ray should be taken. This may show shadowing of the lung, which is more likely to represent pneumonia than leukemic infiltrates. Mediastinal lymph nodes are often enlarged, especially in

Table 17-9. Acute Lymphoblastic Leukemia (ALL)—Immunologic Classification

Characteristic	Null Type (Non-T, Non-B)	T Type	B Type
Frequency	70%–80%	20%–25%	5%
Age	7 yrs	Older	Older
M:F	Equal	M > F	M > F
Morphology	Lymphoblastic (L1 or L2)[a]	Lymphoblastic (L1 or L2)[a]	Burkitt-like (L3)[a]
Cytochemistry	PAS +	PAS + Acid phosphatase +	PAS –
Surface markers	E–[b], SIg–[c] Anti-null +[d] Anti-ALL +[d] Anti-Ia +[d]	E +[b] Anti-T +	SIg +[c] Anti-Ia +[d]
Response to treatment	Excellent	Fair	Fair
Survival (1978)	85%—3 yrs	25%—2 yrs	1 yr

[a]See Table 17-11.
[b]Sheep red cell rosettes.
[c]Surface immunoglobulin.
[d]Antisera for leukemic antigens.

327

ALL. Osteolytic bone lesions are seen frequently in children, particularly in the bones of the limbs and pelvis. In adults and in patients with AML, the skull and the vertebral bodies may occasionally show lytic lesions indistinguishable from multiple myeloma.

FEBRILE EVALUATION

Fever in a patient with leukemia should be assumed to be caused by infection until proven otherwise. The incidence of infection in acute leukemia increases with the degree of neutropenia. In addition, the cellular and humoral immunity are frequently abnormal as a result of leukemia and antileukemic medications. The patient should be examined for localizing symptoms and signs of infection; urine and sputum should be examined and blood cultures obtained. Infections caused by *Pseudomonas*, *Staphylococcus aureus*, and gram-negative enteric organisms are particularly common. In addition, infections with opportunistic organisms such as *Candida* and *Aspergillus* occur. *Pneumocystis carinii* infection of the lung is seen with increasing frequency. The diagnosis is made by identifying the organism by biopsy of the lung.

SERUM BIOCHEMISTRY

Serum uric acid is frequently elevated, especially with high white cell counts and during chemotherapy. Uric acid is the end product of nucleic acid degeneration. Patients with high leukemic counts should be protected against the possibility of uric acid nephropathy before receiving chemotherapy. Elevated serum levels of calcium and magnesium may also be seen in acute leukemia. Levels of serum lactic dehydrogenase (LDH) are usually increased.

COAGULATION STUDIES

Bleeding in leukemia is usually caused by thrombocytopenia. In patients with severe bleeding, however, disseminated intravascular coagulation (DIC) should be considered. DIC is particularly associated with acute promyelocytic leukemia and probably caused by thromboplastic material released from leukemic promyelocytes. In addition to thrombocytopenia, low levels of fibrinogen, Factors II, V, X, and VIII, and secondary fibrinolysis with fibrin and fibrinogen degradation products are seen (see Chapter 27).

BIOPSY OF TISSUE OTHER THAN BONE MARROW

Even though the diagnosis of acute leukemia is usually made by examining blood and bone marrow, occasionally the leukemia may present initially as a tumor. Such tumors are made up of lymphoblasts or myeloblasts, depending on the type of leukemia, and may occur in the skin, testicles, ovaries, bone, lymph nodes, orbit, gastrointestinal tract, and breast. Tumors occur particularly in AML and are called granulocytic sarcoma or chloroma. These tumors may precede the development of acute leukemia by weeks to over a year, and unless granulocytic sarcoma is considered, they are frequently misdiagnosed as a histiocytic lymphoma (reticulum cell sarcoma). A specific esterase stain (chloroacetate esterase) of the paraffin section identifies the cells as granulocytic precursors. The initial site of relapse of acute leukemia may be in an extramedullary location, and a biopsy of the lesion will demonstrate the leukemic infiltrate.

SPECIAL DIAGNOSTIC CONSIDERATIONS

FAB Classification of Acute Leukemia

Numerous classifications of acute leukemia have been proposed (13,14). All have been based predominantly on the cytomorphologic features of leukemic cells as seen in Romanovsky-type stained smears. Cytochemistry, cell surface markers, electron microscopy, and other special studies as described previously may, in addition, be necessary for accurate classification.

Basically, acute leukemia can be divided into two biologically distinct groups, namely lymphocytic and nonlymphocytic leukemia. However, a wide range of morphologic variations occur within these two groups. The purpose of subclassifying the acute leukemias has been to ascertain if any relationship exists between the specific type and clinical and laboratory features, response to treatment, and prognosis. Recently, a French, American, and British (FAB) group described a morphologic and cytochemical classification of AML and ALL to allow comparisons of cooperative leukemia study groups (Tables 17-10 and 17-11). Some preliminary evidence suggests that the prognosis in the different types of ALL described correlate with morphology (Table 17-9). The L1 type of ALL may have a better prognosis than L2 and both L1 and L2 have a better prognosis than L3. No convincing evidence has yet been found that subclassification of nonlymphoid leukemia is of value in selecting treatment or in predicting prognosis. An exception is hypergranular promyelocytic leukemia, which is frequently associated with DIC. The various types of acute leukemias described in the FAB classification are illustrated in Figures 17-1–17-11.

In addition to the types of leukemias described in the FAB classification, one group of leukemias is unclassifiable. In this type the blood and bone marrow show only blasts with no evidence of cell differentiation, and a distinction between ALL and AML cannot be made. The percentage of unclassifiable leukemias varies considerably from investigator to investigator (5%–10%) and depends very much on the extent of the examination, that is, whether tests with cytochemistry, surface receptors, electron microscopy, and so forth are performed.

The classification must be made on the basis of examination of the blood and bone marrow before any treatment is performed. Chemotherapy may rapidly produce considerable changes in cell morphology and complicate the examination.

PRELEUKEMIA (MYELODYSPLASTIC SYNDROMES)

Acute myeloblastic leukemia develops in a certain percentage of patients who have anemia, neutropenia, and/or thrombocytopenia

(Text continues on page 338.)

Table 17-10. **Acute Myeloid Leukemia—FAB[a] Classification[b]**

Type	Characteristic Features
Myeloblastic leukemia without maturation (M1)	Blasts that are nongranular or contain a few azurophilic granules and/or Auer rods
Myeloblastic leukemia with maturation (M2)	Maturation beyond promyelocyte stage observed
Hypergranular promyelocytic leukemia (M3)	Majority of cells are abnormal promyelocytes with numerous bizarre granules and Auer rods; high incidence of DIC
Myelomonocytic leukemia (M4)	Granulocytic and monocytic differentiation; percentage monocytes and promonocytes exceeds 20%
Monocytic leukemia (M5)	Divided into poorly differentiated (monoblastic) and well differentiated (monocytes, promonocytes, and monocytes); cytochemistry with nonspecific esterase and NaF inhibition, necessary for the diagnosis of monoblastic type
Erythroleukemia (M6)	Nucleated red cells exceed 50% of cells in marrow; erythroblasts show bizarre features with multinucleation, giant forms, and megaloblastic features; usually progress to M1, M2, or M3

[a]FAB, French–American–British Cooperative Group.
[b]Modified with permission from information provided in Bennet JM, Catovsky D, Daniel MT, et al: Proposal for the modification of the acute leukaemias. French-American-British (FAB) Cooperative Group. Br J Haematol 33:451–458, 1976.

Table 17-11. Acute Lymphoblastic Leukemia—FAB Classification[a]

Cell Characteristics	L1	L2	L3
Cell size	Predominantly small cells, homogenous	Large, heterogenous	Large, homogenous
Nuclear chromatin	Homogenous in any one case	Heterogenous	Stippled, homogenous
Nuclear shape	Regular, round, occasional clefting	Irregular, clefting	Regular, round to ovoid
Nucleoli	Inconspicuous	One or more, may be large	One or more, prominent
Cytoplasm	Scanty	Variable, moderately abundant	Moderately abundant
Cytoplasmic vacuolation	Variable	Variable	Prominent

[a]Modified with permission from Bennet JM, Catovsky D, Daniel MT, et al: Proposal for the modification of the acute leukaemias. French-American-British (FAB) Cooperative Group. Br J Haematol 33:451–458, 1976.

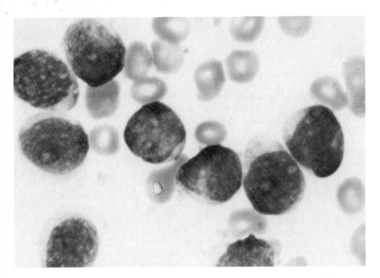

Figure 17-1. Myeloblastic leukemia without cell maturation (M1).

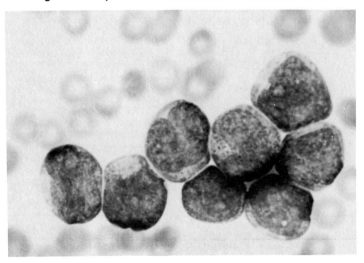

Figure 17-2. Myeloblastic leukemia with maturation (M2).

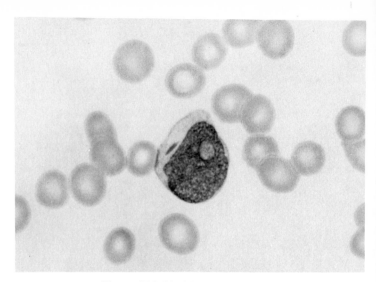

Figure 17-3. Myeloblast with Auer rod.

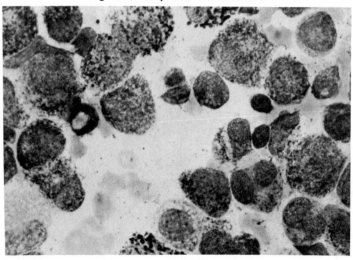

Figure 17-4. Hypergranular promyelocytic leukemia (M3). Note heavy granulation.

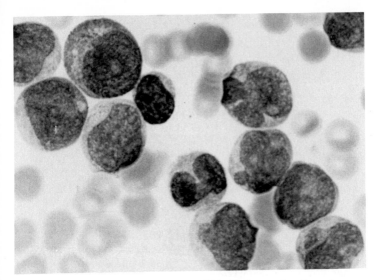

Figure 17-5. Myelomonocytic leukemia (M4). Both granulocytic and monocytic differentiation is evident.

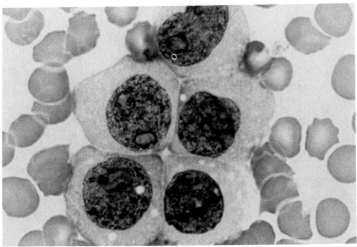

Figure 17-6. Monocytic leukemia (M5), poorly differentiated (monoblastic).

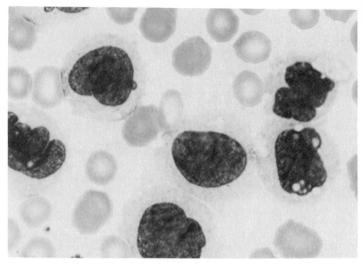

Figure 17-7. Monocytic leukemia (M5), well differentiated. Promonocytes and atypical monocytes are seen.

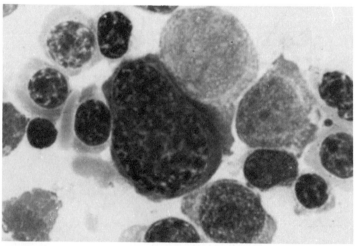

Figure 17-8. Erythroleukemia (M6). Several atypical erythroblasts are seen including a giant form in the center.

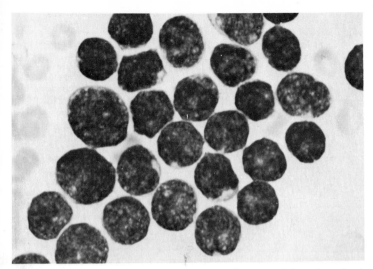

Figure 17-9. Lymphoblastic leukemia (L1). Uniform population of predominantly small blasts with scanty cytoplasm.

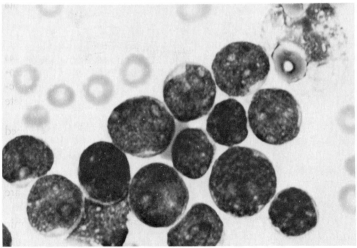

Figure 17-10. Lymphoblastic leukemia (L2). Heterogeneity in cell size and nucleoli are readily seen.

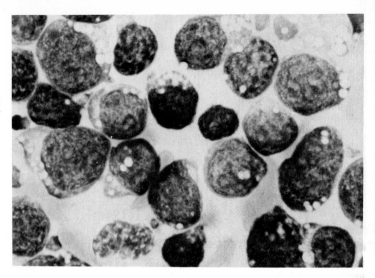

Figure 17-11. Lymphoblastic leukemia (L3). The cells have moderate amounts of cytoplasm with prominent vacuolization.

within a period of months to years (15). The term preleukemia has been given to this phase. Since this diagnosis is only made retrospectively and since the manifestations may disappear spontaneously or remain stable, the term preleukemia is considered obsolete by some investigators.

The term myelodysplastic syndromes was recently introduced and may be defined as a state of abnormal division, maturation, and production of erythrocytes, granulocytes, monocytes, and platelets. It is characterized by qualitative and quantitative abnormalities of hematopoietic cells. Myelodysplastic syndromes are mainly observed in patients more than 50 years of age.

Anemia is the major manifestation and is usually normochromic normocytic with reticulocytopenia. Neutropenia is common, and the granulocytes that are present are often poorly granulated with decreased peroxidase and LAP activity. Pseudo-Pelger-Huët anomaly is frequently present. Thrombocytopenia is common and platelet morphology may be abnormal.

The bone marrow is usually hypercellular and morphologic abnormalities such as megaloblastoid features, cytoplasmic vacuolization, and ring sideroblasts are often observed. In addition, a variety of cytogenetic abnormalities have been described. Refractory anemia with excess blasts (RAEB), which has been described by such terms as atypical leukemia and smoldering leukemia, is the most common form of myelodysplastic syndromes. Acute leukemia develops in approximately 30% of patients with RAEB. Since no absolute definition of the number of blasts in the bone marrow or blood necessary to make a diagnosis of leukemia has been determined, distinguishing RAEB from acute leukemia may be difficult when the blast count approaches 20%–30%. Repeated bone marrow examinations will, however, resolve this, since acute leukemia is usually a rapidly progressive disease.

REFERENCES

1. Yam LT, Li CY, Crosby WH: Cytochemical identification of monocytes and granulocytes. Am J Clin Pathol 55:283–290, 1971

2. Bennet JM, Reed CE: Acute leukemia cytochemical profile: Diagnostic and clinical implications. Blood Cells 1:101–108, 1975

3. Catovsky D, Galetto J, Okos A, et al: Cytochemical profile of B and T leukemic lymphocytes with special reference to acute lymphoblastic leukemia. J Clin Pathol 27:767–771, 1974

4. Kreig AF: Cerebrospinal fluid and other body fluids. In Henry JB (ed): *Todd-Sanford-Davidsohn Clinical Diagnosis by Laboratory Methods*, ed 16. Philadelphia, W. B. Saunders Co, 1979, pp 635–679

5. Kung PC, Long JC, McCaffrey RP, et al: Terminal deoxynucleotidyl transferase in diagnosis of leukemia and malignant lymphoma. Am J Med 64:788–794, 1978

6. Beutler E, Kuhl W: An assay for terminal deoxynucleotidyl transferase in leukocytes and bone marrow. Am J Clin Pathol 70:733–737, 1978

7. Belpomme D, Borella L, Braylan R, et al: Immunological diagnosis of leukemia and lymphoma: A world health organization international union of immunological societies technical report. Br J Haematol 38:85–98, 1978

339

8. Brouet JC, Seligman M: The immunological classification of acute lymphoblastic leukemias. Cancer 42[Suppl]:817–827, 1978

9. Bottomley RH: Cytogenetic heterogeneity of the acute leukemias. Semin Oncol 3:253–257, 1977

10. Bloomfield LD, Peterson LC, Yunis JJ, et al: The Philadelphia chromosome (Ph^1) in adults presenting with acute leukemia; a comparison of Ph^1- and Ph^1+ patients. Br J Haematol 36: 347–358, 1977

11. Golomb HM, Vardimann JM, Rowley JD, et al: Correlation of clinical findings with quinacrine–banded chromosomes in 90 adults with acute nonlymphocytic leukemia. N Engl J Med 299:613–619, 1978

12. Glick AD: Acute leukemia: Electron microscopic examination. Semin Oncol 3:229–241, 1976

13. Bennet JM, Catovsky D, Daniel MT et al: Proposal for the classification of the acute leukaemias. French-American-British (FAB) Cooperative Group. Br J Haematol 33:451–458, 1976

14. Gralnick HR, Galton DAG, Catovsky D, et al: Classification of acute leukemia. NIH Conference. Ann Intern Med 87:740–753, 1977

15. Bessis M (ed): Hemopoietic dysplasia (preleukemic states). Blood Cells, vol. 1, 1976 [Excellent source for review articles.]

chapter 18

Chronic The chronic leukemias arise from either granulocytic or lympho- **Leukemia** cytic cell lines and differ morpho- logically from the acute leuke- mias in that the leukemic cells show more differentiation (1). While in acute leukemia the leukocyte count is variable, in chronic leukemia it is almost always elevated. Thrombocytopenia and ane- mia are usually less prominent in chronic leukemias than in acute leukemias and lymphadenopathy and splenomegaly are more com- mon and pronounced. Patients with chronic leukemia have a more prolonged course than untreated patients with acute leukemia.

Chronic granulocytic leukemia (CGL) is found primarily in pa- tients 30–50 years old; it is rare in children. The other chronic leukemias are usually confined to middle-aged and elderly indi- viduals. Males are more commonly affected than females.

The onset of chronic leukemia is usually insidious and the dis- ease may be discovered by chance during a routine blood test. Fatigue, anorexia, weight loss, fever, lymphadenopathy, and spleno- megaly are other clinical features that may cause the patient to seek medical attention.

DIAGNOSTIC EVALUATION

The approach to the laboratory diagnosis of chronic leukemia proceeds in the following sequence:

1. Hematologic evaluation
   a. Complete blood count. This should include hemoglobin, white

cell count, and platelet count. A well-prepared blood smear should be reviewed and a differential white cell count made.

b. Bone marrow study. Since chronic leukemia (particularly CGL) is frequently associated with varying degrees of fibrosis, a bone marrow biopsy and aspirate is recommended, preferably from the posterior iliac crest. A reticulin stain should be performed on the biopsy to evaluate the presence or absence of fibrosis. If no marrow can be aspirated, touch preparations of the biopsy must be made and stained with a Romanovsky stain and other special stains as necessary. If CGL is suspected, a sample of bone marrow aspirate should be submitted for cytogenetic analysis in search of the Philadelphia chromosome.

2. Special studies to confirm the presence of CGL include the leukocyte alkaline phosphatase (LAP) stain and cytogenetic studies of bone marrow in search of the Philadelphia chromosome.

3. Ancillary studies to determine the extent of leukemia and the presence of complications include serum immunoglobulin levels, Coombs antiglobulin test in patients with chronic lymphocytic leukemia (CLL) who have anemia, and blood biochemistry.

LABORATORY STUDIES

Hematologic Tests

GENERAL FEATURES

The initial laboratory findings that suggest chronic leukemia are leukocytosis and anemia. The anemia is usually mild at the onset of the disease and is normochromic normocytic. The platelet count is initially normal or may be increased, as is often seen in CGL.

BLOOD

The white cell count is invariably increased. In CGL, the white cell count is usually more than $50 \times 10^3/\mu l$ and may be above $200 \times 10^3/\mu l$. The entire spectrum of granulocytic precursors is seen (Figure 18-1). In contrast to AML, there is no hiatus, or discontinuity of cell maturation. Mature granulocytes and metamyelocytes predominate. Myelocytes and promyelocytes are easily found, and a

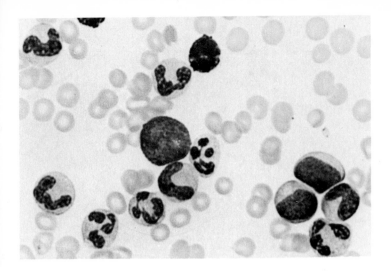

Figure 18-1. Blood smear from patient with chronic granulocytic leukemia showing neutrophils at varying stages of maturation and two basophils.

small number (less than 10%) of myeloblasts are seen. An increased number of eosinophils and basophils is typical in CGL and is a useful marker in distinguishing CGL from a leukemoid reaction.

In CLL, the white cell count ranges from $20 \times 10^3/\mu l$ to over $200 \times 10^3/\mu l$, and 70%–90% of these cells are a uniform population of small, normal-appearing lymphocytes (Figure 18-2). Occasionally, the cells may be larger, have more cytoplasm, and a single nucleolus. In contrast to lymphoblasts, however, the chromatin is coarse and clumped. Many smudged cells are seen. Leukocyte counts obtained with automated electronic counting instruments may be spuriously low because the leukemic cells are fragile (smudged) and may not all be counted.

BONE MARROW

In CGL, the marrow is invariably markedly hypercellular with all granulocytic precursors represented. Myeloblasts, promyelo-

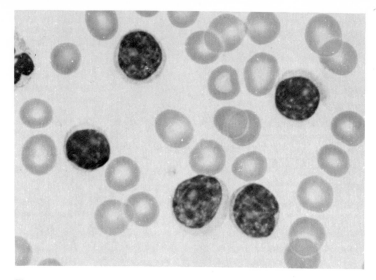

Figure 18-2. Lymphocytes in blood smear from patients with chronic lymphocytic leukemia.

cytes, and myelocytes are prominent, and the number of basophils and eosinophils is usually increased. The megakaryocytes are often increased in number and are not infrequently abnormal in appearance; this is a common feature of the myeloproliferative disorders (see Chapter 19). The number of erythroid precursors is often decreased. It should be emphasized that in the early stage of CGL, the bone marrow is not diagnostic, and the disease may be confused with a reactive granulocytic inflammatory response.

The bone marrow biopsy may show fibrosis as revealed by a reticulin stain. Later in the course of the disease, the fibrosis may be pronounced and the biopsy may resemble myelofibrosis with myeloid metaplasia.

In CLL, the marrow may initially show only slight lymphocytosis. Histologic sections of aspirate or a biopsy is usually more helpful than smears of aspirate at the early stage of the disease and will show islands with sheets of small lymphocytes separated by normal

Table 18-1. **Leukocyte Alkaline Phosphatase (LAP)**

Low Activity	High Activity
CGL	Myelofibrosis with myeloid metaplasia (rarely low)
PNH	PV
Hypophosphatemia	Leukemoid reaction
	Pregnancy and oral contraceptives
	Hodgkin's disease
	Multiple myeloma

marrow. Later in the course of the disease, the lymphocytes gradually replace the normal marrow.

Other Useful Tests

LEUKOCYTE ALKALINE PHOSPHATASE (LAP)

Purpose

The LAP score is a simple confirmatory test in CGL (2).
For sections on *Principle*, *Procedure*, and *Specimen*, see Chapter 14.

Interpretation

In CGL, the LAP score is zero or markedly decreased. The value of a low score in patients with CGL is increased by the fact that the LAP scores are usually elevated in the conditions with which it is most commonly mistaken (Table 18-1). Thus, LAP scores are usually increased in polycythemia vera, granulocytic leukemoid reaction, and myelofibrosis with myeloid metaplasia. However, the LAP score in CGL may be increased in the presence of infections. During the accelerated or malignant phase of CGL, the LAP may be normal or elevated. Decreased LAP scores may also be seen in patients with paroxysmal nocturnal hemoglobinuria or hereditary phosphatemia (see also Chapter 14).

Elevated LAP scores may be seen in patients with bacterial infections, in pregnancy, in women taking oral contraceptives, and in patients with Hodgkin's disease and multiple myeloma. Serum and neutrophil phosphatase levels have no relationship to one another. A control must always be used when any cytochemical stain is performed.

CYTOGENETIC STUDIES

Purpose

Chromosome charts are prepared by examining metaphase spreads of leukocytes from blood and/or bone marrow (1). The Philadelphia (Ph^1) chromosome is present in the majority of patients with CGL.

Principle

The Ph^1 abnormality results from translocation of the greater part of the long arm of chromosome 22 to another chromosome, usually chromosome 9.

Procedure and specimen

A variety of techniques are available by which chromosomes can be studied. The simplest type is termed a direct study. A cell suspension is made of leukocytes from blood or bone marrow and incubated with colchicine to arrest cell division at the metaphase stage. The cells are then swollen by hypotonic saline treatment and fixed. The fixed cells are placed on a slide, flattened, and dried. The metaphase spreads are then stained, examined under the microscope, and photographed.

Cell culture techniques are employed when the cells have a low mitotic index. Malignant leukocytes grow in vitro without stimulation, and peak cell division occurs at 24–48 hours after inception of cell culture.

Specimen

Bone marrow is the tissue of choice. A buffy coat of peripheral blood may be used if no bone marrow can be obtained and if the peripheral blood contains an adequate number of cells at the myelocytic stage or younger.

Interpretation

The Ph^1 chromosome is present in 90% of patients with CGL, both in relapse and in apparent remission of the disease. During so-called blast crisis or accelerated phase of CGL, other chromosome abnormalities may develop in addition to the Ph^1 chromosome.

In patients with CGL who do not have the Ph^1 chromosome, the white cell and the platelet counts are lower. Their clinical course is more acute and response to therapy is usually poor.

The Ph^1 abnormality has also occasionally been observed in acute leukemia (see Chapter 17).

Notes and precautions

Cell culture techniques using antigenic or mitogenic stimulation of leukemic leukocytes are apt to be normal since the metaphases obtained may reflect predominantly normal T-lymphocytes. The major disadvantage of the in vitro culture methods is that the conditions may selectively favor growth of one cell line and give false impressions of the prevalence of the cell type present. Also, cell cultures may possibly induce chromosome abnormalities.

Special Procedures

TERMINAL DEOXYNUCLEOTIDYL TRANSFERASE (TDT)

In approximately 30% of patients with CGL in blast crisis, TDT is present. These patients appear to respond better to treatment with vincristine and prednisone, which are drugs normally used for treatment of acute lymphoblastic leukemia. The blast cell morphology (i.e., lymphoblastic versus myeloblastic) does not, however, appear to be helpful in predicting which case will be TDT positive. (See also Chapter 17.)

CELL SURFACE MARKERS

In the majority of patients with CLL, the lymphocytes have surface receptors for immunoglobulins (usually IgM) and are thus B-lymphocytes. The concentration of surface immunoglobulins is, however, less than what is seen in patients with lymphosarcoma cell leukemia, which consists of leukemic cells from poorly differentiated (small cleaved) lymphocytic lymphoma.

A small number of patients (2%) with T cell CLL have been described. In these patients, the leukemic cells often have prominent purple granules and skin involvement is common.

Ancillary Studies

SERUM IMMUNOGLOBULIN

Hypogammaglobulinemia is seen in the majority of patients with CLL, and it increases in severity as the disease progresses. The hypogammaglobulinemia together with neutropenia account for the increased susceptibility of infection in CLL. In approximately 5% of patients with CLL, a monoclonal hypergammaglobulinemia is present. Since this is usually IgM the disease may be difficult to distinguish from Waldenström's macroglobulinemia.

COOMBS ANTIGLOBULIN TEST

Approximately 10% of patients with CLL develop autoimmune hemolytic anemia, which may be severe. The Coombs direct antiglobulin test is usually positive and the antibody is of the IgG type. The peripheral blood will show spherocytosis and polychromatophilia, and the reticulocyte count will be elevated.

SERUM BIOCHEMISTRY

Serum uric acid may be elevated in CGL and CLL and may increase dramatically when chemotherapy is given. In order to prevent uric acid nephropathy, dehydration should be corrected and the patient given allopurinol, which inhibits production of uric acid. Serum lactic dehydrogenase (LDH) may be nonspecifically increased. In patients with CLL who have associated hemolytic anemia, the LDH levels are usually more markedly elevated.

LYMPH NODE BIOPSY

Lymphadenopathy is commonly seen in CLL and may also be present in CGL, particularly in blast crisis. In CLL, biopsy of the lymph node shows complete replacement of the normal architecture with small, well-differentiated lymphocytes. The morphology is indistinguishable from that seen in well-differentiated lymphocytic lymphoma (3).

In CGL in blast crisis, the lymph node may resemble a malignant lymphoma, particularly histiocytic (large cell) lymphoma. Specific esterase stain is usually necessary to confirm that the cells are of the granulocytic cell line (see Chapter 17). However, few, if any, indications are found for a lymph node biopsy in chronic lymphocytic leukemia or in the blast phase of chronic granulocytic leukemia.

SPECIAL DIAGNOSTIC CONSIDERATIONS

Chronic Granulocytic Leukemia (CGL)

The onset of CGL is insidious (1). There is usually progressive enlargement of the spleen. The laboratory features, including the peripheral blood, bone marrow, and chromosome abnormalities, were described earlier in this chapter, and they are summarized in Table 18-2.

As long as CGL remains chronic, it is usually well controlled without relapses by varying doses of chemotherapy. Difficulty of control with standard chemotherapy usually indicates transformation of the disease. The latter is usually associated with an increase

Table 18-2. Characteristic Features of Chronic Granulocytic Leukemia (CGL)

Age	30–50 years
Leukocyte count	50–200 × 10^3/μl
Blood findings	Granulocytosis with entire spectrum of precursors from myeloblasts ($<$ 2%) to mature neutrophils, eosinophilia and basophilia, platelet count normal or increased
Bone marrow findings	Granulocytic hyperplasia, eosinophilia, and basophilia; megakaryocytic hyperplasia sometimes present
LAP	Decreased
Chromosome analysis	Ph^1 present in 90% of patients
Course	After 2–3 years, disease terminates in an acclerated phase with an increase in blasts (blast crisis) and/or myelofibrosis

in myeloblasts and basophils, thrombocytopenia or thrombocytosis together with increasing anemia and splenomegaly. In addition, bone marrow failure with variable degrees of marrow fibrosis may be seen. This is the so-called accelerated or malignant phase of CGL and occurs on the average of two to three years after the initial diagnosis. The disease is then usually resistant to therapy. The development of so-called blastic crisis is observed in about one-third of the patients. The peripheral blood and bone marrow may then be indistinguishable from acute myeloblastic leukemia, with more than 30% blasts in the blood and/or bone marrow. Rarely, patients appear to be in blastic crisis when they first seek medical advice.

In the majority of patients with blastic crisis, the morphologic feature closely resembles acute myeloblastic leukemia (4). However, a significant number of patients have blasts that are indistinguishable from those seen in acute lymphoblastic leukemia (ALL). These patients may respond to treatment normally used for ALL. As mentioned earlier, the terminal transferase assay may be more useful in predicting which patients will respond to ALL therapy. Monoblasts, erythroblasts or megakaryocytes rarely predominate.

In most patients, the diagnosis of CGL is clear. The combination of splenomegaly, leukocytosis comprised mainly of neutrophils, and immature granulocytic cells and thrombocytosis is typical. Additional studies such as LAP and the presence of the Ph[1] chromosome confirm the diagnosis. Rarely, the diagnosis is not clear-cut. The differential diagnosis of CGL includes other types of myeloproliferative disorders, such as myelofibrosis with myeloid metaplasia, late polycythemia vera, atypical AML, chronic myelomonocytic leukemia, and leukemoid reactions secondary to an infection or malignancy.

Chronic Myelomonocytic Leukemia (CMML)

Chronic myelomonocytic leukemia is not common and mainly affects patients over the age of 60 years (5). The onset of the disease is slow but progressive and the most common presenting feature is anemia. Splenomegaly and moderate enlargement of the lymph nodes in the neck may be present.

The leukocyte count may be normal, moderately increased, or rarely decreased. The peripheral blood shows monocytosis, and the morphology of the monocytes is often abnormal with hypersegmented or horseshoe-shaped nuclei (Figure 18-3). The nonspecific esterase stain helps in identifying the cells as monocytes (see Chapter 17). A varying number of immature granulocytes are also seen. The bone marrow is hypercellular, and monocytes appear less prominent than in the blood. There is a moderate increase in myelocytes, promyelocytes, and myeloblasts (< 30%). The erythroid precursors may show dyserythropoiesis and ring sideroblasts may be seen.

Serum lysozyme levels are increased as in acute monocytic leukemia (see Chapter 17). The LAP score is variable and may be low as in CGL.

In the differential diagnosis of CMML, other diseases associated with monocytosis, such as malaria, tuberculosis, Hodgkin's disease, and carcinoma, must be considered. Acute myeloblastic leukemia,

351

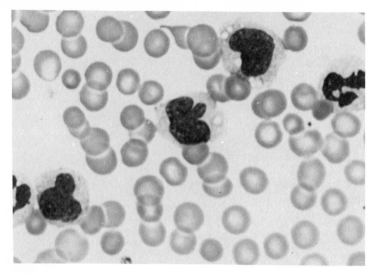

Figure 18-3. Atypical monocytes and neutrophils in blood smear from patient with chronic myelomonocytic leukemia.

particularly the acute myelomonocytic variety (M4), CGL, and refractory anemia with excess of myeloblasts (RAEB) may cause difficulties in the differential diagnosis.

Some authorities consider CMML to be part of the so-called myelodysplastic syndromes (preleukemia) (see Chapter 17). It is important to recognize this disorder since patients suffering from this disease tolerate aggressive chemotherapy poorly.

Chronic Lymphocytic Leukemia (CLL)

The majority of patients with CLL are over 60 years of age and the disease is more common in males than females (1,3,6–8). The disease may be discovered by chance, by blood examination or by the finding of an enlarged lymph node or spleen during examination for an unrelated complaint. Other patients may seek advice because of enlarged lymph nodes or complaints related to anemia.

Table 18-3. Rai's Staging System for Chronic Lymphocytic Leukemia (CLL)

Stage	Criteria
Stage 0	Absolute lymphocytosis of $> 15 \times 10^3/\mu l$
Stage I	Absolute lymphocytosis plus enlarged lymph nodes
Stage II	Absolute lymphocytosis plus enlarged liver and/or spleen
Stage III	Absolute lymphocytosis plus anemia (Hb $< 11 g/dl$)
Stage IV	Absolute lymphocytosis plus thrombocytopenia (platelet count $< 100 \times 10^3/\mu l$)

The laboratory features including blood and bone marrow findings were described earlier in this chapter. A staging system has been suggested based on the degree of lymphocytosis, hemoglobin level, platelet count, and the presence of lymphadenopathy and hepatosplenomegaly (Table 18-3). There is a significant relationship between stage and survival (6).

The diagnosis of CLL is usually not difficult except in recognition of early CLL and in the distinction from lymphocytic lymphoma. Hairy cell leukemia (leukemic reticuloendotheliosis) and Waldenström's macroglobulinemia may also have to be considered in the differential diagnosis.

Well-differentiated lymphocytic (small lymphocytic) lymphoma, Waldenström's macroglobulinemia, and CLL are histologically and cytologically similar and differ primarily by the presence or absence of peripheral lymphocytosis and monoclonal immunoglobulins in the serum or urine (Chapter 20). Most likely these are variants of the same pathologic process. In general, leukemia is diffuse and generalized in distribution, and lymphoma is a more localized process.

A few patients with malignant lymphoma become leukemic; this disease is termed lymphosarcoma cell leukemia. In well-differentiated lymphocytic lymphoma, the leukemic cells are similar to those of CLL. In poorly differentiated lymphocytic (small cleaved) lymphoma, nodular (follicular) type, a leukemic phase is seen in 5%–10%

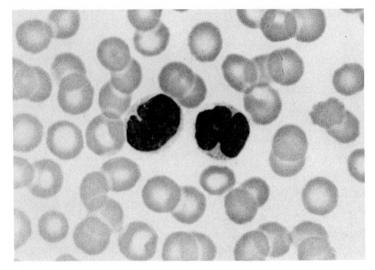

Figure 18-4. Blood smear from patient with nodular, poorly differentiated lymphocytic leukemia showing lymphocytes with notched or clefted nuclei (lymphosarcoma cell leukemia).

of patients. The leukemic cells have a characteristic notched or clefted nucleus with scant cytoplasm (Figure 18-4). Diffuse histiocytic lymphoma (reticulum cell sarcoma) develops in approximately 3% of patients with CLL (Richter's syndrome) (7).

Prolymphocytic Leukemia (PL)

Prolymphocytic leukemia is a rare variant of CLL. It is characterized by marked splenomegaly, absent or minimal lymphadenopathy, marked leukocytosis (usually $> 150,000/\mu l$) consisting predominantly of prolymphocytes, and patients do not respond to treatment that is usually effective in CLL (9,10). The prolymphocytes are larger and have more cytoplasm than small lymphocytes in CLL. Their nuclear chromatin pattern is moderately coarse and a prominent nucleolus is seen (Figure 18-5).

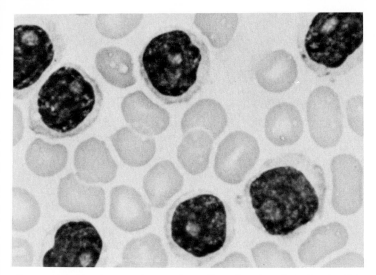

Figure 18-5. Blood smear from patient with prolymphocytic leukemia. Note nuclei with clumped chromatin and a prominent nucleolus.

Hairy Cell Leukemia (Leukemic Reticuloendotheliosis)

Hairy cell leukemia is a rare form of leukemia characterized by splenomegaly, absent or minimal lymphadenopathy, pancytopenia, and the presence of atypical mononuclear cells in the blood and bone marrow (11,12). The mononuclear cells (hairy cells) as seen in blood smears have features of both lymphocytes and monocytes (Figure 18-6). The nuclear chromatin pattern has a ground-glass or spongy appearance. The light, gray-blue cytoplasm is moderately abundant and usually has characteristic hairy projections.

The leukemic cells in hairy cell leukemia have tartrate-resistant acid phosphatase activity. This can be demonstrated with a special cytochemical stain and is quite specific for this disorder.

A bone marrow aspirate often reveals a dry tap, but biopsy of the bone marrow reveals a focal or diffuse infiltrate of mononuclear cells, which are characteristically less densely packed than the

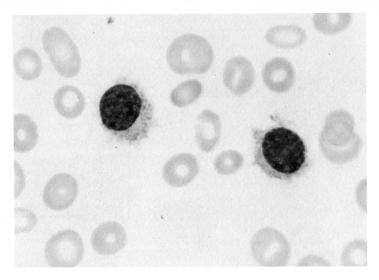

Figure 18-6. Irregular cytoplasmic processes are seen in the mononuclear cells from a patient with hairy cell leukemia.

malignant cells in other leukemias or lymphomas. The infiltrate in the bone marrow biopsy consists of a bland, uniform population of mononuclear cells with well-defined nuclei and a clear cytoplasm giving a halo appearance (Figure 18-7). Since the leukemic cells in the peripheral blood may be few and difficult to recognize and because a bone marrow aspirate frequently reveals a dry tap, the bone marrow biopsy is the most useful examination for the diagnosis of hairy cell leukemia (12).

Hairy cell leukemia has been in the past and probably still is frequently misdiagnosed as chronic lymphocytic leukemia, malignant lymphoma, aplastic anemia, or, rarely, chronic monocytic leukemia. It is important to recognize patients with this disease, because they usually do not respond to conventional chemotherapy used in CLL and most do not tolerate aggressive chemotherapy. Splenectomy, however, appears to be of benefit in many patients.

Table 18-4.   Clinical and Laboratory Features of Chronic Lymphoproliferative Disorders

Type	Leukocyte Count × $10^3/\mu l$	Cell Morphology	Lymph-adenopathy	Spleno-megaly	Special Features
CLL	50–150	Similar to normal, small lymphocytes	1–2+	1–3+	Hypogammaglobulinemia and Coombs-positive hemolytic anemia common
Prolymphocytic leukemia	150–500	Moderate to large lymphocytes with clumped chromatin and prominent nucleolus	0–1+	2–3+	
Lymphocytic lymphoma (lymphosarcoma cell leukemia)	< 30; leukemia develops in 5%–10%	Medium to large lymphocytes often with cleft ed nucleus	2–3+	1–2+	Primarily lymph node disease; diagnosis of type made by lymph node biopsy
Waldenström's macroglobulinemia	< 30; leukemia rarely develops	Small- to medium-sized lymphocytes, some with plasma-cytoid features	0–1+	0–2+	Monoclonal IgM; hyperviscosity
Hairy cell leukemia	< 5.0	Small- to medium-sized mononuclear cells with moderate to abundant cytoplasm and hair-like projections	0–1+	2–3+	Cells contain tartrate-resistant acid phos-phatase; bone mar-row biopsy diagnostic

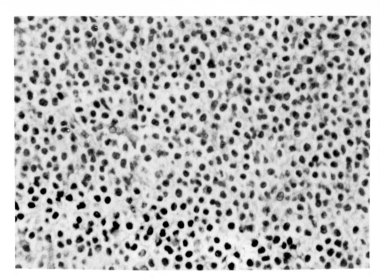

Figure 18-7. Bone marrow biopsy from patient with hairy cell leukemia. Note a uniform population of mononuclear cells with clear cytoplasm giving a halo appearance.

A summary of the characteristic clinical and laboratory features of chronic lymphoproliferative disorders are seen in Table 18-4.

REFERENCES

1. Galton DAG: The chronic leukemias. Clin Haematol, vol 6. Philadelphia, W.B. Saunders Co, 1977. [An excellent source for review of articles with comprehensive bibliographies.]
2. Kaplow LS: Leukocyte alkaline phosphatase in disease. CRC Crit Rev Clin Lab Sci 2: 243–278, 1971
3. Dick F, Maca RD: The lymph node in chronic lymphocytic leukemia. Cancer 41:283–292, 1978
4. Marks SM, McCaffrey R, Rosenthal DS, et al: Blastic transformation in chronic myelogenous leukemia: Experience with 50 patients. Med Pediatr Oncol 4:159–167, 1978

5. Zittoun R: Subacute and chronic myelomonocytic leukaemia: A distinct haematologic entity. Br J Haematol 32:1–7, 1976

6. Rai KR, Sawitsky A, Cronkite EP, et al: Clinical staging of chronic lymphocytic leukemia. Blood 46:219–234, 1975

7. Armitage J, Dick FR, Corder MP: Diffuse histiocytic lymphoma complicating chronic lymphocytic leukemia. Cancer 41:422–427, 1978

8. Silver RT, Sawitsky A, Rai K, et al: Guidelines for protocol studies in chronic lymphocytic leukemia. Am J Hematol 4:343–358, 1978

9. Galton D, Goldman J, Wiltshaw E, et al: Prolymphocytic leukemia. Br J Haematol 27:7–23, 1974

10. Bearman RM, Pangalis GA, Rappaport H: Prolymphocytic leukemia. Clinical, histopathological and cytochemical observations. Cancer 42:2360–2372, 1978

11. Turner A, Kjeldsberg CR: Hairy cell leukemia: A review. Medicine 57:477–499, 1978

12. Burke JS: The value of the bone marrow biopsy in the diagnosis of hairy cell leukemia. Am J Clin Pathol 70:876–884, 1978

chapter 19

Myelo-proliferative Disorders

The term myeloproliferative disorders was introduced to describe closely related syndromes such as chronic granulocytic leukemia, polycythemia vera, myelofibrosis with myeloid metaplasia, essential thrombocythemia, and Di Guglielmo syndrome (erythroleukemia, erythremic myelosis) (1–5) (Table 19-1). The diseases usually occur in those over the age of 50 and rarely in children. These disorders have similar clinical and hematologic manifestations at some stage in the disease process (Tables 19-2 and 19-3). Evidence supports the concept that myeloproliferative disorders are clonal in nature and appear to have arisen from single pluripotent hematopoietic stem cells. The fibrosis that is so commonly seen is thought to be reactive. In all the myeloproliferative disorders, probability of the development of acute leukemia is increased. Several of these entities were described in Chapters 13, 17, and 18, and this chapter will be confined to a discussion of two entities, namely myelofibrosis with myeloid metaplasia and essential thrombocythemia.

A large number of synonyms have been used for myelofibrosis with myeloid metaplasia, including agnogenic myeloid metaplasia, aleukemic megakaryocytic myelosis, leukoerythroblastic anemia, and so forth. These names usually indicate the feature of the disease that appears most striking to the observer. The characteristic features of this disease are listed in Table 19-4 (6,7).

The diagnosis of essential thrombocythemia should be made only when thrombocythemia is the predominant feature of the

Table 19-1. Classification of Myeloproliferative Disorders

Polycythemia vera

Chronic granulocytic leukemia

Myelofibrosis with myeloid metaplasia

Essential thrombocythemia

Di Guglielmo syndrome (erythroleukemia, erythremic myelosis)

Table 19-2. Myeloproliferative Disorders: Common Features

Similar clinical manifestations

Panmyelosis at some stage

Frequent occurrence of myelofibrosis

Apparent transitional forms between types

Blastic crisis common in terminal stages

hematologic picture and is occurring together with bleeding and thrombosis. The essential features of the disease are listed in Table 19-5 (8). Several synonyms have been used for this entity, including idiopathic thrombocythemia, hemorrhagic thrombocythemia, and primary thrombocythemia.

The myeloproliferative disorders usually have an insidious onset, the patient presents with a long history of weakness, and the physical examination reveals splenomegaly. The blood count shows anemia, leukocytosis, and a variable platelet count.

DIAGNOSTIC EVALUATION

After a clinical history and physical examination have been completed, the laboratory diagnosis of myeloproliferative disease proceeds in the following sequence:

Table 19-3. **Myeloproliferative Disorders: Characteristic Features**[a]

	Erythroid Proliferation	Megakaryocytic Proliferation	Granulocytic Proliferation	Fibroblastic Proliferation	LAP	Ph¹ Chromosome	Spleno-megaly
Polycythemia vera	↑↑	↑	↑	↑	↑	−	↑
Chronic myelocytic leukemia	N[b]	↑N	↑↑	↑	↓	+	↑
Myelofibrosis with myeloid metaplasia	↓N	↓↑	↓↑	↑↑	↑N	−	↑↑
Essential thrombo-cythemia	N	↑↑	↑	↑	↑N	−	↑

[a]Modified and reproduced with permission from Gilbert HS, Dameshek W: The myeloproliferative disorders. In Dowling HF, et al (eds): *Disease-A-Month.* Copyright © 1970 by Year Book Medical Publishers, Inc., Chicago.

Table 19-4. Myelofibrosis with Myeloid Metaplasia: Characteristic Features

Insidious onset with weakness, weight loss, pallor

Splenomegaly

Normochromic anemia

Red cell morphology—prominent poikilocytosis (tear drop forms) and anisocytosis

Nucleated red cells common in blood

White cell count elevated ($< 30 \times 10^3/\mu l$), normal or rarely decreased; occasional myeloblasts

Platelet count increased, normal, or decreased; giant platelets

Bone marrow—panhyperplasia with increasing fibrosis

Table 19-5. Primary Thrombocythemia: Characteristic Features

Bleeding and thromboembolic phenomena

Splenomegaly

Platelet count—sustained thrombocytosis $> 1000 \times 10^3/\mu l$

White cells—mature neutrophilic leukocytosis ($< 40 \times 10/\mu l$

Microcytic hypochromic anemia

Bone marrow—marked megakaryocytic hyperplasia

---

1. Hematologic evaluation
   a. Complete blood count, which should include hemoglobin, hematocrit, white cell, and platelet count. In addition, the peripheral blood smear must be reviewed carefully to evaluate the red cells, leukocytes, and platelets.
   b. Bone marrow aspirate frequently gives a dry tap and biopsy must always be performed to evaluate the presence of myelofibrosis or osteosclerosis. Imprints of the biopsy must always be made.

363

2. Studies to differentiate chronic granulocytic leukemia (CGL) from other myeloproliferative disorders include leukocyte alkaline phosphatase (LAP) and cytogenetic studies (Philadelphia chromosome).

3. Ancillary studies such as radiologic tests, bleeding studies, and blood chemistries may be useful in determining the extent of disease and in disclosing any complications.

LABORATORY STUDIES

Hematologic Tests

GENERAL FEATURES

The initial laboratory findings that suggest a myeloproliferative disorder are anemia, neutrophilic leukocytosis, and abnormal platelets (3,7). Rarely it may present as a bleeding problem. The anemia may be normochromic or hypochromic and microcytic if the patient has been bleeding. A hemolytic component is not unusual.

BLOOD

The white cell count is often increased but is usually less than $30 \times 10^3/\mu l$. The whole spectrum of granulocytic precursors may be seen, and the blood smear closely resembles a leukemoid reaction or CGL. The frequency of eosinophilia and basophilia is considerably less in myelofibrosis, polycythemia vera, and essential thrombocythemia than in CGL. In addition to immature granulocytes, a small number of nucleated red cells are usually present, which together with the immature granulocytes constitute the so-called leukoerythroblastic picture (Figure 19-1). As the disease progresses, leukopenia may develop together with the appearance of many blasts whose presence may justify a diagnosis of acute myeloblastic leukemia.

The platelet count is usually initially increased. In essential thrombocythemia, it often exceeds $1000 \times 10^3/\mu l$. In addition, the platelets often have abnormal morphology and may be extremely large. Fragments of megakaryocytes may also be seen.

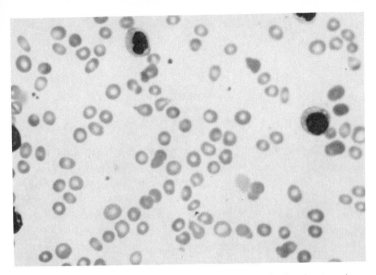

Figure 19-1. Blood smear from patient with myelofibrosis showing tear drop-shaped red cells, normoblast, and immature granulocytes.

The red cell morphology usually reveals a significant degree of anisocytosis, poikilocytosis, and polychromatophilia. Tear drop forms and ovalocytes are common. The anemia in myelofibrosis is usually normochromic but may be hypochromic in patients who are bleeding. Hypochromic microcytic anemia is particularly common in patients with essential thrombocythemia because these patients frequently have bleeding problems.

BONE MARROW

Bone marrow aspirate frequently results in a dry tap and a biopsy must be performed (9). Early in the course of myelofibrosis, the bone marrow may not show striking abnormalities. Usually, however, by the time of diagnosis, the marrow is hypercellular with hyperplasia of all cell lines. All stages of maturation are represented. This is the so-called cellular phase of myelofibrosis (Figure 19-2). The megakaryocytes often occur in clusters and are

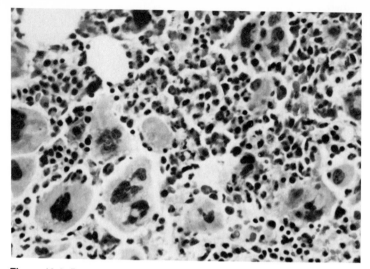

Figure 19-2. Bone marrow biopsy from patient with early myelofibrosis showing panhyperplasia and a cluster of megakaryocytes.

frequently abnormal in size and shape. They may then be difficult to recognize.

A reticulin stain is necessary to detect early myelofibrosis. Reticulin content is increased as the disease progresses. The bone marrow becomes less cellular and the megakaryocytes are usually the last to disappear as myelofibrosis becomes the predominating feature (Figure 19-3). Formation of collagen in the marrow is associated with the appearance of extramedullary hematopoiesis in spleen, liver, and, not infrequently, lymph nodes.

In essential thrombocythemia, the bone marrow also shows panhyperplasia with marked increase in megakaryocytes (Figure 19-4). The bone marrow findings are difficult to separate from myelofibrosis or polycythemia vera. As the disease progresses, there is frequently a transition to myelofibrosis.

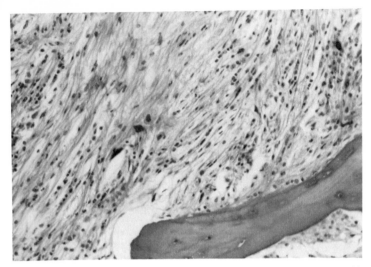

Figure 19-3. Extensive fibrosis of bone marrow biopsy from a patient with myelofibrosis.

Other Useful Tests

LEUKOCYTE ALKALINE PHOSPHATASE (LAP)

Purpose

The LAP score may be useful in differentiating CGL from other myeloproliferative disorders.

For sections on *Principle*, *Procedure*, and *Specimen*, see Chapter 14.

Interpretation

In CGL the LAP score is characteristically zero or markedly decreased. It is usually elevated in the other myeloproliferative disorders (Table 18-1) (see Chapter 18). In myelofibrosis with myeloid metaplasia, the LAP score may, however, be low. A low LAP

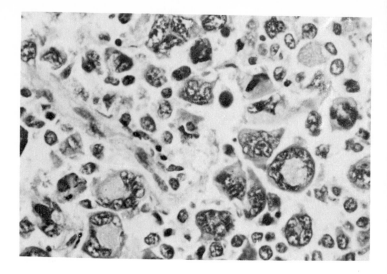

Figure 19-4. Bone marrow biopsy from a patient with essential thrombocythemia showing many atypical and bizarre megakaryocytes.

score, therefore, does not rule out myelofibrosis with myeloid metaplasia.

CYTOGENETIC STUDIES

Purpose

Cytogenetic studies may be useful in distinguishing CGL from the other myeloproliferative disorders.

For sections on *Principle*, *Procedures*, and *Specimen*, see Chapter 18.

Interpretation

The Philadelphia (Ph[1]) chromosome, which is present in approximately 90% of patients with CGL, is seen only in an extremely rare case of polycythemia vera, myelofibrosis with myeloid metaplasia, or essential thrombocythemia. Several chromosome changes have been observed in these disorders, but none are specific.

Ancillary Studies

BLEEDING TESTS

Bleeding problems may occur in myeloproliferative disorders, particularly in essential thrombocythemia and less frequently in myelofibrosis with myeloid metaplasia and polycythemia vera (10). The bleeding may be caused by thrombocytopenia or by a defect in platelet function. When the latter is present, often bleeding time is prolonged and in vitro platelet aggregation is impaired. The most frequent abnormality of in vitro platelet aggregation is failure to aggregate in response to epinephrine. Platelet adhesiveness may also be reduced. Platelet function tests have been suggested as useful in separating benign, reactive thrombocytosis from essential thrombocythemia. In the former, the platelet function tests usually show normal results.

RADIOLOGY

Osteosclerosis has been demonstrated in approximately 50% of patients with myelofibrosis with myeloid metaplasia; it is not seen in CGL. The bones that are most frequently affected are, in the order of frequency, femur, pelvis, humerus, vertebrae, radius, tibia, and sternum. Foci of rarefaction may also be seen.

BLOOD BIOCHEMISTRY

Serum uric acid is frequently elevated, especially in patients with high leukocyte counts. Serum alkaline phosphatase may also be elevated and may be a reflection of extramedullary hematopoiesis in the liver.

BIOPSY OF TISSUE OTHER THAN BONE MARROW

Extramedullary hematopoiesis may be associated with lymph node enlargement. Biopsy of the lymph node usually reveals the normal architecture to be maintained and the sinuses to contain a mixed proliferation of hematopoietic cells. Atypical megakaryocytes may predominate. Rarely, in myelofibrosis with myeloid metaplasia, extramedullary tumors develop. These tumors may occur in pleura, spinal cord, spleen, liver, mesentery, or retroperitoneal cavity. They are composed of immature hematopoietic cells and, unless megakaryocytes are prominent, such tumors may be mistaken for a lymphoma. A specific esterase stain is helpful in confirming the presence of granulocytic cell precursors (see Chapter 17). Biopsy of the lymph node is, however, rarely indicated.

SPECIAL DIAGNOSTIC CONSIDERATIONS

Acute Myelofibrosis (Myelosclerosis)

Acute, or malignant, myelofibrosis is a very rare disease characterized by pancytopenia, minimal poikilocytosis and anisocytosis (in contrast to myelofibrosis with myeloid metaplasia), bone marrow fibrosis, and hyperplasia of all three cell lines (11). Most of the cells present are immature and megakaryocytes are prominent. Also, in contrast to myelofibrosis with myeloid metaplasia, splenomegaly is minimal or absent. The disease is rapidly fatal.

REFERENCES

1. Gilbert HS: The spectrum of myeloproliferative disorders. Med Clin North Am 57:355–393, 1973
2. Videback A (ed): Polycythemia and myelofibrosis. Clin Haematol, vol 4, 1975. [An excellent source for review articles with comprehensive bibliographies.]
3. Laszlo J: Myeloproliferative disorders (MPD): Myelofibrosis, myelosclerosis, extramedullary hematopoiesis, undifferentiated MPD, and hemorrhagic thrombocythemia. Semin Hematol 12:409–432, 1975
4. Adamson JW, Fialkow PJ: Annotation: The pathogenesis of myeloproliferative syndromes. Br J Haematol 38:299–303, 1978
5. Rosenthal DS, Moloney WC: Occurrence of acute leukaemia in myeloproliferative disorders. Br J Haematol 36:373–382, 1977
6. Ward HP, Block MH: The natural history of agnogenic myeloid metaplasia (AMM) and a critical evaluation of its relationship with the myeloproliferative syndrome. Medicine 50:375–420, 1971

7. Takácsi-Nagy L, Graf F: Definition, clinical features and diagnosis of myelofibrosis. Clin Haematol 4:291–308, 1975

8. Gunz FW: Hemorrhagic thrombocythemia: A critical review. Blood 15:706–723, 1960

9. Buyssens N, Bourgeois NH: Chronic myelocytic leukemia versus idiopathic myelofibrosis. A diagnostic problem in bone marrow biopsies. Cancer 40:1548–1561, 1977

10. Weinfeld A, Branehög I, Kutti J: Platelets in myeloproliferative syndrome. Clin Haematol 4:373–392, 1975

11. Bearman RM, Pangalis GA, Rappaport H: Acute ("malignant") myelosclerosis. Cancer 43:287–301, 1979

chapter 20

Non-Hodgkin's Lymphoma

Malignant lymphoma is the generic term for malignant neoplasms of lymphoid tissue. Recent immunologic studies have revealed that they are neoplasms of the immune system and arise from their normal cell counterparts within the lymphoreticular system. The cells involved are lymphocytes and histiocytes. The neoplastic cell proliferation occurs in lymph nodes and lymphoid components of other tissues. The disease usually starts in lymph nodes, but when the patient is first seen, there is frequently evidence of lymphoma in other sites such as spleen, liver, and bone marrow. Less common are extranodal lymphomas, where the disease is initially confined to areas such as alimentary tract, thyroid, breast, gonads, or bone.

Malignant lymphoma differs from leukemia mainly in the distribution of the cell proliferation. Leukemia implies involvement of the bone marrow and the peripheral blood, while lymphoma denotes a malignant neoplasm initially confined to lymphoid tissue. As the lymphoma spreads, however, involvement of the bone marrow and occasionally lymphoma cells may often be seen in the peripheral blood. The term lymphosarcoma cell leukemia has been used for the latter occurrence.

In this chapter, all the malignant lymphomas other than Hodgkin's disease will be discussed. The latter, which differs considerably from the other lymphomas, will be described in Chapter 21. Disorders that may be mistaken for malignant lymphoma will also be discussed briefly.

The malignant lymphomas are a heterogenous group of disorders consisting of many subtypes. Over the years, numerous classifications of malignant lymphoma have been introduced. In contrast to Hodgkin's disease, there is unfortunately no international agreement with regard to staging or histopathologic classification. As a direct consequence of advances in immunology, our understanding of the function and morphology of the lymphoid system is changed. Thus, many of the lymphoid neoplasms can be divided into B and T cell proliferations, and we have learned to appreciate the wide range of morphologic expressions that lymphocytes and histiocytes may have. Thus, the histiocyte in Rappaport's classification is now recognized as being a transformed lymphocyte and not a true histiocyte (1). The controversy regarding the correct classification will undoubtedly continue as more information becomes available regarding the function and morphology of lymphocytes and histiocytes. Rappaport's classification is not biologically correct, but it remains the only classification that has been tested thoroughly for its clinical usefulness.

The clinical manifestations of malignant lymphoma are varied, but the most common presenting complaint is the discovery of enlarged, usually pain-free lymph nodes or an abdominal mass. Extranodal disease brings about one-third of patients to the physician. Fever, weight loss, or anorexia are less common manifestations. Lymphomas may have atypical clinical presentations such as symptoms secondary to compression of vital organs, for example, spinal cord compression, ureteral compression, or thoracic outlet syndrome.

A careful investigation of the patient as to the extent of the disease before treatment is extremely important for proper management. It is recommended that an extensive clinical staging be performed. The decision as to how extensive the staging procedure should be should ideally involve the primary physician, an oncologist, a radiotherapist, a surgeon, a pathologist, and a radiologist. The clinical staging includes physical examination, bone marrow aspiration and biopsy, radiologic studies to detect disease in the

Table 20-1. Recommended Procedures in Staging

Careful clinical history

Thorough physical examination with description of all superficial lymph nodes

Complete blood counts

Liver and renal function tests, serum uric acid, and calcium

Serum protein electrophoresis

Bone marrow biopsy (bilateral needle or open)

Lymph node biopsy to establish diagnosis, reviewed by hematopathologist

Radiologic studies (chest x-ray, lymphangiography, IVP, skeletal survey, as clinically indicated)

Cytologic examination of any effusion

Radioisotopic evaluation as clinically indicated

Exploratory laparotomy and splenectomy if information to be provided is likely to affect therapy

---

mediastinum, retroperitoneum, and bones; certain laboratory tests; and, in selected cases, exploratory laparotomy.

The physician must perform a detailed physical examination, listing and measuring all enlarged lymph nodes and noting the size of the spleen. The clinical staging procedures are summarized in Table 20-1.

The staging sequence is also important. After bone marrow biopsy in nodular, poorly differentiated lymphocytic lymphoma, 50%–70% of the patients will be shown to have marrow involvement, placing them in stage IV. Therefore, except for the histiocytic lymphomas, laparotomy is rarely necessary. The clinical classification of the extent or stage of disease is shown in Table 20-2.

Table 20-2. **Stages of Lymphoma**[a]

Stage	Criteria
Stage I	Disease limited to one anatomic region or to two contiguous anatomic regions, on the same side of the diaphragm
Stage II	Disease in more than two anatomic regions or in noncontiguous regions on the same side of the diaphragm
Stage III	Disease on both sides of the diaphragm, but limited to involvement of the lymph nodes and spleen
Stage IV	Disease of any lymph node region with involvement of liver, lung, or bone marrow.

[a]Modified from Peters MV, Hasselback R, Brown TC: The natural history of the lymphomas related to the clinical classification. In Zaratonetes CJD (ed): *Proceedings of the International Conference on Leukemia–Lymphoma.* Philadelphia, Lea & Febiger, 1968, pp. 357–370.

DIAGNOSTIC EVALUATION

The results of treatment of malignant lymphoma have recently been significantly improved. Good management requires a team approach. The clinician, oncologist, radiotherapist, and pathologist should communicate in planning the evaluation of the patient and in the management.

After a clinical history and physical examination have been completed, the evaluation of a patient with possible malignant lymphoma should proceed in the following fashion (Table 20-1):

1. Hematologic evaluation
   a. Complete blood cell count including platelet count, to establish baseline figures prior to treatment. Evaluation of peripheral blood smear is essential to detect lymphoma cells in the peripheral blood and may be important for the differential diagnosis.
   b. Bone marrow aspirate and biopsy examination are required in the evaluation, since certain types of malignant lymphomas have a high incidence of bone marrow involvement.

2. Tissue biopsy is required for a diagnosis of malignant lymphoma. Such a diagnosis is one of the most difficult problems in surgical pathology, and consultation from a hematopathologist is desirable. The major reason for difficulties in interpretation of lymph nodes is technical and arises from improper handling of the biopsy specimen. Too frequently, a wrong lymph node is biopsied or an inadequate specimen is obtained. Biopsy of inguinal, parotid, and submandibular lymph nodes should be avoided if possible, since they frequently show reactive changes. The biopsy should be performed with the intent of removing the lymph node that appears to be most involved rather than the node that is most accessible. The lymph node must be delivered to the pathologist intact immediately after removal. Before putting the specimen in fixative, touch imprints should be made of a section from one end of the lymph node. The remaining portion of the node should be put in fixative such as 10% buffered formalin or a formalin-mercury fixative (B 5) for one hour. It should then be cut into 2–3 mm sections and further fixed for another 24 hours. The sections should have a thickness of only one cell in order to evaluate the cytologic features. Also, too-thick sections may mask a nodular pattern. Finally, the tissue must be well stained to enable evaluation of the cytologic features. The diagnosis and subclassification of malignant lymphoma should be made on the basis of the histopathologic features in a lymph node biopsy before any treatment is performed. The initial diagnosis should not be made on the basis of a bone marrow biopsy or liver biopsy alone. In true extranodal lymphomas, the diagnosis will have to be made from biopsy of the organ involved; however, every attempt should be made to find a lymph node that can be biopsied.

a. Cytologic examination of any effusion is mandatory to establish the presence of malignant cells in pleural or peritoneal cavity or in the cerebrospinal fluid.

b. Liver involvement is common in non-Hodgkin's lymphoma and can be documented by percutaneous or peritoneoscopic guided liver biopsy.

c. Immunologic and cytochemical studies of malignant cells from biopsy material and/or blood and other body fluids may be of help in establishing a correct diagnosis.

d. Terminal deoxynucleotidyl transferase (TDT) determinations may be performed on fresh or frozen tissue or cellular suspensions.

3. Radiologic studies should include a chest x-ray, inferior venocavagram, intravenous pyelogram, and bilateral lymphangiogram of the lower extremity. Bone and liver scans and gastrointestinal studies are indicated in symptomatic patients. These procedures should be used selectively and only if there is clinical suspicion of involvement of an anatomic area or organ, if the result is likely to influence therapy, or if an investigative study requires it. The procedures are expensive and some are not without morbidity.

4. Evaluation of renal function and liver function should be made before any therapy is performed.

5. Exploratory laparotomy and splenectomy are of value in staging the extent of disease in selected patients.

6. Special procedures include serum protein electrophoresis and immunoelectrophoresis, Coombs test, and serum uric acid and calcium tests.

7. Ancillary studies include estimate of patient's delayed hypersensitivity and chromosome studies. Chromosome studies, however, are expensive and unless an investigative study is being carried out, the information obtained from this procedure is of little practical benefit in non-Hodgkin's lymphoma.

LABORATORY STUDIES

Tissue Biopsy

The histologic features of a lymphoma are characterized by a proliferation of malignant lymphocytes or histiocytes that partially or completely obliterate the normal lymph node architecture. The non-Hodgkin's lymphomas are separated into those with a nodular (follicular) architectural pattern and those with a diffuse pattern. It is important to be able to differentiate a nodular from a diffuse pattern, because the former has a considerably better prognosis. Further classification depends on the predominant cell type present.

In recent years, many new classifications have been added to this complicated and controversial field of pathology (Tables 20-3 and 20-4). Thus, clinicians and pathologists are now in the unenviable position of having at least six major classifications from which to choose. In this chapter, Rappaport's classification, with minor

Table 20-3. Classification of Non-Hodgkin's Lymphoma[a]

Nodular (follicular)
  Lymphocytic, well differentiated (rare)
  Lymphocytic, poorly differentiated
  Mixed cell
  Histiocytic

Diffuse
  Lymphocytic, well differentiated
  Lymphocytic, intermediate differentiation
  Lymphocytic, poorly differentiated
  Mixed cell
  Histiocytic
  Undifferentiated, Burkitt's
  Undifferentiated, pleomorphic (non-Burkitt's)
  Lymphoblastic
  Non-Hodgkin's lymphoma with epithelioid histiocytic reaction (Lennert's
    lymphoma)
  Unclassifiable

[a]Modified Rappaport.

Table 20-4. Classification of Non-Hodgkin's Lymphoma[a]

U cell (undefined)

T cell types
  Small lymphocyte
  Convoluted lymphocyte
  Sézary syndrome—mycosis fungoides
  Immunoblastic sarcoma
  Lennert's lymphoma

B cell type
  Small lymphocyte
  Plasmacytoid lymphocyte
  Follicular center cell types (follicular or diffuse, with or without sclerosis)
    Small cleaved
    Large cleaved
    Small transformed (noncleaved)
    Large transformed (noncleaved)
  Immunoblastic sarcoma

Histiocytic

[a]Modified from Lukes RJ, Collins RD: The Lukes-Collins classification and its significance. Conference on non-Hodgkin's Lymphomas, San Francisco, September 30–October 2, 1976. Cancer Treat Rep 61:971-979, 1977.

modifications, has been used (Table 20-3). The advances made in immunology, cytochemistry, and electron microscopy have produced several changes in our understanding of the function and morphology of the lymphoreticular system. It has been shown that all nodular lymphomas arise from follicular (germinal center) B-lymphocytes, and the histiocytic lymphomas are rarely true histiocytes but are instead transformed B-lymphocytes. The histiocytic lymphoma in Rappaport's classification now appears to be a heterogenous group of lymphomas. Despite these shortcomings, this classification is the one most commonly used in the United States. It has proven to be clinically useful and is reasonably reproducible by pathologists.

The correct histopathologic diagnosis must be established before any treatment is performed because the pathologic findings will predict several histologic and clinical factors. Thus, a patient diagnosed as having poorly differentiated lymphocytic lymphoma or mixed cell lymphoma has an 80% probability of having a nodular lymphoma and only a 20% chance of having diffuse lymphoma. In contrast, less than 10% of malignant lymphomas of the histiocytic type are nodular. About 90% of patients with poorly differentiated lymphocytic or mixed cell lymphomas have stage III or IV disease.

If a lymphoma is first diagnosed in an extranodal site (e.g., bone marrow or liver) and an assessment of the histologic pattern is to be performed (i.e., nodular or diffuse), a careful search should be made for a lymph node that can be biopsied. This is important because the greatest influence on prognosis is the presence of nodularity.

Sequential biopsies may show a change in histologic type over a period of time. This change is almost always toward a more malignant form, such as nodular to diffuse or poorly differentiated lymphocytic lymphoma to histiocytic lymphoma. Unless an investigative study is being carried out, however, sequential biopsies are of little practical value.

Nodular (follicular) lymphomas

The nodular lymphomas account for 50% of all non-Hodgkin's lymphomas in the United States. They occur predominantly in the older age group and occur with equal frequency in both sexes. Gastrointestinal involvement is less common in nodular lymphomas than in the diffuse. Patients with nodular lymphomas have a considerably better prognosis than those with diffuse lymphoma, even though the disease is more frequently disseminated at the time of diagnosis.

The nodular lymphomas are characterized by a nodular growth pattern and must be distinguished from reactive follicular hyperplasia (Figure 20-1). They are neoplasms of B-lymphocytes originating in the germinal centers and are divided into three main subtypes (Table 20-3). Those made up of predominantly small cleaved lymphocytes are called *malignant lymphoma, poorly differentiated lymphocytic type* (Figure 20-2). The term malignant lymphoma, *histiocytic type,* is used for those nodular lymphomas that are composed mainly of large cells. Finally, the term *mixed cell type* is used for those lymphomas that have a mixture of small cleaved and large lymphocytes.

Nodular histiocytic lymphomas have a poorer prognosis than the other two types and are more prone to progress into a diffuse lymphoma. Not infrequently, both a nodular and diffuse pattern occur in the same lymph node. In patients with poorly differentiated lymphocytic or mixed cell lymphoma, this does not imply a poorer prognosis. In histiocytic lymphoma, however, a nodular and diffuse pattern indicates a significantly poorer prognosis than a pure nodular type.

Patients with nodular, poorly differentiated lymphocytic lymphoma or mixed cell type usually have involvement of bone marrow and liver, and lymphoma cells may be seen in the blood (lymphosarcoma cell leukemia). In contrast, the nodular histiocytic

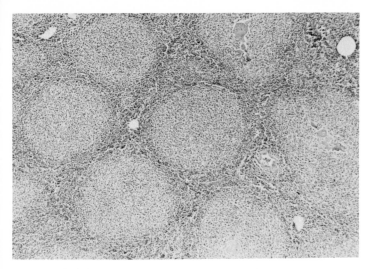

Figure 20-1. Malignant lymphoma with nodular pattern.

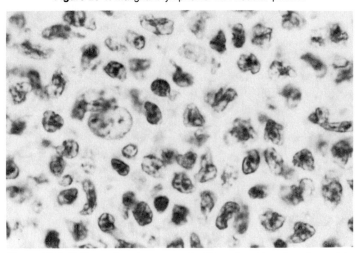

Figure 20-2. Malignant lymphoma, poorly differentiated lymphocytic, nodular. Many cells have small, twisted, and cleaved nuclei and scant, indistinct cytoplasm.

lymphoma, which is a more aggressive tumor, is rarely seen in the blood.

Diffuse lymphomas

The diffuse lymphomas are a heterogenous group of tumors occurring in young as well as older individuals and are twice as common in men as in women. In contrast to the nodular lymphomas, constitutional symptoms are common. The diffuse lymphomas often present with intra-abdominal disease. This is particularly so with diffuse histiocytic lymphoma. Except for the well-differentiated lymphocytic lymphoma, the prognosis in diffuse lymphomas is considerably less favorable than with the nodular lymphomas

Well-differentiated lymphocytic lymphomas (WDL) characteristically reveal diffuse infiltration of the lymph node by small, normal-appearing lymphocytes (Figure 20-3). The histologic features are indistinguishable from those observed in chronic lymphocytic leukemia (CLL). This type of lymphoma may be mistaken for Hodgkin's disease, lymphocyte predominance type. The latter disease should be suspected in any patient less than 40 years of age who has a lymph node showing diffuse involvement by small, normal-appearing lymphocytes, and a careful search for Reed-Sternberg cells must be made.

The majority of well-differentiated lymphocytic lymphomas are composed of B-lymphocytes. In a small percentage of patients with well-differentiated lymphocytic malignancies, the cell proliferations consist of a mixture of lymphocytes, plasma cells, and plasmacytoid lymphocytes. If, in addition, the cells secrete monoclonal IgM into the serum, the disease is referred to as Waldenström's macroglobulinemia.

The *diffuse, poorly differentiated lymphocytic lymphomas* are composed of small cleaved lymphocytes (Figure 20-4). Many of these tumors may have originated as nodular, poorly differentiated lymphocytic lymphomas and most are composed of B-lymphocytes.

The *diffuse, mixed cell lymphomas* are less common and are composed of an equal mixture of small cleaved lymphocytes and

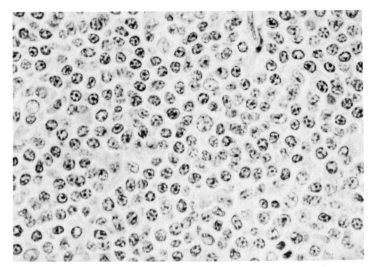

Figure 20-3. Malignant lymphoma, well-differentiated lymphocytic.

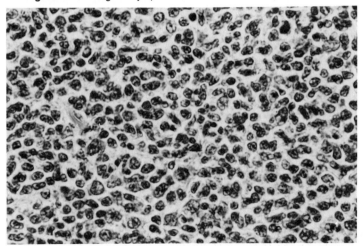

Figure 20-4. Malignant lymphoma, poorly differentiated lymphocytic, diffuse. Compare the appearance of the small cleaved lymphocytes in this figure with the small, normal-appearing lymphocytes in Figure 20-3.

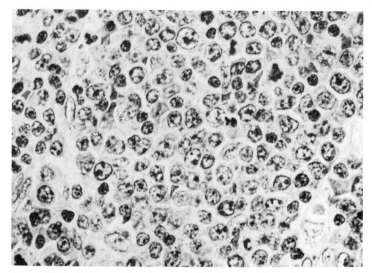

Figure 20-5. Malignant lymphoma, histiocytic type. The cells have round, large nuclei and nucleoli are seen in some cells.

large lymphocytes, which have vesicular nuclei and prominent nucleoli. Immunologic studies have shown that most of these tumors also are B cell malignancies.

The *diffuse histiocytic, or large cell,* lymphomas are characterized by a proliferation of large mononuclear cells (Figure 20-5). The histiocytic lymphoma classified by Rappaport consists of a heterogenous group of lymphomas, the majority of which are composed of lymphocytes at various stages of transformation, and is associated with subtle morphologic variations. Only a small percentage is composed of true histiocytes.

In contrast to nodular lymphomas, the diffuse histiocytic lymphomas are frequently limited to one side of the diaphragm. About 30% of patients are found to have localized disease (i.e., stage I or stage II). The histiocytic lymphomas are more frequently present in extranodal sites than the other lymphomas and are usually found in the gastrointestinal tract, skin, or bone. In addition, the pattern of involvement in the spleen and liver is different in the histiocytic lymphomas. While the poorly differentiated lymphocytic lymphomas are distributed in small, uniform nodules throughout, the histiocytic lymphomas produce large, irregular, often destructive tumors in the spleen and liver.

About 50% of histiocytic lymphomas are composed of B-lymphocytes, approximately 30% are null cells, 5%–15% have T cell markers, and about 5% are true histiocytic tumors. The prognosis in most histiocytic lymphomas is still poor, but significant progress has been demonstrated in certain subtypes.

The so-called *Lennert's lymphoma* is associated with a prominent epithelioid histiocytic reaction and is now realized to be a heterogenous group of disorders that includes non-Hodgkin's lymphoma, Hodgkin's disease, and angioimmunoblastic lymphadenopathy. Only non-Hodgkin's lymphoma with an epithelioid histiocytic reaction appears to be a distinct clinicopathologic entity. Lymph nodes from patients with this disease reveal a proliferation of small, intermediate, and large lymphocytes together with scattered epithelioid histiocytes (Figure 20-6). The lymphocytes have slightly irregular nuclear contours but considerably less than what is seen in poorly differentiated lymphocytic lymphoma. The major reason for separating the non-Hodgkin's lymphoma with epithelioid histiocytic reaction as a distinct entity is that the disease is usually disseminated at the time of diagnosis (stage III or IV) and the prognosis is poor.

The *undifferentiated, Burkitt's type of lymphoma* is composed of primitive-appearing cells (Figure 20-7). The nuclei of these cells are about the same size as the nuclei of the benign starry-sky macrophages frequently observed in this tumor. The cytoplasm often contains fat vacuoles, which are most readily seen in Romanovsky-type stained imprints of the tumor. Burkitt's tumor cells are B-lymphocytes and may be derived from B cells of germinal centers. The cells from Burkitt's lymphoma have a characteristic cytochemical triad consisting of negative periodic acid-Schiff stain and positive oil red-O and methyl green-pyronine stains.

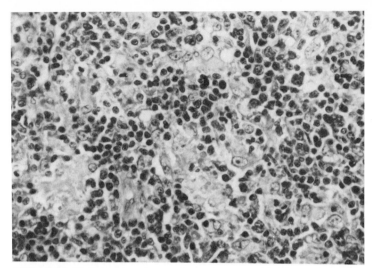

Figure 20-6. Malignant lymphoma with an epithelioid histiocytic reaction (Lennert's lymphoma).

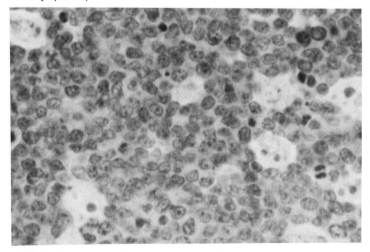

Figure 20-7. Undifferentiated, Burkitt's lymphoma. Note starry-sky macrophages and a uniform population of tumor cells.

In central Africa, where the Burkitt's tumor is endemic, the disease frequently presents as a maxillomandibular lesion. American patients with Burkitt's tumor frequently have disease localized in the abdomen, ileocecal region, retroperitoneum, or ovaries. A leukemic phase is unusual. Burkitt's lymphoma is seen most commonly in children, but it may also be present in adults.

The undifferentiated, non-Burkitt's lymphoma differs histologically from Burkitt's lymphoma, with cells that vary considerably more in size and shape. These tumors may be more appropriately classified with the histiocytic lymphomas and are characterized by an aggressive clinical course with poor prognosis.

The *lymphoblastic lymphomas* were recently separated from the diffuse, poorly differentiated lymphocytic lymphomas as a distinct clinicopathologic entity. The disease was previously called Sternberg's sarcoma or lymphosarcoma of childhood. Lymphoblastic lymphomas are composed of a uniform population of cells similar to those seen in acute lymphoblastic leukemia (Figure 20-8). The nuclei may be convoluted or nonconvoluted and have a fine chromatin pattern. A high mitotic rate is a consistent finding.

The lymphoblastic lymphomas are seen most frequently in children but may also be seen in adults. Mediastinal tumors are seen in at least 50% of patients, and the disease spreads rapidly to involve bone marrow, peripheral blood, and central nervous system. Immunologic studies have revealed that most of the lymphoblastic lymphomas are composed of T-lymphocytes. This tumor is generally very responsive to therapy, including ALL therapy, but it tends to recur rapidly and becomes resistant to subsequent treatment. The optimal treatment program at present is unknown. However, the disease is different from most other non-Hodgkin's lymphomas and requires CNS prophylaxis and continuous vigorous chemotherapy for a prolonged period.

Mycosis fungoides and Sézary syndrome

Mycosis fungoides and Sézary syndrome are closely related diseases. Both are T cell disorders, primarily involving the skin. Clini-

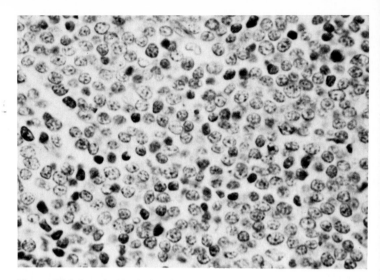

Figure 20-8. Lymphoblastic lymphoma composed of a uniform population of cells with scant cytoplasm and delicate chromatin pattern.

cally, mycosis fungoides presents as a scaly or eczematous lesion that progresses through a plaque stage to eventually form tumors in the skin. Sézary syndrome is characterized by exfoliative erythroderma. Biopsies of the skin reveal lymphocytic infiltrates in the upper dermis, frequently with infiltrates in the epidermis (Pautrier's abscesses). The nuclei of the lymphocytes have deeply indented or convoluted contours. As the disease progresses, neoplastic cells may be seen in lymph nodes, lung, liver, spleen, and other organs. Atypical lymphocytes with convoluted or cerebriform nuclei may also be seen in the peripheral blood. In mycosis fungoides, the presence of these cells in the peripheral blood is frequently associated with progressive disease. Sézary syndrome may be considered a leukemic phase of mycosis fungoides when lymphocytosis exists.

Malignant histiocytosis is a rare disease of true histiocytes. It is characterized by rapid onset, fever, pancytopenia, hepatospleno-

Table 20-5. Surface Markers in Lymphoreticular Neoplasms

Well-differentiated lymphocytic lymphoma	B cell
Chronic lymphocytic leukemia (98%)	B cell
Waldenström's macroglobulinemia	B cell
Nodular (follicular) lymphomas	B cell
Burkitt's lymphoma	B cell
Histiocytic lymphoma	Heterogenous (majority B or null cells, some T cells and, rarely, true histiocytic)
Lymphoblastic lymphoma	T or null cell
Mycosis fungoides and Sèzary syndrome	T cell
Chronic lymphocytic leukemia (5%)	T cell
Malignant histiocytosis	Histiocytic

megaly, and lymphadenopathy. The disease is usually rapidly fatal. Histologically, atypical histiocytes proliferating within sinusoids of lymph nodes, liver, and spleen are seen.

SPECIAL TESTS

In addition to the routine histologic examination of the tissue biopsy, it may be necessary to perform special studies on the malignant cells to subclassify the tumor (Table 20-5). Thus, cell surface markers on live cell suspensions from tissue biopsy may be used to separate the malignant lymphocytes into B, T, and null cells. Evidence exists that in the diffuse, poorly differentiated lymphocytic lymphomas, the patients with B cell tumors have a considerably better prognosis than patients who have tumors composed of null or T cells.

Immunofluorescent studies on frozen tissue specimens or the *immunoperoxidase technique* on paraffin sections may be used to identify immunoglobulins within the cytoplasm of cells. These techniques may also be used to separate poorly differentiated carcinomas from histiocytic lymphomas.

Cytochemical studies, such as the nonspecific esterase stain performed on imprints from tissue biopsy or on frozen sections of tissue, help in differentiating lymphocytic tumors from true histiocytic tumors (see Chapter 17). The specific esterase stain may be used to differentiate granulocytic cells, as in granulocytic sarcomas (chloromas) from lymphocytes and histiocytes.

Finally, the TDT assay may be of use in identifying the lymphoblastic lymphomas, since this enzyme only appears to be elevated in lymphoblastic lymphomas and not in the other lymphomas (see Chapter 17). TDT assays can be performed on fresh or frozen tissue or on cellular suspensions.

Hematologic Tests

GENERAL FEATURES

The majority of patients with non-Hodgkin's lymphoma have normal blood counts. Anemia develops during the course of the disease in about 50% of patients. The causes of anemia may be one or several of the following: (a) bone marrow insufficiency resulting from marrow replacement lymphoma; (b) therapy-induced bone marrow hypoplasia; (c) hypersplenism; (d) autoimmune hemolytic anemia; (e) bleeding from lymphoma in the gastrointestinal tract or from low platelet count.

BLOOD

Circulating lymphoma cells (lymphosarcoma cell leukemia) is seen in a few patients with non-Hodgkin's lymphoma. This is not a specific clinicopathologic entity and may be seen in any of the subtypes of lymphoma. In nodular, poorly differentiated lymphocytic lymphoma, a leukemic phase may be observed in 5%–10% of patients. The leukemic cells have a characteristic notched or clefted nucleus (see Chapter 17).

BONE MARROW

Bone marrow aspiration and particularly a bone marrow biopsy should be performed early in the evaluation. A bilateral, posterior iliac crest bone marrow biopsy increases the chance of finding lymphoma by more than 20%. Positive results on biopsy, which indicate stage IV disease, allow curtailment of much of the staging evaluation. A bone marrow examination should, therefore, always be performed prior to any extensive radiologic examination or laparotomy.

The bone marrow is involved at the time of diagnosis in 70%–85% of patients with nodular, poorly differentiated lymphocytic lymphoma and in 50% of patients with diffuse, poorly differentiated lymphocytic lymphoma and mixed cell lymphoma. The histiocytic lymphomas are associated much less frequently with bone marrow involvement.

The pattern of bone marrow involvement is usually focal or nodular rather than diffuse. No good correlation can be made between the pattern of involvement (i.e., diffuse versus nodular) in lymph nodes and in the bone marrow. Nodules of lymphoma in the bone marrow must be differentiated from benign lymphoid nodules, which are commonly seen in older individuals. Nodules of malignant lymphoma are not as well circumscribed as benign lymphoid nodules, and in lymphoma the infiltrate is frequently located adjacent to bone trabeculae (paratrabecular position). Furthermore, in benign lymphoid nodules, the lymphocytes are small and normal appearing.

Special Procedures

RADIOLOGIC STUDIES

In addition to establishing the specific diagnosis, the anatomic extent of the disease must be determined. Various radiologic techniques are used to detect disease in the mediastinum, retroperitoneum, and bones. Mediastinal and hilar lymph nodes are evaluated primarily by standard posteroanterior and lateral radiographs of the chest. For detecting disease below the diaphragm, a bilateral lymphangiogram of the lower extremity is used. Splenic hilar, celiac, porta hepatis, and mesenteric nodes are, however, not demonstrated by lymphangiogram. An inferior venacavogram is useful in demonstrating enlarged lymph nodes high in the para-aortic chain. When positive, it is thought to be accurate in 90% of cases and the lymphangiogram in 80%. Liver and spleen scans, when positive, are considered accurate in 50% and 75% of cases respectively. Computed tomographic (CT) scanning techniques may provide additional information as to the extent of abdominal disease. An intravenous pyelogram may demonstrate ureteral obstruction.

RENAL AND LIVER FUNCTION TESTS

Evaluation of renal and liver function by routine serum chemistries and urinalysis should be performed on every patient. It may be helpful in detecting disease in those organs and must be performed as part of the evaluation before the patient is given chemotherapy and/or radiotherapy.

LAPAROTOMY

Controversy still exists regarding the need for exploratory laparotomy with splenectomy in staging of non-Hodgkin's lymphomas. Its use is probably rarely necessary except in some patients with diffuse, histiocytic lymphoma. In such individuals, it may be used to determine if there is limited disease that may be cured by radiotherapy. If a laparotomy is to be performed, a preoperative lymphangiogram should be taken as a guide to direct surgical sampling of the lymph nodes. In addition, a wedge biopsy of the liver and an open surgical biopsy of the iliac crest bone marrow should be obtained.

CYTOLOGY OF EFFUSIONS

Pleural effusions are not uncommon in malignant lymphomas, and cytologic examination of fluid specimens is an essential part of the clinical evaluation.

Ancillary Studies

SERUM AND URINE PROTEIN ELECTROPHORESIS AND IMMUNOELECTROPHORESIS

The non-Hodgkin's lymphomas may sometimes be associated with a monoclonal gammopathy (usually IgM) or occasionally hypogammaglobulinemia.

SERUM BIOCHEMISTRY

Serum calcium levels may be elevated in malignant lymphoma, and uric acid levels may increase dramatically during treatment.

CYTOGENETIC STUDIES

Chromosome studies of lymphoma tissue have revealed that a 14 q translocation is the single most frequent abnormality. However, specific patterns related to subtypes of lymphomas are not yet apparent and chromosome studies are of little practical benefit in non-Hodgkin's lymphoma.

SPECIAL DIAGNOSTIC CONSIDERATIONS

Diseases Simulating Malignant Lymphoma

A variety of disorders other than malignant lymphomas may cause enlargement of lymph nodes and may be mistaken histologically for lymphoma (Table 20-6). Such conditions include infectious mononucleosis, toxoplasmosis, giant lymph node hyperplasia, sinus histiocytosis with massive lymphadenopathy, postvaccinal lymphadenitis, certain drug (hydantoin) reactions, cat-scratch disease, and metastatic, poorly differentiated carcinoma. Rheumatoid arthritis, lupus erythematosus, and secondary syphilis may also be associated with lymphadenopathy. Pathologists must be provided with an accurate clinical history, and they must be familiar with the changes in lymph nodes produced by these disorders.

Table 20-6. **Causes of Lymph Node Enlargement Simulating Malignant Lymphoma**

Reactive follicular hyperplasia
Infectious mononucleosis
Toxoplasmosis
Cat-scratch disease
Viral lymphadenitis (herpes zoster)
Syphilis
Phenylhydantoin (Dilantin) lymph node hyperplasia
Rheumatoid arthritis
Dermatopathic lymphadenopathy
Giant lymph node hyperplasia
Sinus histiocytosis with massive lymphadenopathy
Immunoblastic lymphadenopathy
Leukemia
Metastatic carcinoma and melanoma

Immunoblastic lymphadenopathy is a recently described entity associated with enlarged lymph nodes, fever, hemolytic anemia, and polyclonal gammopathy. Frequently, there is history of a drug reaction. Biopsy of the lymph node shows effacement of normal architecture, with marked vascularity and a proliferation of immunoblasts, plasma cells, eosinophils, and epithelioid histiocytes. In some patients, the disease may progress into a malignant lymphoma (immunoblastic lymphoma or sarcoma).

So-called *pseudolymphoma* is a lymphoreticular proliferation that forms benign or reactive tumors. The most common sites are the skin, stomach, intestine, and lung. Occasionally, only the passage of time will allow differentiation of a pseudolymphoma from a malignant lymphoma. The presence of germinal centers, a mixed cell population, and no involvement of regional lymph nodes are features that support the presence of a pseudolymphoma. A regional lymph node biopsy should, therefore, be obtained if possible.

REFERENCES

1. Rappaport H: Tumors of the hematopoietic system. In *Atlas of Tumor Pathology*. Washington DC, Armed Forces Institute of Pathology, 1966, Section III, Fascicle 8

SUGGESTED READING

Dorfman RF, Warnke R: Lymphadenopathy simulating the malignant lymphomas. Hum Pathol 5:519–550, 1974

Lukes RJ, Parker JW, Taylor CR, et al: Immunologic approach to non-Hodgkin lymphomas and related leukemias. Analysis of the results of multiparameter studies of 425 cases. Semin Hematol 15:322–351, 1978

Mann RB, Jaffe ES, Berard CW: Malignant lymphomas—a conceptual understanding of morphologic diversity. Am J Pathol 94:105–192, 1979 [An excellent up-to-date review of the histopathologic, immunologic, and cytochemical aspects of malignant lymphomas.]

Jones SE, Godden J (eds): Proceedings of the Conference on Non-Hodgkin's Lymphomas. San Francisco, 1976. Cancer Treat 61:935–1230, 1977

Rosenberg SA (ed): Hodgkin's disease and other lymphomas. Clin Haematol, vol 3, 1974. [An excellent source for review of articles with comprehensive bibliographies.]

chapter **21**

Hodgkin's Disease

Hodgkin's disease is a complex disorder of the immune system composed of neoplastic mononuclear cells mixed with variable numbers of presumably reactive lymphocytes, plasma cells, eosinophils, and histiocytes. The exact nature of the malignant cell population is still unsettled. Controversy exists as to whether the neoplastic cells are transformed lymphocytes or histiocytes.

Hodgkin's disease differs from non-Hodgkin's lymphomas in patterns of organ involvement and requires a slightly different approach to staging the extent of disease. The spread of Hodgkin's disease is more predictable and is generally from lymph node to lymph node by contiguity. Patients with Hodgkin's disease have less frequent involvement of Waldeyer's ring, gastrointestinal tract, mesenteric lymph nodes, bone marrow, and less advanced disease when seen initially. In addition, they more often have involvement of the mediastinal lymph nodes than patients with non-Hodgkin's lymphoma.

Today, the majority of patients with Hodgkin's disease can be cured if managed properly. The management should be a team approach and should ideally include the primary physician, an oncologist, a surgeon, a radiotherapist, a radiologist, and a pathologist. The biopsy specimen should preferably by reviewed by a hematopathologist.

The clinical presentation of Hodgkin's disease is usually a progressive, painless enlargement of a lymph node(s) in the neck. A few patients present with a mediastinal mass that may be discovered on a routine radiograph of the chest or on a film taken to diagnose respiratory symptoms. Hodgkin's disease is associated more frequently with constitutional symptoms such as fever, night sweats, pruritis, and weight loss than is non-Hodgkin's lymphomas. Physical examination may reveal, in addition to enlarged lymph nodes, splenomegaly and hepatomegaly. All enlarged lymph nodes must be noted and measured. Right supraclavicular or cervical involvement suggests mediastinal disease, and left supraclavicular, left cervical, and inguinal lymphadenopathy often correlate with abdominal disease.

DIAGNOSTIC EVALUATION

After a clinical history has been taken and careful physical examination made, the approach to the diagnosis of Hodgkin's disease proceeds in a similar fashion to that of non-Hodgkin's lymphoma (Table 20-1). (See Chapter 20).

1. Tissue biopsy. The diagnosis and subclassification of malignant lymphoma should be made on the basis of the histopathologic features in a lymph node biopsy before any treatment is performed. The initial diagnosis must not be made on the basis of a bone marrow biopsy or liver biopsy alone. Every attempt should be made to find a lymph node biopsy. The histologic examination of a lymph node biopsy is considered one of the most difficult areas of surgical pathology. The major reason for difficulties in the interpretation of lymph node biopsies is improper handling of the biopsy specimen (see Chapter 20).

2. Hematologic evaluation
   a. Complete blood cell count should include hemoglobin, white cell, and platelet count. A well-prepared blood smear should be reviewed and a differential white cell count made.
   b. Bone marrow study. A bone marrow aspirate rarely demonstrates involvement by Hodgkin's disease. The involvement is usually focal and is associated with fibrosis. Biopsy of the bone marrow is therefore mandatory.

3. Special studies to determine the extent of disease include chest roentgenography, intravenous pyelography, bilateral lower extrem-

Table 21-1. Classification of Hodgkin's Disease

Lukes and Butler	Rye Modification
Lymphocytic and/or histiocytic predominance Nodular Diffuse	Lymphocytic predominance
Nodular sclerosis	Nodular sclerosis
Mixed cellularity	Mixed cellularity
Lymphocytic depletion Diffuse fibrosis Reticular type	Lymphocytic depletion

ity lymphangiography, skeletal survey, and exploratory laparotomy with splenectomy in selected patients.

4. Ancillary studies that may aid in the management of Hodgkin's disease include serum alkaline phosphatase, uric acid and calcium, urinanalysis, and evaluation of renal function.

LABORATORY STUDIES

Tissue Biopsy

The lymph node that appears to be most involved should be removed rather than the node that is most accessible. The biopsy material should be reviewed by an experienced hematopathologist.

In contrast to the non-Hodgkin's lymphomas, one histopathologic classification is generally accepted for Hodgkin's disease, namely the one proposed by Lukes and Butler and modified at the Rye symposium into four subcategories (1) (Table 21-1). Three of the types (lymphocytic predominance, mixed cellularity, lymphocytic depletion) differ mainly in the relative proportions of malignant mononuclear and Reed-Sternberg cells to reactive cells. Correlation is good between the ratio of lymphocytes to neoplastic cells in the lymph node biopsy and biologic behavior of the tumor.

Thus, when lymphocytic proliferation is prominent, Reed-Sternberg cells are rare, the disease is more likely to be localized, and the prognosis is better.

The Reed-Sternberg cell, which is required for the pathologic diagnosis of Hodgkin's disease, is a large binucleated or multinucleated cell. It has a characteristic clear halo around a large nucleus and a prominent eosinophilic or amphophilic nucleolus. Mononuclear variants with the nuclear features of Reed-Sternberg cells are also observed. Even though the presence of Reed-Sternberg cells is required for a pathologic diagnosis of Hodgkin's disease, similar if not identical cells may be observed in a variety of other disorders, including infectious mononucleosis and metastatic carcinoma. Therefore, the appropriate architectural and cellular environment is required in addition to Reed-Sternberg cells to make a diagnosis of Hodgkin's disease.

TYPES OF HODGKIN'S DISEASE

In the *lymphocytic predominant* type, the lymph node is completely or partially obliterated by small, mature-appearing lymphocytes and varying numbers of histiocytes (Figure 21-1). The pattern is usually diffuse but may be vaguely nodular. Reed-Sternberg cells are few and multiple sections may have to be examined in order to find them. Most patients with this type of Hodgkin's disease are in clinical stage I or II and are asymptomatic; the majority can be cured.

The *mixed cellularity* type is characterized by a greater number of abnormal mononuclear cells, and Reed-Sternberg cells are readily observed (Figure 21-2). A variable number of eosinophils, plasma cells, and histiocytes are usually present. This type of Hodgkin's disease has a prognosis that is intermediate between lymphocytic predominance and lymphocytic depletion type. Patients usually have stage III or IV disease and are symptomatic.

The *lymphocytic depletion* type reveals a paucity of lymphocytes with increased numbers of abnormal mononuclear cells; Reed-

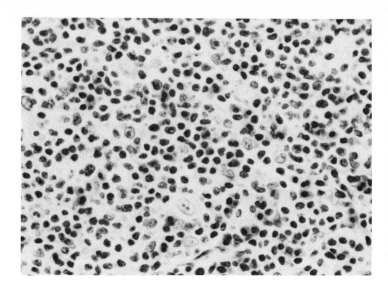

Figure 21-1. Lymph node section from patient with Hodgkin's disease showing numerous normal-appearing lymphocytes and some atypical mononuclear cells. Reed-Sternberg cells were rare and are not seen in this field.

Sternberg cells are often numerous (Figure 21-3). Fibrosis and necrosis may be prominent. The lymphocytic depletion type is the least favorable form with respect to prognosis, since it is the most likely to present with invasion of bone marrow. The patient is usually older with stage III or IV disease and is symptomatic.

The *nodular sclerosis* category has two distinctive histologic features. The lymph node is divided into nodules by thick bands of collagen, and the Reed-Sternberg cells are present in lacunar spaces (so-called lacunar cells) (Figure 21-4). This form of Hodgkin's disease occurs equally in both sexes, while in all the other types, it predominates in males. Its occurrence is unusual in patients over 50 years of age. Nodular sclerosis is usually associated with lower cervical, supraclavicular, and mediastinal lymph node involve-

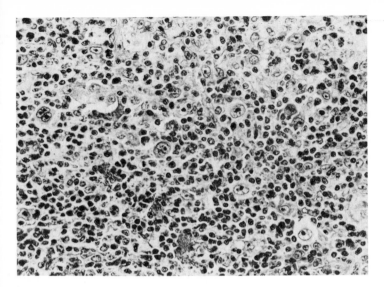

Figure 21-2. Hodgkin's disease, mixed cellularity type. Binucleated Reed-Sternberg cells and mononuclear variants are easily seen.

ment. It is the type most commonly affecting the lungs. The majority of patients have clinical stage II disease and most can be cured.

Simultaneous biopsies from different anatomic sites in patients with Hodgkin's disease usually reveal similar histology. Sequential biopsies, however, may show a change in histologic type over a period of time. This is almost always toward a more malignant form of Hodgkin's disease, such as a change from lymphocytic predominance to mixed cellularity or lymphocytic depletion type. On the other hand, nodular sclerosis rarely changes to another histologic type.

It should be noted that the prognostic differences described for the four subcategories of Hodgkin's disease are becoming less important because of improved methods of therapy.

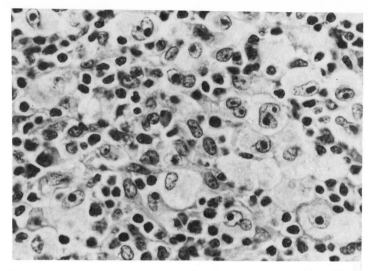

Figure 21-3. Hodgkin's disease, lymphocytic depletion type. Many Reed-Sternberg cells and mononuclear variants are seen.

Hematologic Tests

PERIPHERAL BLOOD

A mild to moderate anemia is frequently present in patients with Hodgkin's disease. It is usually normochromic normocytic, with low or normal reticulocyte count. Hemolytic anemia occasionally occurs in Hodgkin's disease, which will then be associated with an elevated reticulocyte count and, rarely, positive results on a Coombs test. This anemia is usually of the type that is associated with chronic disease. Rarely, severe anemia or pancytopenia may be observed resulting from extensive involvement of the bone marrow or hypersplenism. Neutropenia, monocytosis, and/or eosinophilia are not uncommon features, and lymphopenia is common in patients with extensive disease.

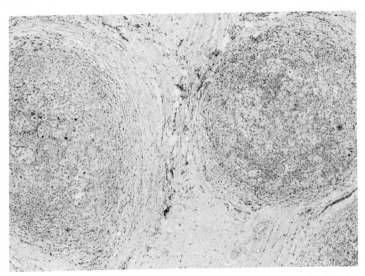

Figure 21-4. Hodgkin's disease, nodular sclerosis. Broad bands of trabecular fibrosis are seen around nodules of lymphoid tissue. The latter contain lacunar variants of Reed-Sternberg cells.

BONE MARROW

A bilateral posterior iliac crest bone marrow biopsy should be performed routinely in staging patients with Hodgkin's disease. When the marrow is involved, the lesion is usually focal and associated with fibrosis, and it may resemble a granuloma. Reed-Sternberg cells may be difficult to identify. The presence of mononuclear cells with nuclear features of Reed-Sternberg cells in the characteristic cellular environments of Hodgkin's disease should be regarded as consistent with marrow involvement, provided that typical Reed-Sternberg cells have been identified in a lymph node biopsy.

Elevated levels of serum alkaline phosphatase and unexplained anemia may indicate that the bone marrow is involved. The frequency of bone marrow involvement varies according to the type of Hodgkin's disease. It is rarely present in lymphocytic predominance type but occurs in approximately 8%, 20%, and 65% of nodular sclerosis, mixed cellularity, and lymphocytic depletion types respectively.

Biopsy of bone marrow containing Hodgkin's disease obviates the need for extensive radiologic studies, such as lymphangiography, intravenous pyelography, and so forth, as well as eliminating the need for surgical staging. The presence of bone marrow involvement indicates stage IV disease.

Special Procedures

RADIOLOGIC STUDIES

Accurate staging is essential in management of Hodgkin's disease and other lymphomas (Table 21-2). The radiographic evaluation plays a crucial role in determining the extent of disease.

The radiologic examination should start with routine radiographs of the chest. If any abnormalities are found, tomography is performed. The latter procedure gives a better appreciation of the extent of mediastinal lymphadenopathy.

Bilateral lower extremity lymphangiography is essential in detecting disease in abdominal lymph nodes. However, it does not demonstrate splenic, hilar, celiac, porta hepatis, and mesenteric nodes. Inferior venacavography is helpful in demonstrating enlarged lymph nodes high in the para-aortic chain. Ultrasonography is useful in detecting both celiac and mesenteric nodal disease. Intravenous pyelography may demonstrate ureteral obstruction by tumor. Skeletal surveys on bone scans should be included in search of lytic or, less commonly, osteoblastic lesions. [67]Gallium scan may be helpful in detecting disease in a variety of sites and should be used in patients unable to undergo lymphangiography. Isotope liver and spleen scans may add useful information but are inaccurate in one-third of patients.

Newer techniques such as computed tomography (CT) appear to be useful in the evaluation of abdominal lymphadenopathy.

While a lymphangiographic study is almost always indicated in

Table 21-2   Hodgkin's Disease: Ann Arbor Modification of Rye Staging System (1971)

Stage	Criteria
Stage I	Involvement of single lymph node region (I) or of a single extralymphatic organ or site (I_E)
Stage II	Involvement of two or more lymph node regions on the same side of diaphragm (II) or localized involvement of extralymphatic organ or site and one or more lymph node regions on the same side of diaphragm (II_E)
Stage III	Involvement of lymph node regions on both sides of diaphragm (III), which may also be accompanied by localized involvement of extralymphatic organ or site (III_E) or by involvement of the spleen (III_S), or both (III_{SE})
Stage IV	Diffuse or disseminated involvement of one or more extralymphatic organs or tissues with or without associated lymph node enlargement

staging of Hodgkin's disease (unless bone marrow biopsy has shown Hodgkin's disease), the other radiologic procedures mentioned, such as inferior venacavography, intravenous pyelography, isotope scanning, and CT scanning are not used routinely. Such techniques are used only under special clinical circumstances and only when the results will affect the therapeutic plan. The cost and morbidity of such procedures should be considered carefully in relation to their yield.

LAPAROTOMY

Surgical staging often detects abdominal disease not detected by clinical evaluation. Therefore, exploratory laparotomy with splenectomy and open liver biopsy have been used to detect Hodgkin's disease in the abdomen and pelvis. The decision to use laparotomy should, however, be individualized and should only be performed when the information is likely to affect treatment.

Before laparotomy is performed, stage IV disease should be excluded. Thus, the presence of bone marrow involvement obviates the need for laparotomy. Lymphangiography should be performed before laparotomy since the findings will guide the surgeon in locating lymph nodes. At operation, surgeons should biopsy all major lymph node groups regardless of their size and macroscopic appearance. Application of clips to tumors and lymph node areas will assist the radiotherapist later in port design. The spleen and splenic hilar lymph nodes are removed and a wedge biopsy is taken of the liver. In addition, an open iliac crest bone marrow biopsy should be performed.

The pathologist must examine the removed spleen carefully since correlation between splenic involvement and the probability of hepatic involvement is excellent. It is extremely rare to have Hodgkin's disease in the liver without splenic involvement. The spleen must be cut into thin sections and inspected carefully; multiple sections should be examined microscopically.

ANCILLARY STUDIES

Serum Biochemistry

Hypercalcemia is found in about 20% of patients and is often associated with hypophosphatemia and with elevated levels of serum alkaline phosphatase. The cause of hypercalcemia is usually involvement of bone by tumor with mobilization of calcium.

Moderately elevated levels of serum uric acid are common in myeloproliferative and lymphoproliferative disorders caused by rapid turnover of neoplastic cells. Hyperuricemia may become severe during therapy.

Liver function tests are generally not reliable in predicting involvement of the liver. The serum alkaline phosphatase activity, which is frequently elevated in Hodgkin's disease, has been used to indicate involvement of the liver and bone. The test is, however, not specific.

Skin Testing

Skin testing can be used to determine anergy as evidence of immunologic dysfunction in patients with Hodgkin's disease. However, it is not yet of proved value in the management of the patient.

REFERENCES

1. Lukes RJ, Butler JH: The pathology and nomenclature of Hodgkin's disease. Cancer Res 26:1063–1081, 1966

SUGGESTED READING

Lukes RJ: Criteria for involvement of lymph node, bone marrow, spleen and liver in Hodgkin's disease. Cancer Res 31:1755–1767, 1971

Rosenberg SA: (ed): Hodgkin's disease and other lymphomas. Clin Haematol, vol 3, 1974. [An excellent source for review of articles with comprehensive bibliographies.]

Sweet D, Kinnealey A, Ultmann TE: Hodgkin's disease: problems of staging. Cancer 42:957–970, 1978

chapter 22

Malignant Immuno- proliferative Disorders

Malignant immunoproliferative disorders may be defined as neo- plastic clonal proliferations of plasma cells or B-lymphocytes, associated with abnormal produc- tion of immunoglobulin. The immunoglobulin abnormality is used to classify the disease.

Immunoglobulins are composed of two heavy and two light chains linked by disulfide bonds (Figure 22-1). The sequence of amino acids in the heavy chains, molecular weight (MW) 55,000, is specific for the immunoglobulin class, annotated gamma (γ) for IgG, mu (μ) for IgM, alpha (α) for IgA, delta (δ) for IgD, and epsilon (ϵ) for IgE. The shorter sequence of amino acids in the light chains (MW, 22,000) is specific for lambda (λ) or for kappa (κ) chains. The light chains can link to any set of heavy chains, but both light chains are the same on any single molecule. Partial hydrolysis of a globulin molecule with papain separates it into a crystallizable fraction (Fc) and the heavy-light chain residue re- sponsible for antibody activity (Fab).

Each immunoglobulin class has a characteristic structure that determines molecular size. Immunoglobulin G, IgD, and IgE are monomeric (i.e., they have one set of heavy and light chains), whereas IgM is pentameric (with five sets), and IgA varies as mono- mer, dimer, or trimer or in secretions where it has an additional secretory piece. The size of the molecule and its sequence of amino acids determine its electrical charge, and, therefore, its migration

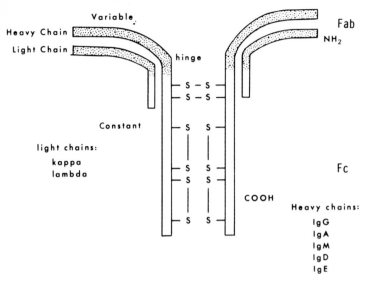

Figure 22-1. Schematic diagram of immunoglobulin monomer. The shaded area is variable in amino acid constitution suggesting multiple gene products. The clear area is relatively constant suggesting a single gene product.

by electrophoresis, as well as other physicochemical characteristics including viscosity or solubility (Table 22-1).

In general one plasma cell produces one type of immune globulin. Thus, neoplastic proliferations of a cell clone will yield a monotonous population of immunoglobulin molecules, defined by a single light-chain type, and migrating to a single narrow zone on electrophoresis, seen as a monoclonal spike. These abnormal molecules are known as M-proteins (for myeloma or monoclonal), or paraproteins. Paraproteins may be abnormal in amount or in structure or configuration. For example, heavy chains with amino acid deficits at the point of light-chain linkage circulate only as heavy chains, and this abnormality becomes a diagnostic feature. The pathologic protein usually proliferates at the expense of normal immunoglobulins. Since antibodies are immunoglobulins, impor-

Table 22-1. Characteristics of Normal Immunoglobulins

Class	Heavy Chain	Sub-types	MW	Configuration	Function	Normal Serum Concentration (mg/dl)
IgG	γ	4	150,000	Monomer	2° phase antibody	800–1800
IgA With secretory piece With J piece	α	2	170,000 390,000	Monomer Dimer Trimer	Secretory antibodies	180–490
IgM	μ	2	900,000	Pentamer	1° phase antibody complement fixing	50–180
IgD	δ	1	150,000	Monomer	? Precursor to IgM, IgG; ? receptor on lymphocyte	3
IgE	ε Fc	1	196,000 53,000	Monomer	Reaginic antibody	0.3

tant antibody function is often lost leading to recurrent infection. The abnormal protein may have antibody activity of one monolithic type.

Normal immune mechanisms involve interaction between monocytes or macrophages and subpopulations of lymphocytes; B-lymphocytes undergo blast transformation and mitotic division to produce clones of plasma cells producing a polyclonal spectrum of antibody or immunoglobulins. The immunoproliferative disorders therefore involve proliferations of B-lymphocytes and plasma cells and are clinically defined by the abnormal immunoglobulin. Because the pathologic cell types are related, a similarity can be seen in the signs, symptoms, and laboratory findings of malignant immunoproliferative diseases, as summarized in Table 22-2. The immunoproliferative disorders are multiple myeloma, macroglobulinemia, light-chain disease, and heavy-chain disease.

Multiple myeloma is a proliferation of plasma cells producing, in most cases, either IgG or IgA paraproteins of either light-chain type. In a few cases IgD is the abnormal protein and, very rarely, IgE is produced.

Waldenström's macroglobulinemia is associated with lymphocytic lymphoma, producing IgM paraproteins that, because of their size, result in marked elevations in serum viscosity and secondary bleeding problems. Light chain disease is a myeloma variant; the light chains conjugate to form dimers, the Bence Jones (BJ) protein, in serum and urine. The dimers form the fibrillar polymers of amyloid, and early renal failure is common. The heavy chain diseases produce pathologic proteins with amino acid deletions in the hinge region, site of usual conjugation to light chains; thus the heavy chain circulates without light chains. Each heavy-chain type produces a different clinical picture: gamma, lymphocytic lymphoma; mu, CLL; and alpha, gastrointestinal lymphoma, which is more common in the young and of increased frequency in the Mediterranean area. Delta and epsilon heavy-chain diseases are presumed to exist but have not been found as yet.

Malignant immunoproliferative diseases are usually found in

Table 22-2. Clinical Characteristics and Laboratory Findings in Immunoproliferative Disease

| Disease | Immunoglobulin | | Electrophoretic Pattern | Urine BJ | Bone X-Ray | Cell Type | Complications |
	Heavy Chain	Light Chain					
Myelomas							
IgG (75%)	γ	κ or λ	Narrow spike	60%	Punched out	Plasma cell	Infection
IgA (15%)	α	κ or λ	Broader spike	70%	Punched out	Plasma cell	Infection
IgD (1%–2%)	δ	Usually λ	Hypogamma	100%		Plasma cell	Amyloidosis
IgE (2 cases)	ε	κ or λ	Narrow spike	Unknown		Plasma cell	Plasma cell leukemia
Light-chain myeloma (10%)	None	κ or λ	Hypogamma	100%	Diffuse osteoporosis	Plasma cell Lymphocyte, mixed	Amyloid kidney Hypercalcemia

Macroglobulinemia	μ	κ or λ	Small spike beta	30%–40%	Minimal	Lymphocytes	Hyperviscosity Bleeding Cold agglutinin in hemolytic anemia
Heavy-chain disease							
Gamma (13)[a]		None	Broad-band polyclonal	γ chain	Normal	Lymphocytes	Palatal edema
Alpha (20)[a]		None	Broad-band alpha$_2$-beta	None	Normal	Plasma cell	GI lymphoma Malabsorption
Mu (3)[a]			None	κ chain, BJ	Osteoporosis	Lymphocyte (CLL)	Amyloidosis

[a] Number of cases.

patients over 40 years old. (See Tables 22-2 and 22-3 for summaries of diagnostic findings in cases of immunoproliferative disorders.) They usually come to attention because of moderate normochromic anemia of undetermined origin and/or one of the following: (a) an abnormal band seen on routine electrophoresis, (b) nephrotic syndrome of undetermined origin, (c) back pain or radiographic evidence of unsuspected fractures of ribs or vertebrae, (d) acute spinal cord compression from vertebral collapse, (e) hypercalcemia.

DIAGNOSTIC EVALUATION

Malignant immunoproliferative diseases are defined by the abnormal protein. Therefore, diagnosis depends on detection of an abnormal globulin, identifying it as monoclonal and characterizing its heavy and light chains, with confirmation of the pathologic cell type by bone marrow or tissue examination.

1. Hematologic findings include a modest normochromic anemia and the peripheral smear should be examined for lymphocytosis. Bone marrow aspirate is necessary to determine the significance of abnormal protein electrophoresis, the pathologic cell type, and the extent of the disease. Sedimentation rate is a nonspecific test of limited usefulness, abnormal in anemia or in the presence of increased globulin.

2. Serum protein electrophoresis is used to detect monoclonal spikes or hypogammaglobulinemia. Protein electrophoresis has supplanted the albumin/globulin ratio. It is a very accurate way of quantitating albumin, and any abnormality of globulins may be seen on the scan pattern. Albumin/globulin ratio, frequently obtained as part of an automated chemistry panel, is unreliable, since hypogammaglobulinemia and small abnormal spikes less than 2 g/dl may neither reverse the ratio nor cause significant elevations of total globulin.

3. Immunoelectrophoresis (IEP) is performed when any clonal peaks or hypogammaglobulinemia are found on routine protein electrophoresis. With hypogammaglobulinemia specific tests should be performed for light chains. Immunoglobulin quantitation is correlative but not diagnostic.

Table 22-3.   Hematologic Characteristics of Immunoproliferative Disorders

Disease	Blood	Marrow	Liver/Spleen	Bone X-Ray
Myeloma	Normochromic anemia Rouleaux Plasma cell leukemia (IgE)	Plasma cells	No increase	Osteolytic lesions
Macroglobulinemia	Normochromic anemia Lymphocytosis Neutropenia, eosinophilia	Lymphocytes, plasma cells	Enlarged	Rare
Light-chain myeloma	Anemia Rouleaux	Plasma cells	No increase	Osteoporosis
Heavy-chain disease				
Gamma	Lymphocytosis	Lymphocytes, plasma cells, eosinophils	Enlarged	No abnormality
Mu	CLL	Lymphocytes	Enlarged	Osteoporosis
Alpha	Normal	Moderate plasma cells	No increase	No abnormality

4. Urine protein electrophoresis and immunoelectrophoresis should replace the antiquated heat tests for Bence Jones protein. Urine tests are performed whenever a monoclonal serum protein or hypogammaglobulinemia is found. Urine immunoelectrophoresis is absolutely necessary to diagnose heavy-chain diseases.

5. Radiographic studies of long bones, ribs, vertebrae, and skull are useful to discern lytic lesions, generalized osteoporosis caused by plasma cell proliferation, or pathologic fractures.

6. Serum viscosity is of prognostic and therapeutic value, particularly when the paraprotein is IgM.

7. Coagulation screening tests can be performed on bleeding patients to categorize the diathesis, as a guide to treatment with blood components. Bleeding diatheses occur most often with IgM paraproteins.

8. Renal function is screened by serum creatinine particularly in light-chain disease where renal amyloidosis is common. Clinical studies that involve dehydration should be avoided to prevent inspissating the abnormal proteins in renal tubules, further compromising renal function.

9. Radiographic studies of the small intestine are helpful in diagnosis of alpha heavy-chain disease.

10. Serum calcium may rise significantly in myeloma causing lethargy and cardiac arrhythmia. Hypercalcemia appears to be closely related to Bence Jones proteinuria.

LABORATORY STUDIES

Hematologic Tests

GENERAL FEATURES

General features are summarized in Table 22-3. In almost all cases of immunoproliferative disease, mild to moderate anemia is present. Leukopenia and thrombocytopenia are uncommon but may result from chemotherapy. Hepatosplenomegaly and lymphadenopathy are unusual in myeloma although they are seen in lymphomas associated with macroglobulinemia or gamma heavy-chain disease. Gastrointestinal lymphoma of alpha chain disease may produce malabsorption. Light-chain disease and some myelomas are associated with amyloid deposition in kidney, ligaments, or tendons (e.g., carpal tunnel syndrome) but rarely in other viscera. Bones are involved focally in some myelomas and more diffusely in others, seen as osteoporosis. Extramedullary plasmacytomas may occur in the nasopharynx or, rarely, in the breast. The majority are followed by disseminated myeloma within a few years. Solitary plasmacytomas of bone are rare but may also disseminate within a few years.

PERIPHERAL BLOOD

Red cell count

Moderate normochromic anemia (Hb, 8–11 g/dl) is present. Rarely, there is a macrocytic anemia unresponsive to B_{12} or folic acid therapy. Hypochromic anemia results from significant gastrointestinal bleeding.

White cell count

The white cell count is normal. Occasionally lymphocytosis is present.

Platelets

Platelets are of normal appearance and numbers unless the patient is undergoing chemotherapy. Abnormal function results from coating with paraprotein, most commonly with IgM.

Morphology

Smears may show rouleaux and background of grey stain representing the paraprotein. Nucleated red cells are seen even early in the disease but become more numerous with progressive anemia resulting from myelophthisis.

Plasmacytoid lymphocytes are usually found late in the course of myeloma. True plasma cell leukemia is rare, appearing late in myeloma, although it may be an initial feature of IgE myeloma. This diagnosis is difficult to make on morphologic grounds unless abnormal plasma cells or plasmablasts are circulating. Lymphocytes

417

with coarsely vacuolated cytoplasm are said to be characteristic of gamma heavy-chain disease. Mu heavy-chain disease is associated with absolute lymphocytosis and CLL.

Sedimentation rate

Sedimentation rate is retarded if anemia is severe and increased when fibrinogen or immunoglobulins are increased. Corrected sedimentation rates are not helpful. The normal range is 0–20 mm for females and 0–10 mm for males. Sedimentation rates greater than 100 mm/hr are rarely seen in any disease except myeloma. Light-chain myeloma may have a normal sedimentation rate.

BONE MARROW ASPIRATE

Cellularity varies from normal to totally replaced. Sampling error is critical in the nodular proliferations of myeloma. Increases in plasma cells (> 10%), lymphocytes (> 20%), or both are usually present. Infiltrates may be nodular or diffuse and there is no morphologic characteristic that will be diagnostic of the associated paraprotein. Nevertheless, some generalizations can be made. In IgG myeloma monotonous sheets of plasma cells are usually found, mostly mature with few plasmablasts. A patient with IgA myeloma may have diffuse infiltration of other marrow elements by immature plasma cells and variable numbers of lymphocytes. Occasionally flamelike discoloration of plasma cell cytoplasm (thesaurocytes) is seen. In light-chain myeloma plasma cells and lymphocytes diffusely infiltrate the marrow. In macroglobulinemia there is diffuse replacement of marrow by poorly differentiated lymphocytes.

Although alcohol abuse and chronic infection may be associated with moderate plasmacytosis, those plasma cells are usually mature, do not appear in aggregates, and, combined with lymphocytes, comprise less than 20% of the total number of cells. Plasmablasts and multinucleated plasma cells are pathologic; if present the disease is not likely to be reactive. Very rarely, plasma cell myeloma is unassociated with a circulating paraprotein, although

418

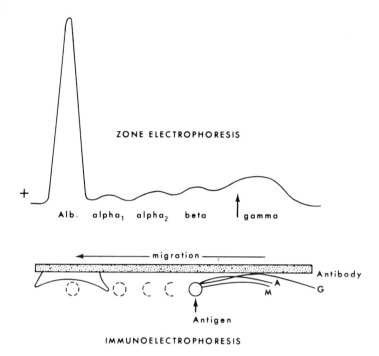

Figure 22-2. Comparison of schematics of protein electrophoretic pattern and immunoelectrophoresis. ↑ = inoculation point.

immunofluorescent studies of air-dried unstained smears may show plasma cells reactive with only one antiserum coinciding with the unsecreted protein.

Other Useful Tests

SERUM PROTEIN ELECTROPHORESIS

Purpose

Serum protein electrophoresis is a screening test for monoclonal spikes or hypogammaglobulinemia (1) (Figure 22-2). Serum

419

proteins are routinely determined in most laboratories by electrophoresis, so that many unsuspected spikes are discovered.

Principle

Proteins, being amphoteric, migrate in an electrical field. A pathologic protein with a monotonous population of similarly charged molecules migrates to one single location creating a dense band, or spike, of paraprotein. In light-chain disease, the small molecules are excreted rapidly in the urine, depleting serum gamma globulin (seen as hypogammaglobulinemia).

Procedure

Serum is inoculated most commonly on transparent cellulose acetate membranes and electrophoresis is performed at pH 8.6, separating the proteins into albumin and the four globulins (alpha$_1$, alpha$_2$, beta, and gamma). The proteins are precipitated on the membrane with glacial acetic acid and stained with Ponceau S, a red dye. The amount of dye absorbed to each band is proportional to the amount of protein. The patterns can be evaluated visually for abnormal bands or quantitated by densitometry. The latter method utilizes the total protein, determined by refractometry or chemically, and divides this value in proportion to the dye absorbance of each protein band. The proportion is translated onto paper as a series of peaks. The area under each peak is calculated and converted to g/dl and is reported alone or with the paper pattern in most institutions. In some cases the cellulose pattern may be attached to the report as well.

Specimen

One ml of serum or plasma is adequate and may be stored refrigerated or frozen. Electrophoretic patterns of plasma yield an additional band between beta and gamma for fibrinogen.

Interpretation

Normal ranges are: albumin, 3.5–6 g/dl; alpha$_1$, 0.1–0.4; alpha$_2$, 0.4–1.2; beta, 0.5–1.1; and gamma, 0.5–1.6.

Abnormal bands are found most often in the beta or gamma zone and may vary from 1.0–12.0 g/dl or higher. Quantitated values may be misleading since small, abnormal bands that are seen easily by inspection of the patterns may not change the g/dl significantly. Since quantitation depends on the relative dye staining of the different zones, high levels of paraprotein result in falsely low levels of albumin, and albumin/globulin ratios may be inaccurate. Although the course of the disease or treatment can be estimated by repeating protein electrophoresis patterns every two to three months, a wide latitude ($\pm$ 0.3 g/dl) must be allowed for quantitation; changes of 0.5 g/dl are probably significant.

Characteristic patterns in neoplastic disorders are hypogammaglobulinemia—light-chain disease, IgD myeloma; spikes in beta or gamma zones—IgG or IgE myeloma, IgM macroglobulinemia; broad-based spikes—IgA myeloma, heavy-chain disease; minimonoclonal spikes ($<$ 0.2 g/dl)—metastatic carcinoma of the stomach, prostate, breast, or colon or other lymphomas. The size, shape, and location of spikes are suggestive but not diagnostic of the paraprotein type. Identification requires immunoelectrophoresis. The small spikes seen with metastatic tumors may be caused by reactive plasmacytosis around necrotic tumor or tumor metastases. Rarely biclonal spikes are found in immunoproliferative or myeloproliferative disease.

A small percentage (3%) of elderly individuals produce monoclonal spikes without immunoproliferative malignancy. These benign idiopathic monoclonal gammopathies may eventually develop into immunoproliferative disease after several years. Benign gammopathies are characterized by monoclonal spikes less than 3.0 g/dl without proteinuria, less than 6% plasma cells in marrow aspirates, and no radiographic abnormalities of bone. The monoclonal protein is usually IgG but may be IgA. Even in these patients, if urine is concentrated 100 times and immunoelectrophoresis is used, 24% will have monoclonal Bence Jones proteins, so concentrated urines cannot be used to distinguish benign from malignant gammopathies. The difference appears to be that patients with benign monoclonal gammopathies excrete less than 50 mg/l protein and do not have gross proteinuria. After initial evaluation such patients are followed with serum and urine protein electrophoresis annually and with complete blood count to detect early appearance of anemia. Bone marrow aspirates are repeated if bone x-rays become abnormal or if anemia or proteinuria appear.

URINE ELECTROPHORESIS AND TESTS
FOR BENCE JONES PROTEIN

Purpose

Monoclonal spikes in unconcentrated urine are diagnostic of immunoproliferative malignancy and confirm the significance of monoclonal spikes or hypogammaglobulinemia seen on serum protein electrophoresis (2). Classic heat precipitation tests for Bence Jones protein are not reliable and should be abandoned.

Principle

As in serum a monolithic population of similarly charged protein molecules migrate as a band on zone electrophoresis and can be quantitated. Excretion of abnormal proteins may damage the kidney and electrophoresis detects a nephrotic pattern of protein loss in addition to the monoclonal spikes. Bence Jones protein is composed of free light-chain dimers with characteristic heat solubility at pH 5.0 so that Bence Jones proteins precipitating at 50–60 C redissolve on boiling. They reprecipitate as the urine cools. However, 30% of patients with myeloma do not excrete abnormal proteins or they excrete both heavy and light chains, which lack the characteristic heat solubility. Thus, electrophoresis has replaced other tests for Bence Jones protein.

Procedure

Urine is inoculated on cellulose membranes and electrophoresis is performed at pH 8.6. Proteins are quantitated by densitometry and reported as grams or mg/dl. The pattern should be attached to the report. Since proteinuria is already an abnormal condition, no normal levels of protein are reported for protein electrophoresis.

Specimen

The first voided morning specimen is refrigerated but not frozen to avoid disruption of light-chain dimers. Specimens may require 50 or 100 times the concentration before electrophoresis is performed, in order to detect minute amounts of protein in early disease. Twenty-four-hour urine samples are difficult to collect and are generally unnecessary.

Interpretation

Urine protein loss reflects benign nephrosclerosis unrelated to myeloma, filtration of myeloma proteins (both heavy and light chains), or myeloma kidney secondary to amyloid deposit. Elderly patients can be expected to show nephrotic loss of proteins mirroring the normal electrophoretic pattern of serum. Monoclonal bands seen on electrophoresis are significant regardless of amount and should be characterized by immunoelectrophoresis.

Notes and precautions

Heat tests, if used, must always be confirmed by electrophoresis since false-positive and false-negative test results are common. Albuminuria frequently results from kidneys damaged by myeloma proteins. Albumin precipitates with Bence Jones protein at 60 C but does not redissolve at 100 C, obscuring the characteristic change if Bence Jones protein is present.

IMMUNOELECTROPHORESIS, SERUM AND URINE

Purpose

Immunoelectrophoresis characterizes protein (as monoclonal, i.e., of one light-chain type) and identifies its specific heavy chain in order to classify the underlying disease (1–3). Absence of light chains is diagnostic for heavy-chain disease.

An initial protein electrophoretic migration on agar or cellulose membranes is followed by application of antiserum along the path of migration. Individual protein molecules diffuse toward the antibody, forming immune precipitin arcs wherever antigen meets specific antibody.

Procedure

Immunoelectrophoresis is available in large hospital laboratories and most local reference laboratories. The test requires at least 72 hours to complete and experience in interpretation. Immunoelectrophoresis is primarily a qualitative procedure that uses agar gel or cellulose as the support medium. It is semiquantitative in that protein arcs may be high, low, or absent. Urine or serum is inoculated into a well and electrophoresed 40–60 minutes at pH 8.6 to separate component proteins. Antiserum from rabbits or goats is then inoculated along the path of migration. The electrophoretically separated albumin and many globulins diffuse toward the antiserum. Wherever antigen and antibody specificity correspond, a precipitin arc is deposited. Antisera to whole human serum or specific sera for each heavy chain and both light chains are available. Specific antiserum for IgD or IgE is in short supply and is not used routinely. The precipitin arcs are denatured with glacial acetic acid, and the agar is evaporated to a film and stained to provide a permanent record. Reports are usually interpretive and may be accompanied by photographs of the precipitin arcs.

Specimen

Aliquots of serum or random urine should be refrigerated rather than frozen to avoid dissociation of trimers or pentamers common to IgA and IgM or dissociation of light and heavy chains. Once paraproteins are identified, specimens may be frozen. Urine specimens frequently require 20–50 times the original concentration to detect minute amounts of light chain. Serums with large amounts of abnormal globulin require dilution to avoid antigen excess, which hinders identification. Saline-diluted specimens should not be frozen.

Interpretation

Paraproteins have characteristic skewing of precipitin arcs rather than the smooth symmetric appearance of a heterogeneous population of molecules. The abnormal immunoglobulin is usually present to the exclusion of the normal, and the presence of a single light-chain type identifies it as monoclonal, as summarized in Table 22-2. A heavy-chain paraprotein without light chains defines heavy-chain disease (HCD). Monoclonal light chains without heavy chain is seen in light-chain myeloma. The association of serum paraproteins with urine Bence Jones protein is seen in Table 22-4. Approximately 70% of IgG myelomas are G-kappa and 30% are G-lambda, which does not appear to be of clinical significance in prognosis. Kappa and lambda chains are equally divided in other classes. In light-chain myeloma, however, the lambda-chain variant has a worse prognosis.

Notes and precautions

Antigen excess produces prozones with antibody that are soluble and may wash away during processing resulting in false-negative results.

Immunoelectrophoresis should not be performed without concurrent standard electrophoresis as a guide to amount and location of the abnormal protein. Routine electrophoresis serves as a guide to specimen dilution needed for testing to avoid prozones.

IMMUNOGLOBULIN QUANTITATION, SERUM

Purpose

Immunoglobulin quantitation has limited usefulness in immunoproliferative malignancy, as opposed to immunodeficiency disorders (4). It may be confirmatory in interpretation of immunoelectrophoresis.

Table 22-4. **Patterns of Abnormal Serum and Urine Proteins in Immunoproliferative Disorders**

Disease	% Occurrence of Serum Protein Constituents	% Occurrence Urine BJ Protein in Pattern Category
Multiple myeloma		
Myeloma globulin only	50%	No BJ protein
Myeloma globulin + BJ	20%	60% in IgG myeloma
		70% in IgA myeloma
		100% in IgD myeloma
BJ protein only	20%–30%	100% in light chain
No myeloma globulin	< 1%	No BJ protein
Macroglobulinemia	10%	40%

Principle

Usually measured in serum only, quantitation of immunoglobulins G, A, M, and D is widely available by radial immunodiffusion. Quantitation of G, A, and M is also available by nephelometry. In radial immunodiffusion, the serum or urine is inoculated into agar impregnated with a single specific anti-immunoglobulin and allowed to diffuse, forming immunoprecipitin rings. The diameter of the ring is proportional to the concentration of immunoglobulin. In nephelometry specific antisera are mixed with serum or urine, and immune precipitate complexes are measured at end point (laser nephelometry) or kinetically (macromolecular nephelometry). IgE is present in such small amounts normally and IgE myeloma is so rare that immunodiffusion plates for it are not available, nor are there plates for light chains.

Procedure

Serum is inoculated into agar for each of the common immunoglobulins, G, A, and M. Diffusion progresses under standard conditions of temperature and humidity for a set length of time (6–24 hours) or to an end point (possibly several days). Standard protein solutions are also diffused and ring diameters are plotted against protein concentration. Using the plot, ring diameters of patient material are converted to mg/dl. Precision is 6%–10%. If the concentration is above the normal range, the specimen is diluted and repeated. The result is then multiplied by the dilution factor.

Specimen

Five microliters of serum are used.

Interpretation

Immunoglobulin concentration is age dependent but since immunoproliferative malignancies are diseases of adults, normal values are:

IgG,	800–1200 mg/dl ± 2 SD
IgA,	180–480
IgM,	50–150
IgD,	3
IgE,	0.3

With paraproteins one globulin will be 5–10 times normal concentration with moderate to severe decreases in the others. Quantitation with abnormal electrophoretic pattern is partial evidence of paraprotein, but quantitation cannot establish the protein as monoclonal. Immunodiffusion of saline-diluted specimens particularly for IgM is often not linear with concentration and may give extraordinary values beyond those quantitated on electrophoresis. The latter technique is more accurate in such cases.

Notes and precautions

Antigen excess may result in prozones with antibody, seen as a haziness, rather than immune precipitate. Repeat testing with diluted specimen may be necessary but with limitations, as already noted.

SERUM VISCOSITY

Purpose

Tests for serum viscosity are used to estimate clinical risk of thrombosis or bleeding in paraproteinemia and to assess the need for plasmapheresis (3). It is used to evaluate therapy as well.

Principle

Normal serum or plasma has a viscosity only slightly greater than water. With marked paraproteinemia of large molecules, such as IgM, or of molecules that conjugate easily with others, such as IgA, marked increases may be seen in serum viscosity. Such increases are often temperature dependent, with cryoglobulins or cryofibrinogens causing gelling of plasma or serum at room temperature or below. Increased viscosity leads to dilatation and sludging of retinal vessels with resultant blindness. Larger vessel thrombosis in limbs leads to Raynaud's phenomenon or cutaneous gangrene; coating of platelets is associated with bleeding. When viscosity is increased markedly it can be relieved by mechanical removal of the plasma by plasmapheresis.

Procedure

Serum or plasma is allowed to flow through glass tubes of narrow diameter, Ostwald viscometers, and the flow between two etched lines is timed. Flow rate is compared with that of water and a serum/water ratio is calculated. Ratios are obtained at 37 C, room temperature, and 4 C.

Specimen

Blood is obtained at 37 C and plasma and/or serum is removed. Serum can be stored in a refrigerator once separated from red cells. Whole blood should not be refrigerated since it may gel in the presence of cryoglobulins or cryofibrinogens.

428

Interpretation

The normal serum/water ratio is 1.0–1.7. Significant elevations are ratios greater than 8 at 37 C. The increase in ratio at room temperature or at 4 C for serum indicates that cryoglobulins are present, and increased ratios or plasma indicate that cryofibrinogen, and possibly cryoglobulin, are present as well. The presence of cryoproteins is of significance in plasmapheresis, which may use a cold centrifuge. Although hyperviscosity is characteristic of IgM, it is also seen with IgA paraproteins, which tend to polymerize easily.

SCREENING TESTS FOR BLEEDING DISORDERS

Purpose

Coagulation screening tests categorize bleeding diatheses in the patient with macroglobulinemia.

Principle

Since bleeding is related to platelet function in the presence of IgM paraprotein, bleeding time and studies of platelet aggregation, adhesion, and platelet factor 3 release are usually abnormal. Occasionally, there is interference with factors II, V, VII, or VIII. Coagulation factor assay and platelet aggregation studies are not available in small laboratories. Screening tests including bleeding time, prothrombin time, and partial thromboplastin time are generally adequate. (See Chapter 23.)

For sections on *Procedure* and *Interpretation*, see Chapter 23.

TESTS OF RENAL FUNCTION

Purpose

Tests of renal function that document decreasing renal function suggest myeloma kidney or amyloid kidney.

429

Principle

Conjugated dimers of light chains precipitate in renal tubular epithelium producing nephrosis. The fibrillar pattern of light chains is seen in amyloid, which is deposited in glomerular loops also resulting in nephrosis. Serum creatinine is an accurate measure of glomerular function.

Procedure

Standard tests for serum creatinine and creatinine clearance are performed.

Interpretation

With decreased renal clearance Bence Jones protein appears in the serum.

SERUM CALCIUM

Purpose

Tests for serum calcium are of therapeutic interest in myeloma since hypercalcemia can be related to lethargy or cardiac arrhythmias.

Principle

Serum hypercalcemia appears in 20%–30% of myelomas, apparently secondary to bone resorption by myelomatous infiltrates.

Procedure

Standard tests for serum calcium are performed.

Hypercalcemia is usually associated with Bence Jones proteinuria. It is uncommon in macroglobulinemia. The normal range for calcium is 9–11 mg/dl. Significant clinical symptoms appear above 14 mg/dl.

DIAGNOSTIC EVALUATION OF MULTIPLE MYELOMA

Multiple myeloma is a multifocal nodular proliferation of plasma cells associated with a paraprotein in all but a few rare cases (less than 1%). It is a disease of people over 40.

Hematologic Tests

PERIPHERAL BLOOD

Normochromic anemia is present with hemoglobin levels of 8–11 g/dl. Rouleaux are seen; nucleated red cells appear late in the course of disease as a result of myelophthisis but may be present early if anemia is present. Rare plasmacytoid lymphocytes are also seen. In plasma cell leukemia the white cell count may be 50,000–100,000/mm^3.

BONE MARROW

Bone marrow is normocellular with hypercellular nodules of plasma cells seen best on sections of marrow clot or with marrow biopsy. Plasma cells appear in variable size aggregates and may be bi- or trinucleate with plasmablasts (Figure 22-3). In light-chain disease and IgA myeloma, plasma cells are mixed with a variable lymphocyte population.

BONE X-RAYS

Bone x-rays show osteolytic lesions in skull, ribs, vertebrae, and long bones in IgG or IgA myeloma. Light-chain myeloma is often associated with diffuse osteoporosis.

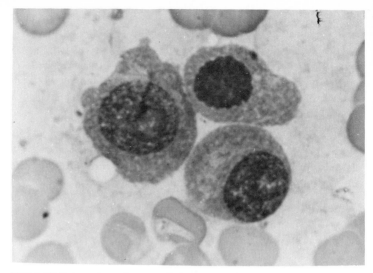

Figure 22-3. Immature plasma cells in marrow aspirate. Reverse pinocytosis seen at cell edge and abnormal protein deposited in background.

Other Useful Tests

SERUM PROTEINS

Protein electrophoresis shows either a monoclonal spike or hypogammaglobulinemia. Immunoelectrophoresis identifies the paraprotein as IgG (75%), IgA (15%), light-chain myeloma (10%), IgD (< 1%), or IgE (rare), with kappa-chain types slightly more common. Light-chain myelomas are associated with hypogammaglobulinemia and no abnormal heavy chain is identifiable by immunoelectrophoresis.

URINE PROTEINS

Only 50% of IgG or IgA myelomas are associated with Bence Jones proteinuria while 100% of light-chain myelomas have Bence Jones proteins. Standard electrophoresis shows a monoclonal band in the same zone as seen on serum. Immunoelectrophoresis usually identifies abnormal heavy chains and light chains, reflecting the serum pattern. Only the pathologic light chain appears in urine, which proves helpful in interpreting the serum proteins. Light chains polymerize as amyloid fibrils in renal tubular epithelium. They can be seen on renal biopsy by electron microscopy or with immunofluorescence.

RENAL FUNCTION TESTS

Renal function tests include serum creatinine, which may be mildly elevated (3.0 mg/dl), an unfavorable prognostic sign. Significant elevations occur early in light-chain myeloma and indicate amyloidosis. With failing renal function Bence Jones protein is retained and appears as small spikes in serum.

SERUM CALCIUM

Serum calcium is elevated in 20%–30% of myelomas and is associated with Bence Jones proteinuria.

DIAGNOSTIC EVALUATION OF MACROGLOBULINEMIA

Macroglobulinemia is a more diffuse involvement of marrow and lymph nodes by poorly differentiated lymphocytic lymphoma. Associated hepatosplenomegaly may be present.

Hematologic Findings

PERIPHERAL BLOOD

Normochromic anemia and marked rouleaux are present. Late in disease immature lymphocytes or lymphosarcoma cells may circulate.

BONE MARROW

Bone marrow is usually hypercellular and often replaced by lymphocytes.

Bone x-rays usually show osteoporosis.

Other Useful Tests

SERUM PROTEINS

Serum proteins by electrophoresis show modest spikes in the beta zone or beta-gamma trough. Immunoelectrophoresis identifies the protein as IgM of either light-chain type. They are often associated with cryoglobulin or cryofibrinogen, which can be semi-quantitated by a cryocrit. A Wintrobe tube is filled with serum or plasma instead of whole blood and refrigerated in ice water 16–24 hours. The percent precipitate is determined after cold centrifugation. Cryoglobulins redissolve at 37 C; they can be responsible for thrombosis of peripheral vessels with resultant gangrene.

IgM paraproteins frequently have rheumatoid factor activity and occasionally have anti-I specificity for red cells. Tests that use latex particles (as for rheumatoid factor, pregnancy, fibrin split products, etc.) must be interpreted with caution, since viscous serum tends to aggregate latex nonspecifically.

URINE PROTEINS

Because of its molecular size, IgM does not usually appear in the urine, although its unconjugated light chains appear in 30%–40% of cases.

BLEEDING STUDIES

Bleeding studies indicate defects in platelet adhesion resulting from coating by paraprotein. This is reflected in prolonged bleeding time, abnormal platelet adhesion and aggregation studies, and a decrease in platelet factor 3 release. Bleeding usually appears in skin or on mucosal surfaces. IgM paraprotein may also form immune complexes with coagulation factors II, V, VII, or VIII inhibiting their function.

LABORATORY STUDIES OF
HEAVY-CHAIN DISEASE (HCD)

Hematologic Findings

GENERAL FEATURES

Heavy-chain disease, originally referred to as gamma heavy-chain disease, is known also as Fc disease or Franklin's disease for its discoverer. It is now apparent that there is a spectrum of lymphocytic disorders in which the pathologic cell product is a partial molecule lacking amino acids at the point of light-chain attachment so that heavy chains circulate alone (Table 22-5). Gamma-chain disease may end in a lymphoma (histiocytic or Hodgkin's) or other malignant disease; it can be associated with hepatosplenomegaly, anemia, eosinophilia, and palatal edema. Lymph node biopsies reveal nonspecific lymphadenitis or follicular hyperplasia. Frequent bacterial infections occur. The disease is distinguished only by its unusual and rare paraprotein. Alpha heavy-chain disease appears in younger individuals of the Mediterranean area, manifested by gastrointestinal lymphoma and malabsorption. It is rare in the United States. Mu-chain disease has been found in only three or four patients with associated CLL. Characteristics are summarized in Table 22-5.

PERIPHERAL BLOOD

Normochromic anemia is seen. Variable lymphocytosis with prominent cytoplasmic vacuolization is present as a result of dissolved immunoglobulin in gamma HCD. Mu HCD resembles CLL; alpha HCD may have normal peripheral blood.

BONE MARROW

In gamma HCD hypercellularity is seen with increased lymphocytes and plasma cells. With alpha HCD slight plasmacytosis is present, and with mu HCD there is hypercellularity with increased lymphocytes.

Table 22-5. Characteristics of Heavy-Chain Disease (HCD)

Class[a]	Serum Electrophoresis	Urine BJ	Blood	Bone Marrow	Other Tissue
γ HCD (12)	Broad-based, fast γ or β, IgA, IgM not decreased	IEP mirror image of serum immunoelectrophoresis	Atypical lymphs, pancytopenia, eosinophilia	Nondiagnostic, pleomorphic with lympho-plasmacytosis	Lymph-adenopathy of nonspecific histology
μ HCD (3)	May be normal or small beta spike; μ and κ chains separate	κ chain	CLL	70%–80% lymphs; few plasma cells	Amyloid
α HCD (20)	Smudged broad $α_2$-β band	No α chain	—	Slight decrease in plasma cells	Small intestine lymphoma

[a]Number of cases appear in parentheses.

436

BONE X-RAYS

Bone x-rays are generally nondiagnostic, although osteoporosis was seen in one case of mu HCD. They are normal in alpha and gamma HCD.

Other Useful Tests

SERUM PROTEINS

An abnormal broad band is seen in the beta or gamma zone. Immunoelectrophoresis classifies only gamma-chain paraprotein. Interpretation may be complicated by residual normal immunoglobulins with their light chains. Alpha HCD may have a flattened band in the alpha$_2$-beta zone. The only cases of mu HCD have had dissociated kappa light chains as well as mu chains.

URINE PROTEINS

Urine electrophoresis and immunoelectrophoresis must be run in parallel. Characteristic of the unattached heavy chain is a migration in serum and urine that is a mirror image. Antisera to light chains do not show any arcs in gamma-chain disease. Lambda-chain antisera are notoriously unreliable so that several lot numbers should be used before it is determined that no light chains are present.

GASTROINTESTINAL X-RAYS

Gastrointestinal x-rays may indicate masses in the small intestine in alpha-chain disease, which should be suspected when the patient is young (under 25) with what initially appears to be IgA paraprotein. Intestinal biopsy shows a variable lymphocyte and plasma cell infiltrate of the lamina propria.

LABORATORY STUDIES OF
AMYLOIDOSIS

Hematologic Tests

GENERAL FEATURES

Amyloidosis has been classified as primary (idiopathic), secondary (following chronic inflammation), and as complicating myelomatosis. The latter category has many similarities to primary amyloidosis. Amyloidosis develops in approximately 10% of patients with myeloma. It is most frequent in light-chain myeloma and does not appear unless Bence Jones protein is present. Its pathogenesis is unknown but circulating immune complexes, possibly involving the paraprotein, are suspected. Amyloidosis complicating myelomatosis has deposits in muscle, lymph nodes, subcutis, or synovia, and, thus, it frequently presents as carpal tunnel syndrome. Such deposits may precede clinical myeloma by years. Primary amyloidosis has a slightly wider spectrum, involving striated and cardiac muscle, kidney, gingiva, and rectal mucosa. Kidney involvement differs markedly between primary amyloidosis and amyloidosis complicating myeloma. In primary amyloidosis large masses of amyloid are deposited in glomeruli resulting in massive nephrotic protein loss. In amyloid complicating myeloma, monoclonal light-chain dimers are deposited in renal tubular epithelium, and urinary proteinuria may be mild until renal failure is present.

HEMATOLOGIC FINDINGS

Hematologic findings in amyloid complicating myeloma are those of the myeloma. In primary amyloidoses 10%–12% plasma cells may be present in the bone marrow without myeloma.

SERUM PROTEINS

Serum proteins in primary amyloidosis may be normal. When spikes have appeared they have been IgG, IgA, or IgM usually with concurrent Bence Jones proteinemia. In amyloidosis of myeloma there may be loss of the previous monoclonal spike with hypogammaglobulinemia as amyloidosis develops. When renal failure occurs a small Bence Jones protein spike appears since it is no longer cleared.

URINE PROTEINS

Bence Jones proteinuria is always present with complicating amyloidosis. It is variable in primary amyloidosis reflecting the serum variability.

REFERENCES

1. Kochwa S: Immunoelectrophoresis (including zone electrophoresis). In Rose NR, Friedman H (eds): *Manual of Clinical Immunology.* Washington, DC, American Society of Microbiology, 1976, pp 22–24

2. Bell CA: Other useful immunologic methods. In Nakamura RM (ed): *Immunopathology: Clinical Laboratory Concepts and Methods.* Boston, Little, Brown, 1974, pp 611–613

3. Bauer JD: White blood cell pathology. In Frankel S, Reitman S, Sonnenwirth AC (eds): *Gradwohl's Clinical Laboratory Methods and Diagnosis: A Textbook on Laboratory Procedures and Their Interpretation,* ed 7. St. Louis, C.V. Mosby Co, 1970, pp 642–643

4. Davis NC, Ho M: Quantitation of immunoglobulins. In Rose NR, Friedman H (eds): *Manual of Clinical Immunology.* Washington, DC, American Society of Microbiology, 1976, pp 4–8

PART C/**BLEEDING DISORDERS**

chapter 23

Diagnosis of Bleeding Disorders

The initial or primary events that stop bleeding from a very small wound are the formation of a platelet plug, which seals the hole in the vessel wall, and arteriolar vasoconstriction. The plug is subsequently fortified by fibrin strands (Figure 23-1). The stimulus that causes the platelets to aggregate and form the primary plug is believed to be exposure to subendothelial components and collagen. Aggregation is probably dependent on the von Willebrand factor and other plasma factors, such as ADP released from lysed red cells or platelets after exposure to collagen. A defect in one of these plasma factors, a qualitative defect in platelets, thrombocytopenia, or a defect in the vascular wall can result in failure of the primary hemostatic mechanism with spontaneous bleeding or purpura. Purpura is not directly attributable to trauma and is exemplified by the type of bleeding seen in severe thrombocytopenia. Such bleeding differs from that resulting from defective fibrin formation, which is referred to as the coagulation or hemophilioid type. The main clinical characteristics of the two types of bleeding are shown in Table 23-1.

Congenital bleeding disorders can characteristically be distinguished from acquired disorders by family history, age, and circumstance of onset and by the presence or absence of an underlying disorder.

The formation of fibrin proceeds in a stepwise manner referred to as a cascade or waterfall (Figure 23-2). Blood clotting in vitro is

443

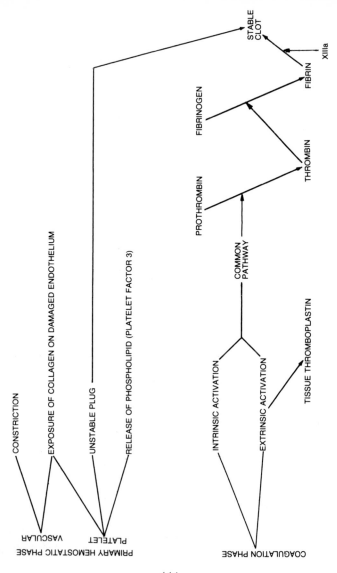

Figure 23-1. Integrated scheme for hemostasis.

Table 23-1. Differentiation of Hemophilioid States and Purpuric States[a]

Clinical Characteristic	Hemophilioid States	Purpuras
Bleeding source	Usually small artery	Usually capillary
Bruises	Often intramuscular, deep and large	Cutaneous and mucosal petechiae and/or ecchymoses, usually small
Preceding trauma	Frequent	Unusual
Venipuncture	No superficial ecchymosis but massive hemorrhage may occur if firm pressure is not maintained long enough	Superficial ecchymoses around venipuncture site despite clean venipuncture
Epistaxis	Seldom a predominant symptom	Often a major source of bleeding
Gastrointestinal bleeding	Rarely a major symptom unless peptic ulceration is also present	Often a major source of bleeding
Hematuria	Common	Uncommon
Menorrhagia	Uncommon, most patients are males	Common
Dental bleeding	Starts hours or even days later and may last several days; not controlled by pressure	Starts immediately, lasts several hours, and is often controlled by pressure
Onset of bleeding after trauma	Usually late (1–4 hours after event)	Usually immediate
Postoperative bleeding	Late bleeding with wound hematomas	Bleeding mainly at the time of operation
Symptoms of mildly affected patients	Large hematomas after injury; persistent and often dangerous bleeding after trauma	Mucous membrane bleeding, e.g., epistaxis and menorrhagia
Hemarthroses	Occur in severe cases	Absent
Inheritance	Often sex linked	No sex-linked hereditary history
Sex incidence	Rare in females	Common in females
Bleeding time	Normal	Usually prolonged

[a]Modified with permission from Biggs R, Macfarlane RG: *Treatment of Hemophilia and Other Coagulation Disorders.* Oxford, Blackwell Scientific Publications, Ltd, 1966.

initiated by contact of the blood with a foreign surface such as glass, kaolin (Celite). The factors involved in this early contact phase are factors XII and XI, high molecular weight kininogen (HMW-k), and Fletcher factor (Table 23-2). However, even patients with severe deficiencies of these factors, with the exception of some patients with factor XI deficiency, are completely asymptomatic. Defective synthesis of any of the other factors shown in Tables 23-3 and 23-4 may give rise to a bleeding disorder, but by far the most frequently encountered are hemophilia A and B, which are attributable to a deficiency of factors VIII and IX respectively. They are both recessive diseases of males and in almost half of the patients a clear-cut sex-linked history is obtained. The clinical manifestations of the milder forms of hemophilia A and B resemble von Willebrand's disease (see Chapters 25 and 26). However, this disease is transmitted as an autosomal dominant or recessive trait. Hereditary deficiencies of the coagulation factors other than factor VIII or IX are usually transmitted in an autosomal recessive manner and are very rare. In moderately severe congenital hemorrhagic states, the bleeding manifestations date from a very early age. However, long remissions may occur and mild cases of hemophilia may present for the first time in the second or third decade. The absence of excessive bleeding following lacerations of the skin or tongue or after relatively minor operations such as tonsillectomy and dental surgery, especially extraction of wisdom teeth, is strong evidence against a congenital hemorrhagic state. On the other hand, excessive bleeding that necessitates blood transfusion is strongly suggestive of this condition.

A secondary bleeding tendency may be a sequela of a systemic disease such as leukemia, acute infection, uremia, and liver disease, or may be drug induced. Scurvy is still seen from time to time. A dietary history points to this diagnosis.

It is not unusual to find severe acquired or hereditary abnormalities in clotting tests of patients who have never bled excessively, even after challenges such as major surgery. More rarely, some patients clearly have a bleeding tendency, yet the abnormality can-

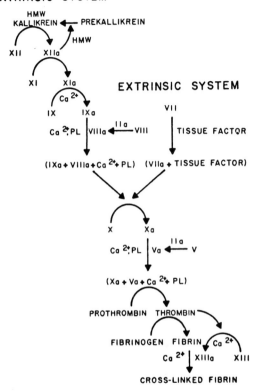

Figure 23-2. Cascade or waterfall mechanism of blood coagulation. Abbreviations: *PL,* phospholipid; *HMW-K,* high molecular weight kininogen. (Adapted from Davie EW, Ratnoff OD: Science 145:1310, 1964.)

Table 23-2. **The Contact Factors**

Preferred Term	Synonyms
XII	Hageman factor
XI	Plasma thromboplastin antecedent (PTA)
Prekallikrein	Fletcher factor
HMW-kininogen	High molecular weight kininogen; Fitzgerald, Williams, Flaujeac factors

Table 23-3. **The Vitamin K-Dependent Clotting Factors**

Preferred Term	Synonyms
Prothrombin	II
VII	Proconvertin
IX	Christmas factor, plasma thromboplastin component (PTC)
X	Stuart, Prower factors

Table 23-4. **The Thrombin-Sensitive Factors**

Preferred Term	Synonyms
Fibrinogen	I
V	Proaccelerin, accelerator globulin (AcG)
VIII	Antihemophilic factor (AHF), VIIIc, antihemophilic globulin (AHG)
XIII	Fibrin stabilizing factor (FST), Laki-Lorand factor

not be detected by currently available tests. A careful history or physical examination, therefore, always takes precedence over laboratory tests.

DIAGNOSTIC EVALUATION

The approach to diagnosis usually begins with the following:

1. Hematologic evaluation to detect anemia and thrombocytopenia.
2. Screening tests for bleeding abnormality. In patients with no personal or family history of bleeding who are to undergo surgery, these should include examination of the peripheral smear to screen for number of platelets (or a platelet count) and a determination of bleeding time, activated partial thromboplastin time (APTT), and prothrombin time (PT) (see Table 23-5). If all of these tests show normal results, no further tests are carried out and surgery may be performed. If an abnormality, however mild, is found, more specialized tests are required. When there is a personal or family history of bleeding, a similar group of screening procedures is carried out, but if these are all normal, additional tests to exclude von Willebrand's disease (Chapter 25), qualitative platelet abnormalities (Chapter 25), factor XIII deficiency, and fibrinogen abnormality are indicated.
3. Specific factor assays and tests for inhibitors are performed if the APTT and PT are prolonged. Assays for Fletcher factor, HMW-K, and factor VII are costly since the deficient plasmas are scarce, and these tests should be performed only when deficiencies of the other factors have been excluded.
4. Tests for qualitative platelet abnormalities are performed when the bleeding time is borderline or prolonged despite a normal platelet count or if all the other blood coagulation tests produce normal results.
5. Evaluation of von Willebrand factor may be performed when factor VIII is decreased and/or the bleeding time is prolonged. This includes determination of von Willebrand antigen and the quantitative ristocetin aggregation test (Chapter 25).
6. Tests for fibrinogen abnormalities are performed when the tests previously described are all normal in a patient with a clear-cut bleeding tendency. The determination of thrombin time is usually adequate for this purpose.

Table 23-5. Routine Coagulation Screening Tests

Disease	APTT	Pro-thrombin Time	Bleeding Time	Platelet Count
von Willebrand's disease	N[a] or ↑	N	N or ↑	N
Hemophilia A and B	↑	N	N	N
Thrombocytopenic purpura	N	N	↑	↓
Liver disease or vitamin K-deficient state	N or ↑	↑	N or ↑	N or ↓

[a]N, normal.

LABORATORY STUDIES

Hematologic Tests

GENERAL FEATURES

Hematologic abnormalities are found primarily in association with thrombocytopenia. Bleeding disorders are also seen in diseases such as polycythemia vera that are associated with thrombocytosis (see Chapter 24).

PERIPHERAL BLOOD

Blood cell measurements

A representative normal range for the platelet count is 180,000–350,000/mm³. In blood smears made from blood collected in EDTA, platelets are discrete, and a rough estimate of platelet numbers can be made by comparative counts of the red cells and platelets in representative fields.

Morphology

Characteristic white cell morphology is seen in thrombocytopenias associated with such disorders as infectious mononucleosis and leukemia. Characteristic red cell changes are often associated with disseminated intravascular coagulation. These include fragmented red cells or schistocytes (helmet cells).

BONE MARROW

Bone marrow study helps to distinguish immune thrombocytopenias from hypoplastic and infiltrative disorders. In the immune thrombocytopenias, megakaryocytes are adequate or increased in number, whereas they are absent or decreased in hypoplastic or replaced marrows.

Other Useful Tests

BLEEDING TIME

Purpose

The bleeding time is used as a screening test for abnormalities of the primary hemostatic mechanism, particularly disorders of platelet function and von Willebrand's disease (1). It is independent of the coagulation mechanism.

Principle

The bleeding time is the length of time it takes for bleeding to cease from a small superficial wound made with a sharp blade under standardized conditions. It is a rough function of the efficacy of the primary hemostatic mechanism. The bleeding time is measured as the interval between puncture of the skin and cessation of bleeding.

Procedure

The best standardized and most reproducible techniques are based on Ivy's method. A blood pressure cuff is placed around the patient's upper arm and the pressure is raised to 40 mm Hg. Two small punctures are made along the outer surface of the patient's forearm. The drops of blood issuing from the bleeding points are absorbed at intervals of 30 seconds into two filter paper disks, one for each puncture wound, until bleeding ceases. The average of the times required for bleeding to stop from the puncture wounds is taken as the bleeding time.

Several modifications of this technique have been devised in attempts to standardize the skin puncture. Perhaps the best and least traumatic of these is a sterile disposable device (Simplate),* which makes a uniform single incision 5 mm in length by 1 mm in depth by means of a spring-loaded blade contained in a plastic housing. The device is placed firmly on the nonhairy part of the skin of the forearm without pressure and positioned so that the incision will be parallel to the fold of the elbow, with care taken to avoid superficial veins, scars, and bruises; the blade is then released by depression of the triggering device. The normal bleeding time with this method is less than seven minutes.

Interpretation

There is a fairly good correlation between platelet count and bleeding time. If the platelets are qualitatively normal, the platelet count usually has to drop to below $80,000/mm^3$ before an abnormality in the bleeding time becomes apparent. The prolongation does not become pronounced until the count falls below $40,000/mm^3$. A prolongation is also seen in some patients with qualitative platelet abnormalities or myeloproliferative disorders. The bleeding time is prolonged in about one-third of patients with von Willebrand's disease. Occasionally a prolonged bleeding time is the sole abnormality that can be found, despite exhaustive tests, in a patient with a lifelong history of bleeding.

Notes and precautions

By far the most common cause of a prolonged bleeding time is the ingestion of a drug that interferes with platelet function. As little as 600 mg of sulfosalicylic acid (aspirin) taken seven days before can result in a significantly prolonged bleeding time. Aspirin

---

*Manufactured by General Diagnostics, Division of Warner-Lambert Pharmaceuticals Co., Morris Plains, NJ.

is not considered to be a drug or medication by many patients and is present in a large number of proprietary preparations (see Table 23-6). If the patient has taken aspirin and bleeding time is normal, the result is significant and valid, but if prolonged, the test must be repeated at a later time.

The Simplate method may leave a small scar, and the patient should be so warned. There is no purpose in performing the bleeding time test on a patient with a platelet count less than 40,000/mm^3.

WHOLE BLOOD COAGULATION TIME AND CLOT OBSERVATION AND RETRACTION

Purpose

The test of whole blood coagulation time and clot observation and retraction monitors heparin therapy and screens for abnormalities in fibrinolysis (2). It is a very insensitive index of clotting function and of little value for the detection of mild to moderate bleeding disorders.

Principle

The time required for blood to clot in a test tube is a crude measure of intrinsic clotting. Failure of the clot to retract may result from a qualitative or quantitative platelet defect. A weak clot or one that breaks down indicates abnormal fibrinolysis, which is usually secondary to DIC.

Procedure

Venous blood obtained by a clean venipuncture is withdrawn into a plastic syringe. To minimize contamination with tissue juice, some coagulation laboratories prefer a two-syringe technique. After 1–2 ml of blood has been withdrawn into the first syringe, it is disconnected from the needle and only blood collected into the second syringe is used. One ml aliquots of the blood are immediately transferred into three 12-mm by 77-mm glass tubes. The tubes are placed in a heating block at 37 C and tilted gently every

Table 23-6. Compounds Containing Aspirin[a,b]

ACA capsules and ACA no. 2
Acetidine capsules
Alka-Seltzer
Allylgesic[c]
Amytal with ASA[c]
Anacin
Anahist
APC
ASA
ASA compound
ASA compound with codeine
Aspirbar
Aspodyne
Bayer aspirin
Buff-A
Buffacetin
Bufferin
Buffinol
Colrex
Coricidin
Darvon with ASA[c]
Darvon-N with ASA[c]
Empiral[c]
Empirin
Excedrin
P-A-C compound[c]
Percodan[c]
Persistin
Phenaphen[c]
Phenergan compound[c]
Robaxisal[c]
Sedagesic
Sine-Off tablets
St. Joseph aspirin

[a]Adapted with permission from Leist ER, Banwell JG: Products containing aspirin. N Engl J Med 291:710, 1974.
[b]For complete list consult Leist ER, Banwell JG: N Engl J Med 291:710, 1974, and Selner J: N Engl J Med 292:372, 1975.
[c]Available through prescription only.

30 seconds until a clot is seen in one of the tubes. The stopwatch is then stopped and the clotting time recorded. The clotting times of the remaining two tubes need not be determined. If no clot is present in any of the tubes after 10 minutes, the clotting time should be recorded as abnormal. The tubes are inspected at the end of one hour and again on the following morning. In the original Lee and White clotting test, the first tube was tilted at intervals of 30 seconds until a solid clot formed. The second and third tubes were then treated similarly in sequence. The clotting time was the time required for a solid clot to form in the third tube.

Specimen

Whole blood is used.

Interpretation

When performed in the manner described previously, normal blood clots appear within seven minutes. If no clot has formed by 10 minutes, a defect in intrinsic coagulation is present and there is no point in determining the exact time of clotting. The test is prolonged when a severe deficiency (less than 6%) of a clotting factor (other than factor VII or XIII) or a circulating anticoagulant including heparin is present.

At the end of one hour, the degree of clot retraction and the general size of the clot is noted. It should be firm and occupy a volume approximately equal to half the total volume of the blood. If it occupies a volume more than this or if it has not retracted at all, the result is considered abnormal. However, the test is not very sensitive and a normal result does not exclude a platelet abnormality. By freeing the clot from the tube and tilting the tube up and down so the clot impinges on the bottom of the tube, some idea of its weight can be gauged. Sometimes the clot will show signs of breaking up, indicating it is weak and defective, and on inspection the following morning it may appear to have completely disintegrated. In a few patients with severe intravascular coagulation and secondary fibrinolysis, the clot may have very ragged margins and

455

be soft and flabby. As it disintegrates red cells form a clearly demarcated layer in the bottom of the tube. When the concentration of fibrinogen is low, the clot may initially be normal in size but after retraction may be so small as to be overlooked. In the past the whole blood clotting time was the test used most often to monitor heparin therapy. However, it is cumbersome and time consuming and the same information can be obtained more conveniently by the use of the APTT.

Notes and precautions

Tubes that have been siliconized some time in the past may extend clotting times, and only disposable tubes or new tubes that have been washed with acid should be used. The whole blood clotting time may be normal in moderately severe cases of hemophilia. It cannot be overemphasized that this test can never be used as the sole screening test for disorders of coagulation.

THE ACTIVATED PARTIAL THROMBOPLASTIN TIME (APTT)

Purpose

The APTT is used as a screening test for deficiencies of plasma coagulation factors other than factors VII and XIII (3). The test is also used to monitor heparin therapy.

Principle

Platelet-poor plasma contains all the coagulation factors necessary for the formation of intrinsic prothrombinase or plasma thromboplastin with the exception of calcium ions and phospholipid. In the APTT test, phospholipid and CA^{++} are added to the plasma, and, therefore, the clotting time is a function of intrinsic prothrombinase formation. The extent of exposure of the plasma to glass surfaces is controlled by exposing the plasma to optimal surface activation by addition of kaolin (Celite) or ellagic acid. Factor VII is not measured, as it is involved in the extrinsic pathway only. Neither is factor XIII measured since it is involved only in clot

456

stabilization. As platelet-poor plasma is used, the test is not influenced by quantitative or qualitative abnormalities in the platelets.

Procedure

The test is performed by mixing the platelet-poor plasma from the patient or healthy subject with phospholipid and an activating agent such as kaolin (Celite) to achieve optimal contact activation. An optimal amount of calcium is then added and the clotting times are recorded.

Specimen

Blood is collected by clean venipuncture using a plastic syringe. Nine parts of the whole blood are mixed with one part anticoagulant but an adjustment in the ratio of anticoagulant to whole blood may be made in cases where the hematocrit is very high. The anticoagulant is 3.2% or 3.8% trisodium citrate. Most specialized coagulation laboratories use a 3.8% (0.1 M) buffered citrate solution; EDTA or heparin should not be used. The blood is best collected in a plastic tube and plastic pipettes are used to process the plasma. However, most general laboratories use plain or silicone-coated glass tubes; the latter are available commercially.*

Interpretation

The normal range for the APTT is dependent on a large number of variables. Semiautomated instruments with photoelectric devices for the determination of the end point give shorter values than when the clotting time is determined visually; however, variability is found from instrument to instrument even of the same type and manufacturer. It is therefore important to know the normal range for the particular laboratory performing the test. Using a coagulyzer† in which the preincubation period is at least five minutes,

---

*Manufactured by Becton and Dickenson, Rutherford, NJ.
†Manufactured by Sherwood Medical Industries, St. Louis, MO.

APTT reagent,* and buffered citrate, the normal range in the University of California Hospital laboratory, San Diego, has usually been between 25–29 seconds, varying somewhat with the particular batch of partial thromboplastin reagent used.

The APTT is prolonged when one or more of any of the factors necessary for the formation of intrinsic prothrombinase is deficient. These include factors XII, HMW-K, prekallikrein, XI, X, IX, VIII, and V, and also prothrombin and fibrinogen (Table 23-7). If the period of contact activation is greater than two or three minutes, the test may become insensitive to prekallikrein. The sensitivity of the test to deficiencies of the other factors varies from factor to factor. As a general rule the level has to decrease to below 40% before the APTT becomes significantly prolonged.

Specific inhibitors of clotting factors may also result in a prolongation of the APTT. The most frequently encountered of these is an antibody against factor VIII. The so-called lupus anticoagulant, which is an antibody that appears to act nonspecifically, is one of the most frequent causes of a prolonged APTT found on routine preoperative screening. In monitoring heparin therapy, when heparin is given continuously by intravenous drip for the treatment of venous thromboembolism, the APTT should be prolonged to 1.5–2.5 times the control level. However, the sensitivity of the method to heparin depends on the type and concentration of the activator and the phospholipid used. The results are not always reliable, particularly when the blood sample has been withdrawn through an intravenous catheter used to infuse the heparin. The test is more helpful than the Lee and White clotting test for the monitoring of heparin therapy, as it is more convenient and less time consuming. However, whether such therapy needs to be monitored at all remains an unsettled question.

---

*Manufactured by General Diagnostics, Division of Warner-Lambert Pharmaceuticals Co., Morris Plains, NJ.

Table 23-7. Factors Measured by Activated Partial Thromboplastin Time (APTT) and Prothrombin Time (PT) Tests

APTT	PT	Both Tests
XII	VII	
HMW-K (Fitzgerald)		
Fletcher (prekallikrein)		
XI		
IX		
VIII		
V	V	V
X	X	X
Prothrombin	Prothrombin	Prothrombin
Fibrinogen	Fibrinogen	Fibrinogen

Notes and precautions

The normal range is sometimes not included on the report, although a normal control value is given. This is because the range tends to vary from time to time depending on variations in the batch of partial thromboplastin reagents used and whether the end point is determined by machine through changes in the sensitivity of the instrument. However, the normal range is quite narrow when individuals with low levels of factors XI or XII or those with the lupus anticoagulants are excluded. Such subjects are encountered quite frequently in the healthy population of individuals with no family or personal history of a bleeding tendency. If the plasma is very turbid or icteric, the change of optical density caused by fibrin formation may be too small to trigger the clot timing device of instruments that use photoelectric devices. The value of the APTT (and also PT) printed by the machine will then be the highest value the instrument is capable of recording; whenever these values are obtained on such an instrument, the test should be repeated using a manual method.

THE ONE-STAGE PROTHROMBIN TIME TEST

Purpose

The one-stage prothrombin time test is used to screen for abnormalities of those factors that are involved in the extrinsic pathway (factors V, VII, and X; prothrombin and fibrinogen) (4). It is used to monitor the effects of the coumarin anticoagulants and to study patients with hereditary and acquired disorders of clotting.

Principle

When tissue extract, loosely referred to as thromboplastin, is added to plasma in the presence of calcium, it reacts with the factor VII to form a product that converts factor X to its activated form, factor Xa; this, in turn, reacts with the factor V and phospholipid present in the tissue extract to form extrinsic prothrombinase, which converts prothrombin to thrombin. Thrombin then converts fibrinogen to fibrin. The rate of fibrin formation is therefore a function of the concentration of factors V, VII, and X and prothrombin and fibrinogen; the test measures the overall activities of these factors (Table 23-7).

Procedure

In Quick's test, one volume of tissue extract is added to an equal volume of plasma. The mixture is then recalcified by the addition of an optimal amount of calcium chloride and the clotting time is recorded. Both the patient's and the healthy control subject's values are reported.

Several different types of tissue extracts or thromboplastins are available. While almost all commercial preparations are acetone extracts of rabbit brain, several large coagulation laboratories prefer saline extracts of human brain. Saline extracts tend to be more sensitive then acetone extracts, while extracts from a human source are more sensitive than their equivalent rabbit counterpart. Therefore, it is important to know the source and type of tissue extract used to perform the test, and before a new batch of tissue extract is used it must be compared with samples from the preceding batch.

Specimen

Tests may be performed on the same specimen of plasma used for the APTT test. It is important to collect the normal control plasma in the same manner as the patient plasma at approximately the same time.

Interpretation

There are several ways to express results of the prothrombin time test. A widely used practice expresses results as a precentage of normal concentration. In Quick's method, the prothrombin times of varying dilutions of normal pooled plasma in saline are determined and a prothrombin dilution curve is constructed by plotting percent concentration against prothrombin time (Figure 23-3). The curve is used to read off prothrombin concentration from the patient's prothrombin time. Percent concentration determined in this manner reflects the concentration of factor V and fibrinogen as well as the vitamin K-dependent factors. Ideally, a test used to monitor oral anticoagulant should reflect only the vitamin K-dependent factors. In the prothrombin-proconvertin (P and P) test of Owren, this is accomplished by diluting the test plasma and the pooled normal control plasma used to prepare the dilution curve with normal $BaSO_4$ or $Al(OH)_3$-absorbed plasma instead of saline, thereby providing a constant amount of factor V and fibrinogen (5). Clotting times with samples diluted with adsorbed plasma are shorter than those diluted with saline at corresponding dilutions, and the desirable therapeutic range of percent concentration for anticoagulant therapy is lower with the P and P test than Quick's test.

For a number of reasons, percent concentration is an inadequate expression of prothrombin time results. The percent values as derived from the dilution curve give distorted representations of the true concentration of coagulation factors, and errors are introduced in preparation and reading of dilution curves. Therefore, a more helpful method for monitoring anticoagulant therapy is use of the ratio of the patient's prothrombin time to that of the healthy control subject. For each type of tissue thromboplastin, there is an optimal

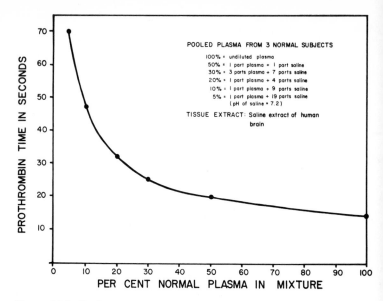

Figure 23-3. Prothrombin dilution curve prepared by diluting pooled normal plasma with buffered normal saline pH 7.2. The prothrombin times were performed using a saline extract of human brain. Note that dilution of the plasma with an equal part of saline (50% concentration) results in little more than a one-second increase in clotting time. As the concentration of plasma falls below 20%, the clotting times increase markedly.

ratio range (Table 23-8), but no general agreement has been reached on the minimum prothrombin time to accomplish effective anticoagulation. The prolongation of the prothrombin time usually indicates defective or decreased synthesis of the vitamin K-dependent clotting factors, with the exception of factor IX, which is also depressed but not measured by this test. The test is also sensitive to decreases in factor V concentration, which are sometimes seen in cirrhosis of the liver and chronic hepatitis.

A hereditary deficiency of one of the factors affecting the prothrombin time test is very rare. The prothrombin time is sometimes

Table 23-8. **Suggested Therapeutic Ranges of Prothrombin Time with Different Types of Tissue Extracts**

Tissue Extract	Range[a]
Saline extract of human brain	$2\frac{1}{2}$–3
OBT (ortho brain thromboplastin)[b]	$1\frac{1}{2}$–$2\frac{1}{2}$
Activated thromboplastin (Thromboplastic C)[c]	$1\frac{1}{2}$–2
Simplastin[d]	$1\frac{1}{2}$–2
Bacto/thromboplastin[e]	2 –$2\frac{1}{2}$

[a]Expressed as the ratio of the patient's prothrombin time to the normal control time: patient PT/normal PT.
[b]Manufactured by Ortho Pharmaceutical Corp., Diagnostic Division, Raritan, NJ.
[c]Manufactured by Dade Reagents, Inc., Miami, FL.
[d]Manufactured by Warner-Chilcott Laboratories, Division of Warner-Lambert Pharmaceuticals Co., Morris Plains, NJ.
[e]Manufactured by DifCo Laboratories, Detroit, MI.

prolonged when a very potent lupus-type anticoagulant is present. It may also be slightly prolonged in disseminated intravascular coagulation associated with decrease in factor V and fibrinogen. Factors measured by the APTT and prothrombin time are compared in Table 23-7. The normal range for the prothrombin time varies according to the tissue extract and technique used to record the clotting time. It is very narrow with a standard deviation of less than 0.5 seconds from the mean.

Notes and precautions

If normal plasma is left at cold temperatures for several hours, the prothrombin time of normal and pathologic plasmas may be shortened significantly; it is believed that the contact factors are involved in this process. Thus, if the patient's blood is drawn in the afternoon while the control plasma was collected in the morning and kept in the refrigerator, the patient's time, although normal, may be significantly longer than that of the control subject. Thus it is important that the control plasma be drawn approximately at the same time as that of the test specimen. In order to obviate the need for fresh normal controls, it is common practice to use commercial standards or aliquots of freshly frozen normal pooled plasma.

The test should not be performed if a small clot is present within the specimen. As discussed earlier, the clot timing devices of photoelectric instruments may fail to detect fibrin formation in very turbid or icteric specimens and a manual technique must then be employed.

THROMBIN TIME

Purpose

The thrombin time is used to screen for abnormalities in the conversion of fibrinogen to fibrin (6). These may be caused by qualitative or quantitative abnormalities of fibrinogen or by inhibitors such as heparin or fibrin/fibrinogen split products.

Principle

The addition of thrombin to plasma converts fibrinogen to fibrin and bypasses both the intrinsic and extrinsic pathways. The time taken for plasma to clot on addition of thrombin, referred to as the thrombin time, is a function of fibrinogen concentration.

Technique

One part of a solution of thrombin is added to a mixture of one part of the patient's citrated plasma and one part of normal saline, and the clotting time is recorded. Two strengths of thrombin should be used. One strength should give a normal clotting time of 9–11 seconds and the other a time of 25–35 seconds with normal pooled plasma.

Interpretation

A prolongation over the normal time of three seconds or more with the stronger solution and five seconds or more with the weaker is considered abnormal. If the plasma does not clot with either strength in five minutes, either the concentration of fibrinogen is less than 5 mg/100 ml or, far more likely, a potent antithrombic substance, almost invariably heparin, is present. A moderate prolongation is also likely to be caused by heparin but occasionally may result from fibrin or fibrinogen split products, hypofibrinogenemia, or dysfibrinogenemia. When a significant abnormality is found, the test must be repeated using the stronger thrombin solution on a mixture consisting of equal parts of patient and normal plasma. If the thrombin time of the mixture is three seconds or more longer than the control's, an inhibitor is present. If the thrombin time is corrected to within two seconds of the control, hypofibrinogenemia or dysfibrinogenemia is likely.

Notes and precautions

A slight prolongation with the weaker strength and a normal value with the stronger is probably not significant. If a potent inhibitor is present, as demonstrated by little or no correction with normal plasma, the cause is almost always heparin medication. Occasionally contamination with heparin occurs when the blood is withdrawn through a catheter through which heparin had previously been infused. However, if contamination of the specimen with heparin can be definitely excluded a new specimen should be withdrawn and the test repeated. If an anticoagulant can still be demonstrated, a protamine titration test for heparin or a reptilase time test should be performed. The principle of the latter test is that reptilase, a snake venom that is available commercially, converts fibrinogen to fibrin directly and its action is not inhibited by heparin. The test is performed similarly to the thrombin time, with reptilase substituted for thrombin. A normal reptilase time with a prolonged thrombin time in this setting is evidence that the patient has received heparin or that heparin contamination has occurred.

REFERENCES

1. Hougie C: Bleeding time. In Williams WJ, Beutler E, Erslev AJ, et al (eds): *Hematology*, ed 2. New York, McGraw-Hill, 1977, p 1655

2. Hougie C: Whole blood coagulation time test and clot observation. In Williams WJ, Beutler E, Erslev AJ, et al (eds): *Hematology*, ed 2. New York, McGraw-Hill, 1977, p 1641

3. Proctor RR, Rapaport SI: The partial thromboplastin time with kaolin: a simple screening test for first stage plasma clotting factor deficiencies. Am J Clin Pathol 36:212–219, 1961

4. Hougie C: One-stage prothrombin time. In Williams WJ, Beutler E, Erslev AJ, et al (eds): *Hematology*, ed 2. New York, McGraw-Hill, 1977, pp 1645–1647

5. Owren PA, Aas K: The control of dicumarol therapy and the quantitative determination of prothrombin and proconvertin. Scand J Clin Lab Invest 3:201, 1951

6. Hougie C: Methods for estimating fibrinogen concentration. In Williams WJ, Beutler E, Erslev AJ, et al (eds): *Hematology*, ed 2. New York, McGraw-Hill, 1977, p 1650

chapter 24

Thrombo-cytopenic Purpura

Thrombocytopenia is the most common cause of major bleeding in children and adults and, with rare exceptions, is an acquired disorder (Table 24-1). It may be caused by decreased production or excessive destruction of platelets; a smaller number of cases result from redistribution of the platelets with splenic pooling. Reduced production occurs in hypoplastic or aplastic anemia from causes such as leukemia, multiple myeloma, myelofibrosis, or infiltration of the bone marrow by carcinoma or lymphoma. It is also seen in vitamin B_{12} or folic acid deficiency, but in such cases the thrombocytopenia is rarely severe enough to result in significant bleeding.

Excessive destruction of platelets can usually be attributed to an autoantibody directed toward a platelet-associated antigen. Such antibodies are found in some patients with systemic lupus erythematosus or lymphoma. Evidence for these diseases may not be apparent at the onset of bleeding. Rarely, an isoagglutinin develops in patients who have received multiple transfusions. Certain drugs may cause an antibody-mediated thrombocytopenia. The best known of these are the sulfonamides, quinine, quinidine, and digitoxin. Antibodies may develop after viral infections such as rubella, measles, or infectious mononucleosis. The demonstration of an autoantibody is difficult to achieve and special techniques that are currently performed in only a few research or reference laboratories are needed. Even with the most sensitive of these techniques, anti-

Table 24-1. Causes of Thrombocytopenia

Decreased platelet production
    Marrow injury
        Drugs, chemicals, or radiation

    Bone marrow infiltration
        Carcinoma, leukemia, lymphoma
        Myelofibrosis

    Congenital abnormalities
        Aldrich-Wiskott syndrome
        Fanconi's syndrome

    B_{12} or folic acid deficiency

Increased platelet destruction
    Autoantibodies
        Postinfectious fever
        Lupus erythematosus
        Lymphomas
        Hemolytic anemia (Evans' syndrome)
        Drugs
        Idiopathic

    Alloantibodies
        Fetal material incompatibility
        After transfusion

    Platelet injury
        Viral or bacterial
        Prosthesis

    Disseminated intravascular coagulation

Sequestration of platelets in spleen

Thrombotic thrombocytopenic purpura

Dilution after massive transfusion

bodies can only be demonstrated in about 90% of cases. The term autoimmune thrombocytopenic purpura is sometimes used to refer to those cases in which an antibody has been demonstrated, and the term idiopathic thrombocytopenic purpura (ITP) is reserved for those cases in which no antibody has been found. This distinction is quite arbitrary, since the relative incidence of each of the two types may merely be a function of the sensitivity of the method used to detect the antibody. Some drugs such as the thiazide diuretics appear to cause thrombocytopenia by suppressing platelet production through a toxic effect on the megakaryocytes of sensitive persons. Viruses can cause thrombocytopenia by interfering with megakaryocytic maturation, but peripheral destruction of platelets by immune mechanisms also occurs in viral infections. Mild subclinical thrombocytopenia is a frequent event in infectious mononucleosis, Rocky Mountain spotted fever, tuberculosis, malaria, and gram-negative infections. In some instances the thrombocytopenia may be attributable to disseminated intravascular coagulation (DIC), but other factors may be operative. Any condition associated with an enlargement of the spleen may cause thrombocytopenia by the sequestration of the platelets in splenic sinusoids.

Thrombocytopenia can be accompanied by qualitative abnormalities in the platelets, in which case the degree of reduction of platelet count correlates only roughly with the severity of the bleeding. Bleeding, even after operation, is rare with platelet counts above $100,000/mm^3$, provided that no qualitative platelet defect is present. When the platelet count falls below $40,000/mm^3$, spontaneous bleeding is common and may reach quite severe proportions when the platelets decrease to below $5000/mm^3$.

The bleeding manifestations resulting from thrombocytopenia include petechiae, spontaneous bruising, and mucosal bleeding and can usually be distinguished from those seen in hemophilioid states (see Table 23-1) (see Chapter 23); in the latter states petechiae are not seen and the hematomas tend to be deeper and more often related to trauma. In acute ITP the onset is usually quite sudden, with severe manifestations such as petechiae and bleeding from the

469

mucous membranes. There is often a history of a preceding viral infection and young children are most often affected. In contrast, the onset of chronic ITP tends to be insidious, adults are more often affected, and the course tends to be protracted. Differentiation between the acute and chronic forms may be difficult if not impossible at the time the thrombocytopenia is first discovered. A history of a recent infection or ingestion of some drugs has special relevance. A complete review of systems may suggest other diseases that may be associated with thrombocytopenia such as a collagen disease, lymphoma, sarcoidosis, or tuberculosis. Particular attention should be given to the type of bruising, whether of the capillary type seen with thrombocytopenia or the small arteriolar or hemophilioid type, and to the presence or absence of adenopathy and splenomegaly. The finding of an enlarged spleen virtually excludes the diagnosis of ITP.

Hereditary thrombocytopenic states are rare and include Fanconi's syndrome and thrombocytopenia with bilateral absence of radii. In both of these conditions megakaryotic hypoplasia is present. Similar hypoplasia may be seen as a result of intrauterine infections with viral organisms such as rubella or exposure of the fetus to drugs such as thiazide diuretics in the maternal circulation. Cyclic thrombocytopenia is a rare condition in which transfusion of normal platelet-free plasma results in the production of platelets in the donor. The Wiskott-Aldrich syndrome, which is inherited as a sex-linked recessive trait, is characterized by thrombocytopenia, recurrent infections, and eczema.

DIAGNOSTIC EVALUATION

Diagnostic evaluation (Figure 24-1) includes:

1. Hematologic evaluation, to confirm thrombocytopenia and exclude thrombocytopenia secondary to leukemia, aplastic leukemia, infiltration of the bone marrow by metastatic carcinoma, multiple myeloma, and lymphoma and/or hemolytic anemia including microangiopathic hemolytic anemia.

470

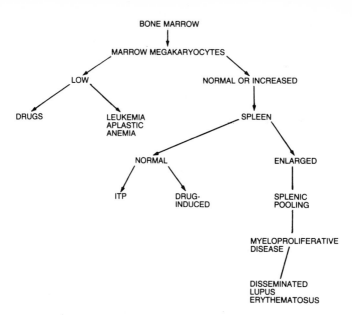

Figure 24-1. Flow diagram for diagnosis of thrombocytopenia.

2. Blood coagulation screening tests. A normal activated partial thromboplastin time (APTT) and prothrombin time (PT) exclude an associated coagulation abnormality such as a lupus anticoagulant. The bleeding time gives an assessment of the severity of the primary hemostatic defect, but this test is not necessary with thrombocytopenia or if purpura is present.

3. Special bleeding tests. A test for the detection of soluble fibrin monomers and fibrin split products should be performed when it is necessary to exclude DIC. In all patients with a normal platelet count and prolonged bleeding time, platelet aggregation studies should be performed. Study of ristocetin-induced aggregation is particularly valuable in suspected von Willebrand's disease.

4. Coombs test is performed to exclude an associated autoimmune hemolytic anemia (Evans' syndrome).

5. Tests for systemic lupus erythematosus (SLE) should be performed and repeated at least twice if the patient has an enlarged spleen.

471

Sometimes during the course of ITP, the tests will become positive for SLE.

6. A test for heterophilic antibodies is carried out when atypical lymphocytes are seen on the peripheral blood smear.

7. Blood and viral cultures are performed whenever a bacterial or viral etiology is suspected.

LABORATORY STUDIES

Hematologic Tests

GENERAL FEATURES

In ITP the peripheral blood is usually unremarkable except for the sparsity or absence of platelets. The diagnosis of ITP is made by excluding all known causes of thrombocytopenia.

PERIPHERAL BLOOD

In thrombocytopenia caused by leukemia, blast cells are almost invariably present in the peripheral blood, while in hypoplastic or aplastic anemia neutropenia with no blast cells is present. Atypical lymphocytes suggest a viral etiology such as infectious mononucleosis. Fragmented red cells or schistocytes (helmet cells), together with some spherocytes, are found in micoangiopathic hemolytic anemia and point to the diagnosis of DIC, thrombotic thrombocytopenic purpura, or the hemolytic uremic syndrome. Oval macrocytes and poikilocytosis with hypersegmented polymorphs are seen in folic acid or vitamin B_{12} deficiency. Spherocytosis and polychromatophilia and a high reticulocyte count suggest an associated immune hemolytic anemia. Heavy bleeding in a thrombocytopenic patient (e.g., a patient with menorrhagia), may result in a normocytic or ultimately a hypochromic, microcytic anemia.

Platelets are diminished on the smear and they may be larger than normal, reflecting a predominance of young forms. Large, bizarre platelets suggest an associated qualitative functional abnormality. Such abnormalities are discussed in Chapter 24.

Accurate platelet counts are important in gauging the progress and severity of the disease. The most reliable counts are obtained by an electronic counter.

BONE MARROW

In ITP the bone marrow is usually normal except for quantitative and subtle qualitative changes in the megakaryocytes. Magakaryocytes are present in normal or increased numbers. They are less granular and more basophilic than normal megakaryocytes, indicating defective maturation or decreased production of platelets. Large megakaryocytes that have an increased number of nuclear divisions may be seen. In aplastic or myelophthisic anemia, megakaryocytes are decreased or absent. Bone marrow examination is necessary to exclude an otherwise unapparent primary bone marrow disease such as leukemia.

Other Useful Tests

BLEEDING TIME TEST

The bleeding time is almost invariably prolonged with platelet counts below $40,000/mm^3$, and this test should not be performed when the patient is known to have a platelet count below this value (see Chapter 23).

PROTHROMBIN TIME AND ACTIVATED PARTIAL THROMBOPLASTIN TIME (APTT)

The prothrombin time and APTT are normal in ITP (see Chapter 23). The APTT may be prolonged if the patient has lupus erythematosus or if some other perhaps coincidental abnormality such as von Willebrand's disease is present. In DIC, the prothrombin time and APTT may be prolonged and a test for fibrin split products and serial fibrinogen determinations help to exclude the condition.

PLATELET FUNCTION TESTS

If the platelet count is above $80,000/mm^3$ platelet aggregation tests may be useful in excluding a qualitative platelet disorder associated with mild thrombocytopenia. However, in autoimmune thrombocytopenia the platelets may be damaged by antibody and they may fail to aggregate normally. Clot retraction is abnormal (see Chapter 23).

DETECTION OF ANTIPLATELET ANTIBODIES

Purpose

This test detects drug-induced or posttransfusional platelet antibodies (1,2).

Principle

In the presence of complement and the suspected drug, if relevant, platelets are damaged by the antibody and clot retraction is impaired.

Procedure

The patient and normal control serum are each incubated with freshly drawn compatible blood. If a drug is suspected, a very low concentration in distilled water is included in the mixture. The two tubes are incubated at 37 C. At the end of one hour, the degree of clot retraction is determined by inspection or by determining the amount of fluid in the tubes after removal of the clots. The test may be modified by substituting platelet-rich plasma for fresh whole blood and adding magnesium to permit complement activity; the mixture is clotted by addition of calcium.

Specimen

Serum is used and no special precautions are required.

Interpretation

The failure of the blood containing the patient's serum to retract as fully as that containing the control serum indicates the presence of a platelet antibody. If the purpura is caused by a drug-induced antibody, impairment of retraction may be seen at very low concentrations of the drug in the tube containing the patient's serum.

Notes and precautions

Some drugs at certain concentrations inhibit clot retraction by a direct action and no retraction will be seen in either tube.

REFERENCES

1. Aster RH: Detection of antiplatelet antibodies: Inhibition of clot retraction. In Williams WJ, Beutler E, Erslev AJ, et al (eds): *Hematology*, ed 2. New York, McGraw-Hill, 1977, p 1660
2. McMillan R: Diagnostic approach to immune thrombocytopenia. In Greenwalt TJ, Jamieson GA (eds): *Blood Platelets in Transfusion Therapy*. NY, Alan R. Liss Inc, 1978, pp 215–227

chapter 25

Functional Platelet Disorders

The primary function of platelets is believed to be the formation of a hemostatic plug. Impairment of this function results in purpura and excessive bleeding from the smallest cuts or wounds with prolongation of the bleeding time. Several other functions or properties have been assigned to the platelet based on in vitro studies, but their relevance to clinical situations is by inference only. In any patient with a history of purpura and a normal platelet count, a qualitative abnormality of platelets or von Willebrand's disease must be considered. In von Willebrand's disease a plasma factor essential for the normal function of platelets is deficient, and the signs and symptoms may be indistinguishable from those of a qualitative platelet disorder (Table 25-1). Hereditary qualitative platelet disorders are transmitted in an autosomal manner, but there is an apparent female sex predilection because heavy menstrual bleeding focuses attention on the bleeding disorder. Normally, except in the rare severe cases, the easy bruising and excessive bleeding from cuts are not severe enough to cause patients of either sex to seek medical attention. Many of the cases are so mild that symptoms are only manifested when some precipitating factor such as ingestion of aspirin or mild associated thrombocytopenia following an infection is present. A careful history of recent medication is essential, with special attention to aspirin or over-the-counter pain relievers containing aspirin. Patients frequently adamantly deny ingestion of aspirin or any medicines containing aspirin, yet on requestioning

Table 25-1. Clinical and Laboratory Findings in von Willebrand's Disease

Autosomal dominant trait but sometimes recessive

Features of both coagulation and purpuric type of bleeding

Ristocetin-induced platelet aggregation decreased or absent

von Willebrand's antigen[a] usually decreased; if normal, the antigen may have an abnormal mobility on crossed immunoelectrophoresis

Factor VIII usually 6%–60%, but may rarely be normal or very low

Bleeding time prolonged in about one-third of cases

Adhesiveness to glass beads decreased (Salzman test)

Factor XII decreased in about one-third of cases

Antithrombin III slightly increased

Immediate and delayed rise in factor VIII after transfusion of preparations containing von Willebrand factor (e.g., cryoprecipitate) indicating de novo synthesis of factor VIII

Levels of both vWf and factor VIII may increase to normal values or even higher in mild cases following stress, exercise, pregnancy, or certain diseases such as hepatitis

Normal platelet aggregation with ADP, epinephrine, and collagen

[a]Sometimes referred to as factor VIII related antigen or factor VIII vWf antigen.

---

after abnormal results on a platelet function test, recall taking an over-the-counter aspirin preparation (see Table 23-6, Chapter 23).

Many other drugs such as the antihistamines interfere with platelet function; a list of the more important of these is shown in Table 25-2. The thrombocytopenia that can accompany an infectious fever such as infectious mononucleosis may precipitate bleeding in a patient with a previously undiagnosed hereditary qualitative platelet disorder or von Willebrand's disease. If in such a case the first platelet count is performed a few days after the bleeding episode, the reduction in the platelet count may seem insignificant, but subsequent platelet counts will show a progressive increase, suggesting that moderate thrombocytopenia may have existed at the time bleeding occurred.

The hereditary qualitative platelet disorders may be classified on the basis of platelet aggregation tests (Table 25-3). They fall into three main groups. Bernard-Soulier disease is characterized by

Table 25-2.   **Drugs that Affect Platelet Function[a]**

Anesthetics
>   Cocaine (local)
>   Procaine (local)
>   Volatile general anesthetics

Antibiotics
>   Ampicillin
>   Carbenicillin
>   Gentamicin
>   Penicillin G
>   Ticarcillin

Anticoagulants
>   Dextran
>   Heparin (?)
>   Warfarin sodium

Anti-inflammatory and analgesics
>   Aspirin
>   Colchicine
>   Ibuprofen (Motrin)
>   Indomethacin (Indocin)
>   Mefenamic acid (Ponstel)
>   Phenylbutazone (Butazolidin)
>   Sulfinpyrazone (Anturane)

Cardiovascular drugs (i.e., vasodilators and antilipemic)
>   Clofibrate
>   Dipyridamole (Persantine)
>   Nicotinic acid
>   Papaverine (Myobid)
>   Theophylline

Genitourinary drugs
>   Furosemide (Lasix)
>   Nitrofurantoin (Furadantin)

Table 25-2. **Drugs that Affect Platelet Function (Continued)**

Psychiatric drugs

    Phenothiazines

    Tricyclic antidepressants—imipramine (Tofranil), Triavil, amitriptyline, (Elavil)

Sympathetic blocking agents

    Phenoxybenzamine hydrochloride (Dibenzyline)

    Propranolol (Inderal)

Miscellaneous

    Antihistamines (diphenhydramine hydrochloride)

    Ethanol

    Glyceryl guaiacolate ether (cough suppressant)

    Hashish compounds

    Hydroxychloroquine sulfate

    Nitroprusside sodium

    Vinblastine sulfate (Velban)

[a]Reprinted with permission from Triplett DA, Harms OS, Newhouse P, et al: *Platelet Function. Laboratory Evaluation and Clinical Application.* Chicago, American Society of Clinical Pathologists, 1978.

a failure of the platelets to aggregate with ristocetin in the presence of normal plasma; aggregation is normal with ADP, epinephrine, collagen, and thrombin (Figure 25-1). Moderate thrombocytopenia may be present and the platelets tend to be very large. The basic defect may be an abnormality of a membrane-specific glycoprotein. Other similar conditions have been described under the term giant platelet syndromes. Bernard-Soulier disease is inherited as an autosomal recessive trait; it is very rare and consanguinity is common among the parents of affected individuals. The hemorrhagic manifestations are severe.

Thrombasthenia, or Glanzmann's disease, is another very rare condition in which there is no aggregation with any concentration

Table 25-3. Congenital Qualitative Abnormalities of Platelet Function

| Giant Platelet Syndromes | Aggregation Response | | | | Special Features |
| | ADP or Epinephrine | | Collagen | Ristocetin | |
	Primary	Secondary			
Bernard-Soulier disease	N[a] or D[a]	N or D	N	Absent	Large platelets seen on smear, clinically severe
von Willebrand's disease	N	N	N	Absent	Patient's platelets aggregate with ristocetin in presence of normal plasma
Thrombasthenia	Absent	Absent	Absent	N	Clot retraction poor or absent; clinically severe
Storage pool disease	N or D	Absent	N or D	N	Electron microscopy shows decreased or absent dense granules
Release defect (aspirinlike disorder)	N or D	Absent	N or D	N	Platelet ATP:ADP ratio increased; ATP:ADP ratio in platelets normal
Intermediate type	N	D	N or D	N	Bleeding time abnormal after aspirin ingestion; very mild

[a]Abbreviations: N, normal; D, decreased.

of ADP, epinephrine, or collagen (Figure 25-2). Clot retraction is poor or absent. The platelets, while failing to aggregate, undergo most of the normal changes including the release reaction when stimulated by collagen or thrombin. However, the platelets do not release platelet factor 3 when exposed to kaolin. The platelets on the peripheral blood film are round and isolated but otherwise unremarkable. Like Bernard-Soulier disease, the condition is associated with severe bleeding manifestations and is inherited as an autosomal recessive trait.

The thrombopathies, abnormalities in the release reaction, are quite common, in contrast to Bernard-Soulier and Glanzmann's diseases. They can be subdivided into two subgroups: storage pool disease, in which there is a deficiency of the specialized pool of ADP, and defects in the mechanism responsible for the release of the storage pool contents, which are normal. Both of these subgroups are characterized by the absence of a secondary wave of aggregation with epinephrine or ADP (Figure 25-3). Aggregation with ristocetin is normal. Differentiation of the two subgroups requires special tests or procedures not usually available in most coagulation laboratories. In storage pool disease dense granules are decreased, as seen by electron microscopy. In the second subgroup, the storage pool and dense granules appear normal but fail to release their constituents when the platelets are exposed to ADP, epinephrine, or collagen. This type is, by far, the most frequently encountered type of hereditary qualitative abnormality of platelets and the platelet defects closely resemble those seen after ingestion of aspirin. It has recently been pointed out that many patients with this condition have normal or borderline results on bleeding tests that are significantly prolonged after aspirin ingestion; this type of case has been referred to as an intermediate syndrome of platelet dysfunction (1). However, for convenience this condition may be considered a very mild type of release defect. Its importance lies in the fact that postoperative bleeding can be avoided in these patients by abstinence from drugs known to interfere with platelet function.

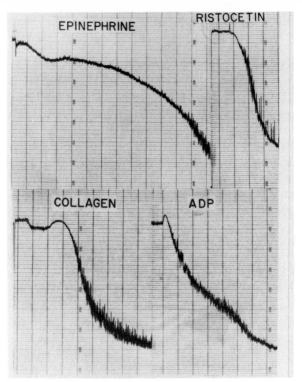

Figure 25-1. Platelet aggregation studies: normal tracing.

The condition may not be recognized with routine screening tests for hemostasis.

Considerable heterogeneity is seen within the groups and sub-groups and forms exist with features of more than one group. In patients with bleeding disorders and an abnormality in platelet factor 3 availability, almost invariably an associated platelet aggregation defect is present and the distinctions that were made previously between disorders of platelet aggregation and impairment of platelet factor 3 availability may be more apparent than real. An isolated

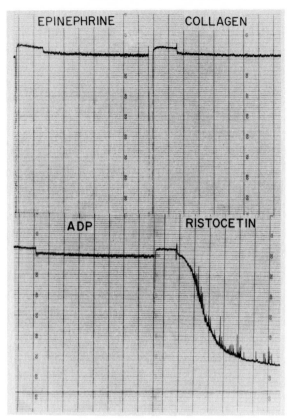

Figure 25-2. Platelet aggregation studies: thrombasthenia. No aggregation with epinephrine, ADP, or collagen. Normal aggregation with ristocetin.

483

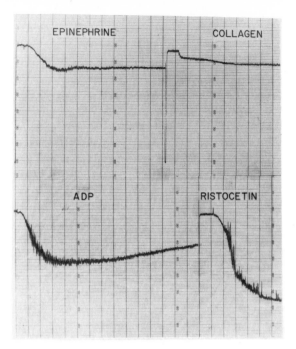

Figure 25-3. Platelet aggregation studies: storage pool disease. Note the absence of secondary wave with epinephrine and ADP and no aggregation with collagen. Platelets react normally with ristocetin. Similar tracings may be seen in platelet membrane defects or after ingestion of drugs such as aspirin and many others.

impairment of platelet factor 3 release probably does not result in a prolonged bleeding time and is asymptomatic.

Qualitative platelet abnormalities have been reported in patients with glycogen storage disease, type I, and Wilson's disease. They have also been observed in some patients with hereditary disorders of connective tissue, including Ehlers-Danlos and Marfan's syndromes (Table 25-4).

Although the primary defect appears to reside in the plasma rather than the platelets, von Willebrand's disease has to be con-

Table 25-4. Hereditary Conditions Associated with Decreased Platelet Aggregation[a]

Glanzmann's thrombasthenia

Essential athrombia

Storage pool defect (decreased content of ADP)
    Chédiak-Higashi syndrome
    Thrombocytopenia with absent radii (TAR syndrome)
    Wiskott-Aldrich syndrome
    Hermansky-Pudlak syndrome

Aspirinlike defect
    Cyclo-oxygenase deficiency
    Thromboxane synthetase deficiency

Inborn errors of metabolism
    Homocystinuria
    Wilson's disease
    Glycogen storage disease, type I

Connective tissue abnormalities
    Ehlers-Danlos syndrome (collagen[b])
    Pseudoxanthoma elasticum (collagen[b])
    Osteogenesis imperfecta (collagen[b])
    Marfan's syndrome
    Constitutional abnormality of collagen (patient's collagen only[b])

Afibrinogenemia

Bernard-Soulier syndrome (ristocetin[b])

von Willebrand's syndrome (ristocetin[b])

Swiss-cheese platelets

Gray platelet syndrome

[a]Reprinted with permission from Triplett DA, Harms CS, Newhouse P, et al: *Platelet Function. Laboratory Evaluation and Clinical Application.* Chicago, American Society of Clinical Pathologists, 1978.
[b]The abnormal aggregation patterns are obtained only when this aggregating reagent is used.

sidered in the differential diagnosis of purpura in a patient with a normal platelet count. The clinical manifestations closely mimic those of a qualitative platelet defect. The disease is characterized by a decreased amount of a plasma factor, referred to as vWf$_{Rist,}$ necessary for the aggregation of platelets in the presence of the antibiotic ristocetin (ristocetin-induced platelet aggregation) (Figure 25-4, Table 25-5). Unlike Bernard-Soulier disease, the isolated platelets in von Willebrand's disease appear normal. Other features of von Willebrand's disease are shown in Table 25-2.

Acquired forms of von Willebrand's disease have been reported. These may result from development of an autoantibody against the von Willebrand factor appearing in a previously healthy individual without any apparent cause. One report has been made of a paraprotein in patients with multiple myeloma that interfered with the action of von Willebrand factor by competitive inhibition. Antibodies that interfere with ristocetin aggregation have also been reported in patients with disseminated lupus erythematosus.

Qualitative abnormalities of platelets are encountered in the myeloproliferative disorders (especially essential thrombocythemia) and, to a lesser extent, in polycythemia vera, myeloid metaplasia, and chronic myelogenous leukemia. Mild abnormalities are found in uremia, cirrhosis, scurvy, and the dysproteinemias (Table 25-6). However, by far the commonest acquired cause is ingestion of aspirin and other medications.

DIAGNOSTIC EVALUATION

Evaluation of functional platelet disorders proceeds with the following:

1. Hematologic evaluation, with particular attention to platelet numbers and morphology.
2. Screening tests for bleeding abnormality, including the activated partial thromboplastin time (APTT), prothrombin time (PT), bleeding time, platelet count, and clot retraction test, performed as part of whole blood clotting and clot observation tests. The hemophilioid or coagulation type of abnormality is excluded if the APTT

Table 25-5. **Factor VIII/von Willebrand Factor Terminology**

Term[a]	Synonyms	Definition
VIIIc	VIII VIII AHF	The factor deficient or defective in hemophilia A and currently measured by conventional 1- or 2-stage factor VIII assay techniques
VIII:C(Ag)	VIII antigen VIII AHF-antigen	The antigen measured using a specific human antibody against VIIIc in IRMA[b]
vWf$_{Rist}$	VIII:WF$_{Rist}$	The factor deficient or defective in all cases of von Willebrand's disease and measured quantitatively by RIPA
vWf$_{Ant}$	VIII:WF$_{Ant}$ VIII R:Ag	The antigen measured by quantitative immunoelectrophoresis[c] using an antibody against vWf$_{Rist}$

[a]Recommended and least confusing term.
[b]Abbreviations: IRMA, immunoradiometric assay; RIPA, ristocetin-induced platelet aggregation.
[c]Can also be measured by IRMA using the same antibody but this technique is only used in research laboratories.

Table 25-6. **Acquired Conditions Associated with Decreased Platelet Aggregation**[a]

Myeloproliferative disorders
    Polycythemia vera
    Myeloid metaplasia
    Hemorrhagic thrombocythemia
    Paroxysmal nocturnal hemaglobinuria
    Di Guglielmo syndrome
    Chronic myelocytic leukemia (?)
    Acute myelomonocytic leukemia
    Sideroblastic anemias

Immunoproliferative disorders
    Waldenström's macroglobulinemia
    Plasma cell myeloma

Cirrhosis

Uremia

Asthma (epinephrine[b])

Platelets in idiopathic thrombocytopenic purpura

Drug induced

Tuberculosis (approximately 15% of cases)

Scurvy

[a]Reprinted with permission from Triplett DA, Harms CS, Newhouse P, et al: *Platelet Function. Laboratory Evaluation and Clinical Application.* Chicago, American Society of Clinical Pathologists, 1978, pp 43–44.
[b]Abnormal aggregation pattern observed only when this reagent is used.

and prothrombin time are normal. If results of one or both of these tests are prolonged, specific assays are performed (see Chapter 26). If factor VIII is found to be decreased or at the limits of normal, von Willebrand's disease must be excluded. If the bleeding time test is normal and a qualitative platelet abnormality is suspected, the test may be repeated two hours after ingestion of 10 grains aspirin (aspirin tolerance test), but this should be performed only when all other types of coagulopathies have been excluded.

3. Platelet aggregation tests, which are nonquantitative, are necessary

for the diagnosis of von Willebrand's disease and the qualitative platelet disorder. If ristocetin-induced platelet aggregation is abnormal and aggregation with the other agents is normal, the patient has von Willebrand's disease or, rarely, Bernard-Soulier disease. A quantitative ristocetin aggregation test is then performed, using the patient's plasma and normal freshly washed or formalin-fixed platelets. This test gives a measure of the vWf_{Rist}. It is normal in Bernard-Soulier disease, since normal platelets are used in the test and the defect in this condition resides in the platelets while the plasma is normal. This is the reverse of von Willebrand's disease in which the vWf_{Rist} is reduced.

4. Determination of the von Willebrand antigen (vWf_{Ant}). Occasionally von Willebrand's disease, which in the mild form is relatively common, may coexist with an intrinsic qualitative platelet disorder.

5. If the von Willebrand antigen is normal or only slightly reduced and the von Willebrand factor as determined by ristocetin-induced aggregation is very low, the patient has a rare variant type of von Willebrand's disease. This is confirmed by crossed immunoelectrophoresis to find an antigen of abnormal mobility.

LABORATORY STUDIES

Hematologic Tests

GENERAL FEATURES

General features are usually unremarkable and abnormal platelets are seen only rarely on the smear. The importance of these studies lies in the exclusion of thrombocytopenic purpura.

PERIPHERAL BLOOD

The number of platelets in the peripheral blood should be estimated and the presence of any large platelets noted. Unless there has been significant bleeding, the red and white cells will be normal. A direct platelet count should be performed.

BONE MARROW

Characteristic changes in bone marrow are seen with acquired platelet defects secondary to myeloproliferative disorders or in association with the dysproteinemias of immune proliferative disorders.

Other Useful Tests

PLATELET AGGREGATION TESTS

Purpose

Platelet aggregation tests are used to detect abnormalities in platelet function (2). Such defects, which may be hereditary or follow the ingestion of certain drugs, can be the cause of bleeding in certain patients.

Principle

When an aggregating agent is added to platelet-rich plasma, which is turbid in the cuvette of an aggregometer, the platelets clump, permitting more light to pass through the plasma. The aggregometer is basically a photo-optical instrument and the amount of light transmitted through the cuvette is recorded on a strip recording chart.

Procedure

Platelet-rich plasma is obtained by the slow centrifugation of whole blood anticoagulated with sodium citrate; this procedure is carried out in plastic tubes at room temperature and at no time should the plasma be cooled. The aggregating agents used are ADP, collagen suspensions (which may be obtained commercially or prepared by homogenizing tissue obtained at operation), epinephrine, and ristocetin; some laboratories also use thrombin. A blank value is obtained by using platelet-poor plasma from the patient. The platelet-rich plasma is placed in the cuvette and warmed to 37 C, the aggregating agent is added, and the contents of the cuvette are kept constantly stirred by means of a small Teflon stirring rod.

Specimen

Platelet-rich plasma prepared from whole blood anticoagulated with sodium citrate is used. The responsiveness of the platelets to aggregating agents is influenced by the time elapsing from collection, and the tests should be completed within one to three hours of collection. The temperature at which the platelet-rich plasma is stirred prior to aggregation studies as well as the temperature at which the actual aggregation tests are carried out have a significant influence upon the rate and extent of aggregation. Platelets stored at room temperature are more sensitive to ADP than platelets stored at 37 C.

Interpretation

The results with each aggregating agent may be recorded as the slope of the curve, the absolute magnitude of the transmittance change, or the percentage change of the transmittance or of the optical density. However, in most laboratories the results are not reported in a quantitative manner but merely in descriptive terms. The results are dependent on the concentration of the aggregating agents and these should be stated in the report. With relatively low doses of ADP (1 μg/ml), two waves of aggregation are seen (Figure 25-5). The first, or primary, wave is induced by the ADP added to the patient's plasma, while the secondary wave is attributed to release of relatively large amounts of intrinsic ADP from the storage pool within the platelets. With lower concentrations of ADP (0.5 μg/ml), the release reaction does not occur, the platelets disaggregate, and only a primary wave is seen, while with relatively large doses of ADP a single broad wave is seen. A biphasic response is seen with epinephrine in about 50%–80% of healthy persons. As collagen acts by inducing release of ADP, a primary wave is not seen. In thrombasthenia there is no aggregation with any concentration of ADP, epinephrine, or collagen but aggregation is seen with ristocetin. In Bernard-Soulier disease, there is normal aggregation with ADP, epinephrine, or collagen, but no aggregation with ristocetin. The findings are similar in von Willebrand's disease, but it is more common to find reduced rather than absent aggregation with ristocetin (Figure 25-4). In storage pool disease and in release defects (aspirinlike disorders), the secondary waves with ADP and

491

epinephrine are absent, and there is reduced or absent aggregation with collagen; ristocetin aggregation is normal.

More subtle changes may be clinically significant when ristocetin is used as the aggregating agent, and the slope should be compared to that of the control. A normal tracing with ristocetin does not exclude a moderate deficiency of the von Willebrand factor. Thus, when this disease is suspected a quantitative ristocetin aggregation test must be performed.

Notes and precautions

Specimens left for more than three hours at room temperature may lose their ability to aggregate. Platelets stored at 0 C sometimes undergo spontaneous aggregation. Occasionally, platelets of healthy individuals who have apparently not taken any drugs appear abnormal. Whenever an abnormal result is obtained, the test should be repeated on another specimen collected some days later.

VON WILLEBRAND FACTOR (vWf) QUANTITATIVE ASSAY (QUANTITATIVE RISTOCETIN AGGREGATION)

Purpose

The test is used to measure the biologic activity of the vWf (3). It is decreased in von Willebrand's disease and in certain acquired disorders.

Principle

The ability of the patient's plasma to aggregate normal platelets in the presence of ristocetin is compared to that of normal pooled plasma.

Procedure

Serial dilutions of plasma in saline are prepared and an aliquot of each is added to a fixed amount of washed platelets in the cuvette of an aggregometer. Ristocetin is then added and the slope

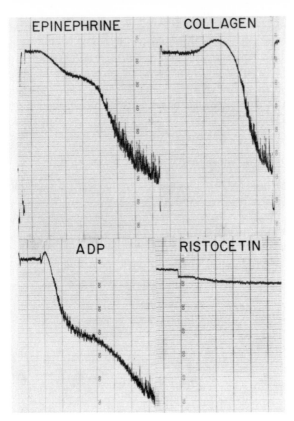

Figure 25-4. Platelet aggregation studies: von Willebrand's disease. Note absence of aggregation with ristocetin. A total lack of aggregation with this reagent is seen only in severe cases. In mild cases aggregation of ristocetin is variable and quantitation is necessary.

of the wave determined (maximum change in light transmittance). By plotting slope against dilution of the plasma on log-log paper, a straight line is obtained. A dilution of the patient's plasma is tested and the equivalent dilution of normal plasma that would give the same slope is read off from the straight-line curve. For example, if a one in five dilution of the patient's plasma gives the same slope as a one in ten dilution of the patient's plasma, the activity of vWf in the patient's plasma is 50% of that of the normal control subject.

Specimen

Plasma used for the performance of the APTT is satisfactory; the plasma may be stored for several weeks at −20 C without losing activity.

Interpretation

A decrease in vWf in a patient with a lifelong history of bleeding is pathognomonic of von Willebrand's disease. Acquired deficiencies caused by antibodies against the von Willebrand factors and certain paraproteins may also result in a decrease in vWf.

IMMUNOPRECIPITATION ASSAY FOR THE VON WILLEBRAND ANTIGEN

Purpose

The immunoprecipitation assay is used for the diagnosis of von Willebrand's disease (4). In this disease the von Willebrand factor antigen (also referred to as the factor VIII related antigen) is usually decreased.

Principle

A precipitating rabbit antibody against the von Willebrand factor is used to quantitate von Willebrand factor. The immunoassay is usually performed by the Laurell technique, which is an electroimmunodiffusion method for the quantitation of proteins in which rocket-shaped anodic immunoprecipitates are formed. The height

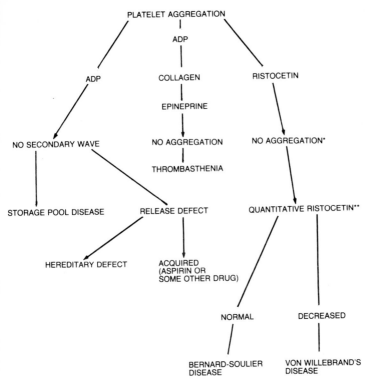

Figure 25-5. Flow diagram for diagnosis of qualitative platelet disorder. * May be decreased or normal in von Willebrand's disease; ** patient's plasma is used with normal platelets.

of the rocket is proportional to the concentration of von Willebrand factor.

Procedure

The antibody is mixed with liquid agarose, which is then poured onto a plate and allowed to solidify by cooling. Holes are punched on one side of the plate, which is then placed in an electrophoresis chamber. The standard is normal pooled plasma. Serial dilutions of this (one in two, one in four, one in eight, etc. in saline) and a one

495

in two dilution of the plasma being tested are prepared and placed in the wells. Electrophoresis of the sample is then performed and when the run is completed the plate is examined. The rocket-shaped immunoprecipitates are sometimes hard to see, but the visibility can be increased by immersing the plates in tannic acid for a few minutes.

Specimen

The patient's plasma or serum may be used, but the former is preferable. Plasma collected for the APTT test is satisfactory.

Interpretation

A value below 50% is consistent with von Willebrand's disease and values between 50% and 60% are borderline. If the quantitative ristocetin aggregation test shows abnormal results and the antigen is normal, cross-immunoelectrophoresis is indicated. The von Willebrand factor antigen and von Willebrand factor as determined by quantitative ristocetin aggregation are both increased by exercise, hepatitis, and during pregnancy, and a corresponding increase is seen in patients with von Willebrand's disease. Thus in these conditions normal values do not preclude the disease.

Notes and precautions

The determination of von Willebrand antigen, often referred to as factor VIII related antigen, should be distinguished from the determination of the factor VIII antigen. The latter is the antigen corresponding to the factor VIII coagulant protein, which is decreased in at least 90% of patients with hemophilia A. The test to determine factor VIII antigen is currently available in only a few laboratories.

REFERENCES

1. Czapek EE, Deykin D, Salzman E, et al: Intermediate syndrome of platelet dysfunction. Blood 52:103–113, 1978
2. Triplett DA, Harms CS, Newhouse P, et al: *Platelet Function. Labo-*

ratory Evaluation and Clinical Application. Chicago, American Society of Clinical Pathologists, 1978

3. Weiss HJ: Abnormalities of factor VIII and platelet aggregation: Use of ristocetin in diagnosing the von Willebrand syndrome. Blood 45:403–412, 1975

4. Zimmerman TS, Ratnoff OD, Powell AE: Immunologic differentiation of classic hemophilia (factor VIII deficiency) and von Willebrand's disease. J Clin Invest 50:244–254, 1971

chapter 26

Hereditary Coagulation Disorders

The characteristic clinical features of a bleeding disorder caused by an abnormality of a blood clotting factor and their differentiation from platelet disorders are outlined in Table 23-1 (Chapter 23). Hemarthroses in a male may be considered the hallmark of a severe coagulation disorder, and if this is sex linked the patient has either hemophilia A or B; exceptions to this rule are rare. All that is then needed to establish the diagnosis is a specific assay of factor VIII and, if this is normal, an assay for factor IX.

The great majority of hereditary disorders of the coagulation type are relatively benign and bleeding only occurs when the hemostatic mechanism is severely challenged. There is usually a history of easy bruising and excessive bleeding after minor surgery such as tonsillectomy or tooth extraction. Such bleeding is troublesome but rarely life-threatening. The clinical differentiation of this type of disorder from a purpuric state is usually not clear-cut, but a history of bleeding from a wound or injury starting after an interval of several hours or days suggests a coagulation type rather than a purpuric disorder. The lifelong nature of the bleeding disorder is usually sufficient to permit categorization of the disorder as a hereditary rather than acquired one. Acquired disorders of clotting are considered in the next chapter.

DIAGNOSTIC EVALUATION

Evaluation of coagulation disorders proceeds as follows:

Table 26-1. Use of Screening Tests in Hereditary Deficiencies of Clotting Factors

Factor	APTT	Prothrombin Time	Thrombin Time
HMW-K (Fitzgerald) Fletcher XII, XI, IX VIII	Increased	Normal	Normal
V, X Prothrombin	Increased	Increased	Normal
VII	Normal	Increased	Normal
Hypofibrinogenemia Dysfibrinogenemia	Increased	Increased	Increased
Factor XIII deficiency	Normal	Normal	Normal

1. Hematologic evaluation to exclude thrombocytopenia and anemia.
2. Screening tests for a bleeding disorder, including the APTT, PT, thrombin time, and bleeding time. Subsequent studies are dependent on the results of these tests (Tables 26-1 and 26-2). Thus if the bleeding time is prolonged, the PT normal, and the APTT normal, tests for a qualitative platelet disorder or von Willebrand's disease should be performed (Chapter 25). The clinical and laboratory findings that enable the differentiation of mild hemophilia A from von Willebrand's disease are shown in Table 26-3. The majority of patients with a coagulation type defect have a prolonged APTT, normal PT, and normal bleeding time. In 95% of cases a deficiency of factor VIII, IX, or XI will be found.
3. If the APTT is prolonged and the PT normal, specific assays for the intrinsic factors are performed (Figure 26-1). Factor VIII is assayed first and, if normal, factor IX is assayed. If both these factors are found to be normal, factor XI is assayed. If all three of these factors are normal, the Passovoy defect should be considered (1,2). Deficiencies of factor XII, Fletcher factor (prekallikrein), or HMW-kininogen result in a prolonged APTT but do not cause a bleeding tendency. Thus a deficiency of any one of these three contact factors can account for the prolonged APTT but not for the bleeding tendency.

Table 26-2. **Use of APTT, Prothrombin Time (PT), and Bleeding Time as Screening Tests in Lifelong Bleeding Disorders**

APTT	PT	Bleeding Time	Further Tests to be Performed
N[a]	N	N or ↑	Platelet function tests, including ristocetin aggregation, vWf factor antigen, VIII assay if APTT is borderline, factor XIII screen
↑	N	↑	VIII assay, vWf$_{Ant}$ quantitative ristocetin
↑	N	N	VIII assay, if normal IX, then XI; if VIII is low perform vWf$_{Ant}$ and quantitative ristocetin, exclude inhibitor
↑	↑	N or ↑	Thrombin time, if normal V, X, and prothrombin assays; if thrombin time is prolonged, assay fibrinogen
N	↑	N or ↑	VII deficiency

[a]N, no change.

4. If both the APTT and PT are prolonged while the thrombin time is normal, specific assays for factors X, V, and prothrombin are performed.

5. If the APTT, PT, and thrombin time are prolonged, dysfibrinogenemia or hypofibrinogenemia should be considered and a fibrinogen determination should be performed using at least two techniques.

6. If the APTT is normal and the PT is prolonged, a deficiency of factor VII should be considered and a specific assay for this factor performed.

7. If the APTT, PT, and thrombin time are normal, a test for clot solubility in 5 M urea should be performed to exclude a deficiency of the fibrin stabilizing factor (Laki-Lorand factor, or factor XIII).

8. Inhibitor screen. When the APTT is prolonged while the PT is normal, the APTT should be repeated on a mixture of equal parts of the patient's and normal plasma. This test is, however, relatively insensitive and nonspecific and in all patients with a deficiency of factor VIII a specific test for the presence of an antibody against factor VIII should be performed. In patients with other types of

Table 26-3. Differential Diagnosis of von Willebrand's Disease from Hemophilia A

Characteristic	von Willebrand's disease	Hemophilia A
Inheritance	Autosomal	Sex linked
Hemarthroses or joint damage	Rare	Present in most severe cases
Clinical severity	Usually mild and rarely dangerous or crippling	Mild to severe
Bleeding time	May be prolonged	Normal if performed correctly
Factor VIII level	Usually 6%–50%	0 to 35%
Factor VIII level following stress, exercise, or severe liver disease	May increase dramatically	No significant change
von Willebrand's factor antigen	< 50%	> 50%
von Willebrand's factor (ristocetin aggregation)	Abnormal	Normal
Effect of transfusion of factor VIII	Immediate response, but factor VIII continues to rise for 24–48 hr	Immediate response followed by rapid decay ($T^1/_2$ = 12 hr)

hereditary deficiencies, with the possible exception of factor XIII, the development of an antibody specifically directed against the deficient factor is excessively rare. Accordingly, unless there is some unusual circumstance, such as failure to respond to treatment with the appropriate concentrate or when the APTT inhibitor screen is positive, a specific search for antibody is not part of the evaluation of hereditary deficiencies of a clotting factor other than factor VIII.

9. von Willebrand factor and antigen determinations. In some patients with von Willebrand's disease, the bleeding time may be normal and the clinical and laboratory findings may mimic those seen in mild hemophilia (Table 26-3). It is therefore necessary to perform tests for von Willebrand's disease in all patients with decreased levels of factor VIII in whom there is no clear-cut sex-linked family history.

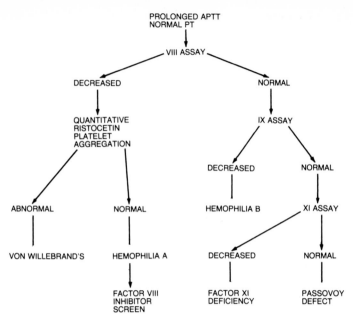

Figure 26-1. Evaluation of patient with lifelong history of bleeding and prolonged APTT.

LABORATORY STUDIES

Hematologic Tests

GENERAL FEATURES

Apart from the exclusion of anemia and thrombocytopenia, the morphology of the formed elements in the blood are usually unremarkable.

BLOOD

Blood counts and red cell morphology can be consistent with a hypochromic anemia in a few patients with very frequent or chronic blood loss.

502

Other Useful Tests

ASSAY FOR FACTOR VIII

Purpose

The determination of the level of factor VIII is necessary for the diagnosis of hemophilia A (3). The level usually correlates well with clinical severity. Assays are also used for monitoring the effect of concentrates.

Principle

The ability of dilutions of the patient's plasma to correct the prolonged APTT of plasma deficient in factor VIII is compared with that of normal pooled plasma. For example, if a 1 in 20 (1:20) dilution of normal plasma shortens the clotting time of the deficient plasma to the same extent as a 1:5 dilution of the patient's plasma, the patient's plasma has 25% of the activity of the normal plasma.

Procedure

The deficient plasma used is obtained from a patient known to have less than 1% factor VIII. It may be kept for several months if stored at −70 C. Dilutions of normal pooled plasma (1:5, 1:10, 1:20, 1:40, 1:80, 1:160) and of the patient's plasma (1:5, 1:10) in saline are prepared. One part of each dilution is added to one part of the deficient plasma and the APTT of the mixture is determined.

Specimen

The plasma collected for the APTT test is used. Factor VIII is fairly stable and the test may be performed on plasma frozen within an hour or two of collection and stored at −30 C.

Interpretation

The 1:5 dilution of the normal pooled plasma is arbitrarily taken as 100% activity, the 1:10 as 50%, the 1:20 as 25%, and so forth. A straight line is obtained on log-log paper when clotting times are

503

plotted against percent concentration of normal plasma. The concentrations of normal plasma that would give the same clotting times as the 1:5 and 1:10 dilutions of the patient's plasma are determined from the graph. The percentage concentration obtained with the 1:5 dilution is the actual concentration of factor VIII in the patient's plasma, while the value obtained with the 1:10 dilution has to be multiplied by two. The mean of the two values is reported. If the value with the 1:10 dilution is significantly higher than that of the 1:5, an inhibitor should be suspected, but the assay should be repeated to exclude an error in technique. The normal range for factors VIII and IX is 60%–150%.

Notes and precautions

The activity of factor VIII may be increased significantly by trace amounts of thrombin that may form if the blood is collected too slowly or if it is incompletely mixed with the anticoagulant. Factor VIII is also sometimes increased in DIC, presumably because of thrombin activation, as well as by exercise. Running for five minutes may double the level, which may remain high for several hours.

ASSAYS FOR OTHER FACTORS INVOLVED IN INTRINSIC PATHWAY ONLY

Purpose

Assays for other factors involved in intrinsic pathway only investigate the nature of a defect resulting in a prolonged APTT but having a normal PT that is not attributable to factor VIII.

Principle

The principle is the same as that underlying the one-stage procedure for the factor VIII assay described previously. The relative ability of the patient's plasma to shorten the prolonged APTT of plasma from a patient deficient in the factor being tested is compared to that of pooled normal plasma.

Procedure

The procedure is the same as that described for the assays of factor VIII, using the appropriate deficient plasma in place of factor VIII-deficient plasma. For the assay of Fletcher factor (prekallikrein), the preincubation period in the APTT test after addition of kaolin should not exceed three minutes; longer incubation periods cause the APTT of Fletcher-deficient plasma to approach the normal value. Accordingly, certain automated instruments in which the preincubation period exceeds three minutes cannot be used. In the HMW-kininogen assay, the 1:20 dilution of normal plasma may be as effective in shortening the APTT of the HMW-kininogen deficient plasma as the 1:5 dilution. Therefore, in performing this assay it is advisable to start at a 1:20 dilution and to continue up to a 1:320 dilution. The unknown is tested at a 1:5 dilution up to 1:20.

Interpretation

The normal range for these factors is 60%–150%.

Notes and precautions

The deficient plasma may be obtained from a commercial source. Fletcher factor and HMW-kininogen-deficient plasmas are very rare and accordingly very few coagulation laboratories are able to perform these assays, although they are technically quite simple. However, in most instances a provisional diagnosis of these two deficiencies may be made by a process of exclusion. Thus, if the patient has a prolonged APTT, normal PT, normal levels of all the intrinsic factors (including factors XI or XII), and a negative bleeding history, a deficiency of Fletcher factor or HMW-kininogen should be considered. Fletcher factor-deficient plasma shortens progressively on incubation with kaolin (Celite) and may be normal after eight minutes of preincubation, thereby differing from HMW-kininogen-deficient plasma.

ASSAYS FOR PROTHROMBIN AND FACTORS V, VII, AND X

Purpose

Assays for prothrombin and for factors V, VII, and X are performed to determine the specific cause(s) of a prolonged prothrombin time (4,5).

Principle

The principle is the same as that for assays of the factors that were described previously, but the prothrombin time is used instead of the APTT.

Procedure

The actual technique using plasma from patients deficient in prothrombin and factors V, VII, and X is very simple; however, these deficient states are very rare and the deficient plasmas are usually prepared artificially and are available commercially. For example, factor V-deficient plasma is prepared for aging plasma at 37 C. The assays are performed in the same manner as the assays for the intrinsic factors (e.g., factor VIII), using the prothrombin time instead of the APTT. The ability of the patient's plasma to shorten the prolonged prothrombin time of plasma deficient in the factor being assayed is compared to that of normal plasma.

Specimen

Blood is collected in the same manner as for the assay of factor VIII. The assay for factor V should be performed within four hours of collection since it is relatively labile. Assays of factor VII are best performed as soon as possible after collection since it may increase in value when the plasma is stored in the refrigerator.

Interpretation

The normal range for prothrombin and for factors V, VII, and X is 60%–150%.

Purpose

The inhibitor screening test is used for detection of inhibitors of clotting, which are usually immunoglobulins.

Principle

The addition of plasma containing an inhibitor of a factor involved in intrinsic clotting prolongs the APTT of normal plasma.

Procedure

One part of the plasma being tested is incubated with an equal part of normal plasma. The APTTs of the mixture are determined immediately and after 20 minutes incubation at 37 C.

Specimen

The same plasma used in the APTT test is used as a specimen.

Interpretation

When one part of plasma congenitally deficient in a clotting factor such as factor VIII is mixed with an equal part of normal plasma, the APTT of the mixture is usually no more than 4 seconds longer than that of the normal plasma alone if this is between 26 and 30 seconds. A difference of six seconds or more is good evidence of an inhibitor, while a difference of five seconds is suggestive of one. Most inhibitors are immediate acting, that is, their action is not enhanced by incubation, but notable exceptions are antibodies to factor VIII.

Notes and precautions

The inhibitor screening test is subject to many technical variations such as differences in the concentration of the sodium citrate used to anticoagulate the normal and patient's plasma. Incubation of normal platelet-poor plasma alone can result in an increase in the APTT because of loss of factor V; on the other hand, if the plasma is not centrifuged at a speed sufficient to convert most of the platelets to sediment, the APTT can actually shorten.

FACTOR VIII ANTIBODY SCREENING TEST

Purpose

Antibodies against factor VIII develop in about 7% of patients with hemophilia A. The titer of the antibody increases after transfusions of plasma or factor VIII concentrates, and their detection is important since the patient may become refractory to treatment.

Principle

If hemophilic plasma is incubated with an equal volume of normal plasma and the hemophilic plasma contains an antibody against factor VIII, the factor VIII concentration of the mixture will be significantly less than the mean of the two.

Procedure

One part of plasma from the patient with hemophilia A is mixed with an equal volume of normal pooled plasma (used as the 100% standard). After incubation for 30 minutes at 37 C, the mixture is diluted in a ratio of one to five in saline and assayed for factor VIII.

Specimen

Plasma collected for the APTT is used as a specimen; the antibodies are remarkably stable and are present in both plasma and serum. The specimen may be adsorbed with aluminum hydroxide and heated to 56 C for 30 minutes without effect on the antibody.

Interpretation

If the factor VIII concentration of the mixture is 35% or more, the patient does not have an inhibitor or the inhibitor is too weak to be significant.

Notes and precautions

In order to detect a low-titer inhibitor, it is advisable to obtain plasma several days after, as well as before, replacement therapy.

FACTOR VIII ANTIBODY TITER

Purpose

This test estimates the potency of an antibody against factor VIII (6).

Principle

Serial dilutions of plasma containing the inhibitor are incubated with normal plasma for a specified period of time and the residual factor VIII is determined. Factor VIII inhibitor titers are commonly expressed in Bethesda units, which are defined as the amount that, when incubated with normal plasma, neutralize half of the factor VIII in two hours.

Procedure

Serial dilutions in saline (1:2, 1:4, etc.) of the plasma being tested are incubated with an equal volume of normal plasma for two hours at 37 C. The residual factor VIII in each of the incubation mixtures is determined. The inhibitor titer in Bethesda units is the reciprocal of the dilution of the test plasma that gives 50% inhibition; this may be determined by drawing a curve relating activity of residual factor VIII to the reciprocal of the dilution or by a rough approximation made by inspection of the data.

Specimen

Blood is collected as for the APTT or factor VIII assay.

Interpretation

A hemostatic level of factor VIII can usually be achieved by replacement therapy using human factor VIII concentrates in patients with two or less Bethesda units. However, after four days the inhibitor titer in a hemophiliac is likely to have increased several fold; in a nonhemophiliac this increase may not occur.

There is considerable heterogeneity between the factor VIII antibodies of different patients. The antibodies seen in nonhemophiliacs may differ strikingly from those seen in hemophilic patients. For example, some of the antibodies seen in nonhemophiliacs may only neutralize 80% of the available factor VIII in normal plasma over a period of 12 hours, reaching a plateau, yet when the factor VIII concentration of the mixture is increased to 100% by addition of factor VIII concentrate, the level again only falls to 20%, indicating that the antibody was only partially neutralized. Moreover, if a factor VIII concentrate is given to a patient with a factor VIII antibody, the factor VIII level determined in the laboratory may not be a true reflection of the level at the time the plasma was withdrawn, as destruction occurs in vitro between the time of collection and actual performance of the assay. Other test systems are used to assay factor VIII antibodies, with different definitions of a unit. The results obtained using different test systems are in general poorly correlated; however each method gives useful information with respect to the relative potency of the antibody in any one patient over a period of time.

REFERENCES

1. Hougie C, McPherson RA, Brown JE, et al: The Passovoy defect: Further characterization of a hereditary hemorrhagic diathesis. N Engl J Med 298:1045–1048, 1978
2. McPherson RA, Hougie C: Passovoy defect. N Engl J Med 299:776–777, 1978 (letter)
3. Biggs R: *Human Blood Coagulation, Haemostasis and Thrombosis,* ed 2. Oxford, Blackwell Scientific Publications, 1975, pp 682–684
4. Hjort P, Rapaport SI, Owen PA: A simple specific one-stage prothrombin assay using Russells' viper venom in cephalin suspension. J Lab Clin Med 46:89–97, 1955
5. Austen DEG, Rhymes IL: *A Laboratory Manual of Blood Coagulation.* Oxford, Blackwell Scientific Publications, 1975
6. Kasper CK, Aledort LM, Counts RB, et al: A more uniform measurement of factor VIII inhibitors. Thromb Diathes Haematol 34:869–872, 1975

Acquired Coagulation Disorders

In contrast to the bleeding of thrombocytopenia, which is purpuric in type, bleeding manifestations associated with acquired deficiencies of clotting factors are of the coagulation type; however, usually there are also purpuric features (see Table 23-1). The liver is the most important site of synthesis of clotting factors and a hemorrhagic diathesis can occur in severe hepatitis or cirrhosis. In these conditions the clotting factors that are depressed the most are those that are vitamin K-dependent, namely prothrombin, and factors VII, IX, and X. In addition, there may be a moderate reduction of factor V and a defect in the polymerization of fibrin monomer. The fibrinolytic potentiality may be increased and the capacity to inactivate partially activated products of blood coagulation may be impaired; these two factors may account for the fairly common occurrence of disseminated intravascular coagulation (DIC). Moderate thrombocytopenia, which can be a result of splenic pooling if splenomegaly is present, or DIC may also frequently be found in these patients.

In the absence of vitamin K, prothrombin and the other vitamin K-dependent clotting factors are synthesized in normal amounts but are inactive. They may actually inhibit their normal counterpart. Naturally occurring vitamin K is fat soluble and bile is essential for its absorption from the gastrointestinal tract. In any condition in which influx of bile into the gut is impeded, a hemorrhagic diathesis may ensue. The absorption of vitamin K occurs in the small intestine and may be deficient in such diseases of the intestinal wall as regional ileitis and nontropical sprue. Since bacterial flora play an important part in the synthesis of vitamin K in the gut, sterilization of the bowel resulting from the oral administration of antibiotics or nonabsorbable sulfonamides such as succinylsulfathiazole (Suflasuxidine) may also result in vitamin K deficiency.

Hemorrhagic disease of the newborn (melena neonatorum) caused by deficiency of vitamin K, which was a common disease four decades ago, has been virtually eliminated as a result of prophylactic vitamin K therapy. The bleeding typically occurs during the second to sixth day after delivery. This disease is an exaggeration of physiologic hypoprothrombinemia, a temporary state that reaches its maximum point of bleeding on the second or third day and usually returns to normal within a week. The onset of bleeding is usually abrupt and the commonest presenting symptoms are melena with hematemesis, umbilical bleeding, epistaxis, submucous hemorrhages affecting the buccal cavity, and urethral and vaginal bleeding. The disease may also present as excessive bleeding at circumcision or persistent bleeding following a heel prick. Multiple ecchymoses may be found. Petechial hemorrhages are exceptional and suggest thrombocytopenia. Premature infants are particularly prone to excessive bleeding, as immaturity of the liver cells results in decreased synthesis of vitamin K-dependent factors; this is enhanced by vitamin K deficiency. The tissue necrosis that accompanies intracranial hemorrhage in these infants may precipitate DIC and thereby aggravate a pre-existing bleeding tendency.

The response of the prothrombin time to administration of parenteral vitamin K in patients lacking the vitamin K-deficient factors is useful in differentiating hepatocellular diseases from biliary obstruction. In hepatocellular disease the prothrombin time remains prolonged, while it returns to normal in biliary obstruction unless some associated liver parenchymal damage is present. The finding of a prolonged prothrombin time with normal liver function tests in a previously healthy individual in whom a bleeding diathesis has developed can often be attributable to accidental ingestion of warfarin. These drugs may have a direct toxic effect on the capillary wall and the type of bleeding seen after an overdose has features of both coagulation and a purpuric type of defect; thus petechiae may be present and hematoma often appears at the site of a clean venipuncture.

The delicate hemostatic balance between the procoagulant factors and the natural inhibitors, which is necessary for the maintenance of the fluidity of the blood, may be disturbed in many disease states (Table 27-1). This can result in the widespread formation of thrombi in the microcirculation, a process referred to as disseminated intravascular coagulation (DIC). This term is usually used to include a paradoxic hypocoagulable state that is its natural sequela and which is attributable to the consumption of platelets, fibrinogen, and other factors in the formation of the thrombi. The bleeding tendency that results is, as a general rule, purpuric in type. The removal of the thrombi essential for the survival of the patient is accomplished by fibrinolysis, and this mechanism, although primarily protective, may in itself aggravate the bleeding tendency. The formation of thrombin is believed to be a sine qua non of DIC, but its neutralization is almost instantaneous. Its presence is presumed by the recognition of the products of its action on fibrinogen. These products include fibrinopeptides A and B and fibrin monomer. While some of the fibrin monomers polymerize, forming fibrin, a proportion form soluble complexes with native fibrinogen and with the degradation products that result from the lysis of formed fibrin. The fibrinopeptides have half-lives of only a few minutes and this limits their usefulness as an index of DIC. On the other hand, the soluble fibrin monomer complexes remain in the circulation for several hours. Fibrinolysis results in formation of several fibrin degradation products of which products D and E are the most stable and readily measured. Fibrinogen is an acute-phase reactant protein and in many of the conditions that can cause DIC the level may be very high. A significant decrease in the concentration may therefore not be apparent from a single fibrinogen determination, as this may be normal or even high depending on the

Table 27-1. **Causes of Disseminated Intravascular Coagulation**

Release of tissue products after necrosis or trauma
  Metastatic carcinoma
  Tissue injury, e.g., brain tissue destruction, lung surgery
  Extensive burn
  Heat stroke

Infections
  Gram-negative endotoxinemia
    Meningococcemia
    Septicemia
  Severe gram-positive septicemia
  Rocky Mountain spotted fever
  Viral infections

Obstetric
  Concealed antepartum hemorrhage
  Amniotic fluid embolism
  Retained dead fetus
  Eclampsia
  Hypertonic saline abortion

Hemolytic reactions

Endothelial damage
  Acute systemic vasculitis
  Trauma

Liver disease
  Severe cirrhosis
  Hepatic necrosis

Antigen-antibody reactions

Promyelocytic leukemia

Giant hemangioma

Snake bites

baseline level. Serial fibrinogen determinations to follow the course of the process should therefore be performed.

Factor VIII is also an acute-phase reactant protein and may remain above normal in DIC despite a significant fall. Thrombin is believed to cause activation of factor VIII, as measured by the one-stage method, and a high factor VIII may also be attributed to this cause. Factor V is usually decreased, but rarely sufficiently to raise the prothrombin time by more than a second or two. Milder depressions of the other factors such as factor XIII also occur, but these changes are of little or no diagnostic value. One of the consequences of the intravascular fibrin deposition is the fragmentation of red cells by strands of fibrin in the microcirculation resulting in red cell fragmentation with schistocytes, or helmet cells. When associated with a significant hemolytic anemia, it is referred to as microangiopathic hemolytic anemia.

An antibody specifically directed against factor VIII or, more rarely, one of the other clotting factors may appear in an individual with previously normal hemostasis, resulting in a bleeding diathesis. Antibodies against specific factors are encountered far less frequently than antibodies that inhibit clotting without demonstrable specificity for any one of the clotting factors (Table 27-2). This type of nonspecific antibody results in a prolongation in the APTT and occasionally the PT and is perhaps the most frequent cause of a prolongation of the APTT. Patients with a nonspecific antibody rarely bleed excessively even while undergoing major surgery. This type of antibody was first found in a patient with disseminated lupus erythematosus and is referred to as the lupus inhibitor even though lupus erythematosus is now known to be a relatively rare cause. The lupus antibody may be seen in individuals who are taking hypotensive drugs such as procainamide and certain tranquilizers but may also be found in some individuals in whom no etiologic factor can be invoked. The VDRL test may give a false-positive result. The so-called lupus inhibitor probably comprises a heterogenous group of antibodies with different actions.

515

Table 27-2. **Acquired Inhibitors of Clotting**

Type	Clinical Associations	Nature of Antibody	Clinical Findings and Course	Laboratory Finding
Specific antibodies against factor VIII	Previously healthy elderly persons Patients with some autoimmune disorder Postpartum	IgG, monoclonal	May be persistent especially in elderly patients; life-threatening bleeding can occur	APTT↑, PT:N, factor VIII ↓ Other factors usually normal or only slightly reduced
Specific antibodies against factor V	Usually preceded by streptomycin administration May develop after massive blood transfusion	IgG or IgM Polyclonal	Bleeding tendency usually disappears in weeks or months	APTT↑, PT↑, factor V ↓
Specific against factor XIII or XIIIa	Therapy with isoniazid	IgG but may not be an immunoglobulin	Bleeding tendency usually disappears in weeks or months	APTT normal; PT normal; clot soluble in 5 M urea
Specific against von Willebrand factor	Myeloma	IgG	Mild bleeding tendency	Bleeding time↑; vWf antigen↑; ristocetin aggregation↓; factor VIII normal
Lupus anticoagulant	Drug ingestion viz chlorpromazine Lupus erythematosus No apparent etiologic agent	Usually IgG, sometimes IgM or both	Bleeding tendency rare; patients may have thromboembolic manifestations	APTT↑; PT usually normal; inhibitor screen +

DIAGNOSTIC EVALUATION

Evaluation of the acquired coagulation disorders proceeds with the following:

1. Hematologic evaluation, with attention to platelet numbers, red cell changes indicative of DIC, and white cell count and differential.
2. Screening tests for bleeding disorders, including platelet count, bleeding time, APTT, PT, and thrombin time. This battery of tests is useful in helping to differentiate the thrombocytopenic purpuras and the acquired diathesis caused by inhibitors, liver disease, or vitamin K deficiencies or DIC (Table 27-3).
3. Screening test for an inhibitor.
4. If the inhibitor screening test produces positive results, more specific tests such as the factor VIII antibody test should be performed.
5. A search for fibrinogen degradation products (FDPs) and for evidence of fibrin monomer, using the protamine sulfate paracoagulation test if the history or screening procedures suggest DIC.
6. Serial fibrinogen determinations.
7. Liver function tests are useful in differentiating a prolongation of the prothrombin time caused by ingestion of sodium warfarin (Coumadin) from that caused by liver disease or biliary obstruction. If it is suspected that the patient has ingested Coumadin or that some failure of absorption of vitamin K has occurred, the prothrombin time should be repeated 4–24 hours after the parenteral administration of this vitamin.
8. Tests for lupus erythematosus (Chapter 24) should be performed whenever a lupus-type inhibitor is suspected. A VDRL determination should also be performed as false-positive results are common in patients with the lupus inhibitor.

LABORATORY STUDIES

Hematologic Tests

GENERAL FEATURES

If platelets are absent or markedly reduced, the patient is evaluated for thrombocytopenic purpura (Chapter 21). However, a mod-

Table 27-3. **Use of Screening Tests in Acquired Hemorrhagic Disorders**

Disorder	Platelet Count	Bleeding Time	APTT	PT	TT
Thrombocytopenic purpura[a]	↓	↑	N	N	N
Liver disease	N[b] or ↓	N or ↑	↑	↑	N or ↑
Vitamin K deficiency	N	N or ↑	↑	↑	N
Factor VIII antibody	N	N	↑	N	N
Lupus-type inhibitor	N	N	↑	N or ↑	N
DIC	↓	↑	↑ N ↓	N	↑

[a]See Chapter 24.
[b]N, no change.

erate reduction is found in DIC and may be associated with schistocytes and spherocytes in the peripheral blood smear.

PERIPHERAL BLOOD

A platelet count is performed and morphology of red cells (schistocytes, etc.) is evaluated.

BONE MARROW

Bone marrow tests are performed only if thrombocytopenia is present (see Chapter 24).

Other Useful Tests

THE PROTAMINE PLASMA PARACOAGULATION TEST (3P TEST)

Purpose

The 3P test detects fibrin monomer in plasma and is used for the diagnosis of DIC (1).

Principle

Soluble complexes of fibrin monomer with FDPs or fibrinogen dissociate on the addition of protamine sulfate and the fibrin monomers then polymerize forming a fibrin web.

Procedure

Ten drops of plasma are placed in a small glass test tube warmed to 37 C and one drop of 1% protamine sulfate is then added and mixed well by gentle shaking.

Specimen

Platelet-poor plasma is used as collected for the APTT test.

Interpretation

Webs or strands of fibrin are considered an equivocally positive result while a finely granular, noncohesive precipitate is usually interpreted as a weakly positive result.

Notes and precautions

False-positive results may be obtained if there is difficulty with venipuncture or delay in mixing the blood with anticoagulant because of the formation of small amounts of thrombin in vitro. A test should not be performed on oxalated or heparinized blood, but the administration of heparin to the patient does not interfere with the test.

LATEX PARTICLE AGGLUTINATION TEST FOR FIBRIN OR FIBRINOGEN DEGRADATION PRODUCTS*

Purpose

The test detects the presence of fibrin or fibrinogen degradation products in serum and is helpful in the diagnosis of disseminated intravascular clotting (2).

---

*Kit manufactured by Wellcome Reagents Division, Burroughs Wellcome Co., Research Triangle Park, NJ.

Principle

Antisera to highly purified preparations of human fibrinogen fragments D and E are absorbed onto latex particles. These clump in the presence of fibrinogen or fibrin degradation products.

Procedure

A drop of serum diluted 1:5 and 1:20 with buffer are each placed on a slide. One drop of latex suspension is then added to each of the diluted serum samples, and the mixtures are stirred with a mixing rod while the slides are rocked gently to and fro for exactly two minutes, with inspection for macroscopic agglutination. This, if present, can be visually observed. Known negative and positive controls are run with each test.

Specimen

Blood obtained by careful and clean venipuncture is placed in a special sample collection tube that contains soybean trypsin inhibitor and bovine thrombin. The blood clots within two seconds and is then incubated at 37 C for approximately 30 minutes before being separated by centrifugation.

Interpretation

The normal serum level of FDP is less than 10 μg/ml and the reagents are so adjusted that serum with less than this concentration will give no agglutination with either 1:5 or 1:20 dilutions of normal serum. In DIC the level of FDP exceeds 10 μg and in acute cases may exceed 40 μg. However, similar increases may be found in other states involving enzymatic (other than thrombin) or nonenzymatic degradation of fibrinogen. Increased levels are sometimes found in deep vein thrombosis and pulmonary embolism, but such increases are very transient.

Notes and precautions

The latex particle agglutination test does not distinguish between fibrinogen and fibrin degradation products.

REFERENCES

1. Rapaport SI: Paracoagulation test for fibrin or fibrinogen degradation products. In Williams WJ, Beutler E, Erslev AJ, et al (eds): *Hematology*, ed 2. New York, McGraw-Hill, 1977, p 1652
2. Hougie C: Latex particle agglutination for fibrin or fibrinogen degradation products. In Williams WJ, Beutler, E, Erslev AJ, et al (eds): *Hematology*, ed 2. New York, McGraw-Hill, 1977, pp 1652–1654

PART D/**APPENDICES**

Blood Cell Values in Normal Adults[a,b]

Test	Men[c]	Women[c]
Red cell count, $\times\ 10^6/\mu$l blood	4.4–5.9	3.8–5.2
Hemoglobin, g/100 ml blood	13.0–18.0	12.0–16.0
Hematocrit, ml/100 ml blood	40–52	35–47
MCV, μm^3/red cell	81–100	81–100
MCH, pg/red cell	26–34	26–34
MCH concentration, g/100 ml red cells	31–36	31–36
White cell count $\times\ 10^3/\mu$l blood	3.9–10.6	3.5–11.0
Platelet count $\times\ 10^3/\mu$l blood[d,e]	156–344	156–344

[a]Based on automated counts using Coulter Counter Model S except for platelet count.

[b]Reprinted with permission from Williams WJ, Schneider AS: Examination of the peripheral blood. In Williams WJ, Beutler E, Erslev AJ, et al: *Hematology*, ed 2. New York, McGraw-Hill, 1977, pp 10–25.

[c]Ranges based on mean ± 2 standard deviations.

[d]By phase microscopy.

[e]Karpatkin S, Garg SK, Siskind GW: Autoimmune thrombocytopenic purpura and the compensated thrombocytolytic state. Am J Med 51:1–4, 1971.

Red Cell Values in Children[a,b]

Age	Red Cell Count, $10^6/\mu l$	Hematocrit, ml/100 ml	Hemoglobin, g/100 ml	MCV, μm^3	MCH, pg	MCHC, g/100 ml Red Cells
1 day	5.1 ± 0.7	61 ± 7	19.0 ± 2.2	119 ± 9	37	32 ± 2
3 months	3.7 ± 0.3	33 ± 3	11.3 ± 0.9	88 ± 8	30	35 ± 2
6–12 months	4.6	35	11.4	76	25	33
3–7 years	4.7	37	12.6	79	27	34
10–14 years	4.8	39	13.4	81	28	34

[a]Reprinted with permission from Altman PL, Katz DD: *Human Health and Disease.* Bethesda, Federation of American Societies for Experimental Biology, 1977, pp 151–153.

[b]Where given, ± 1 standard deviation. Standard deviations given for 3 months closely approximate standard deviations not shown for later ages.

Units Recommended by the Committee for Standardization in Hematology[a,b]

Test	Abbre-viation	Traditional Units[c]	Correction Factor (Multiply By)	Recom-mended Units	Example
Red cell count	RBC	Number/mm³, μ^3 or μl	10^6	Number/l	5.1×10^{12}/l
Hemoglobin concentration	Hb	g/100ml	1.0	g/dl	16.0 g/dl
Hematocrit, packed cell volume	Hct, PCV	% or ml/100 ml	0.01	1/1	0.46 l/l
Mean corpuscular volume	MCV	μm^3 or cμ	1.0	fl	90/fl
Mean corpuscular hemoglobin	MCH	$\mu\mu$g	1.0	pg	30 pg

		% or g/100 ml	1.0	g/dl	34 g/dl
Mean corpuscular hemoglobin concentration	MCHC				
White blood cell count	WBC	Number/mm³, μ^3 or μl	10^6	Number/l	7.2×10^6/l
Platelet count		Number/mm³, μ^3 or μl	10^6	Number/l	200×10^9/l
Reticulocyte count (absolute number)		Number/mm³, μ^3 or μl	10^6	Number/l	50×10^9/l

[a]This complies with International System of Units (SI) except for Hb and its derived indices, MCH and MCHC. Hemoglobin is expressed in molar terms in SI units.

[b]Abbreviations: *fl*, femtoliter (10^{-15} liter); *pl*, picoliter (10^{-12} liter); *nl*, nanoliter(10^{-9} liter); μl, microliter (10^{-6} liter); *ml*, milliter (10^{-3} liter); *l*, liter; *dl*, deciliter (10^{-1} liter); *pg*, picogram; *fg*, femtogram; *ng*,nanogram; *μg*, microgram; *mg*, milligram.

[c]*Traditional Units*

	Equivalent
$\mu^=$ or mm³ = cubic millimeter	(10^{-6}l)
cμ or μm³ = cubic micrometer	(10^{-15}l)
$\mu\mu g$ = micromicrogram	(10^{-12}g)

527

Normal Leukocyte and Differential Counts[a,b]

Age	Leukocytes, Total	Neutrophils		
		Total	Band	Segmented
12 months	11.4(6.0–17.5)	3.5(1.5–8.5) (31%)	0.35 (3.1%)	3.2 (28%)
4 years	9.1(5.5–15.5)	3.8(1.5–8.5) (42%)	0.27(0–1.0) (3.0%)	3.5(1.5–7.5) (39%)
10 years	8.1(4.5–13.5)	4.4(1.8–8.0) (54%)	0.24(0–1.0) (3.0%)	4.2(1.8–7.0) (51%)
21 years	7.4(4.5–11.0)	4.4(1.8–7.7) (59%)	0.22(0–0.7) (3.0%)	4.2(1.8–7.0) (56%)

[a]Reprinted from Altman PL, Dittmer DS (eds): *Blood and Other Body Fluids.* Washington, DC, Federation of American Societies for Experimental Biology, 1961.

[b]Values are expressed as cells $\times 10^3/\mu l$. Mean values are given; ranges are in parentheses. Percent is for mean values.

Eosinophils	Basophils	Lymphocytes	Monocytes
0.30(0.05–0.70) (2.6%)	0.05(0–20) (0.4%)	7.0(4.0–10.5) (61%)	0.55(0.05–1.1) (4.8%)
0.25(0.02–0.65) (2.8%)	0.05(0–0.20) (0.6%)	4.5(2.0–8.0) (50%)	0.45(0–0.8) (5.0%)
0.20(0–0.60) (2.4%)	0.04(0–0.20) (0.5%)	3.1(1.5–6.5) (38%)	0.35(0–0.8) (4.3%)
0.20(0–0.45) (2.7%)	0.04(0–0.20) (0.5%)	2.5(1.0–4.8) (34%)	0.30(0–0.8) (4.0%)

INDEX

540

Evelyn-Malloy method, in bilirubin measurement, 80
Extrinsic prothrombinase, in prothrombin time test, 460

F

FAB classification of leukemia, 329–330, 331(table), 332(table)
Factor II
  in immunoproliferative disorders, 429
  in leukemia, 329
  in macroglobulinemia, 434
Factor V
  acquired coagulation disorders and, 511
  in activated partial thromboplastin time test, 458
  assay for, in coagulation disorders, 506
  in disseminated intravascular coagulation, 515
  in immunoproliferative disorders, 429
  inhibitor screening test and, 507
  in leukemia, 329
  in macroglobulinemia, 434
  in prothrombin time test, 460, 461, 462
Factor VII
  acquired coagulation disorders and, 511
  in activated partial thromboplastin time test, 456
  antibody screening test for, 508–509
  assay for, in coagulation disorders, 506
  clotting mechanism and, 455
  in immunoproliferative disorders, 429
  in macroglobulinemia, 434
  in prothrombin time test, 460, 461
Factor VIII
  in activated partial thromboplastin time test, 458
  antibody titer for, 509–510
  coagulation disorders and, 498, 499, 502(figure)
  in disseminated intravascular coagulation, 515
  hemophilia and, 446, 503–504
  heterogeneity between antibodies of different patients with, 510
  in immunoproliferative disorders, 429
  inhibitor screening test and, 507

intrinsic pathway factors in coagulation disorders and, 504, 505
  in leukemia, 329
  in macroglobulinemia, 434
  von Willebrand factor terminology and, 487(table)
Factor VIII related antigen (see von Willebrand antigen)
Factor IX
  acquired coagulation disorders and, 511
  in activated partial thromboplastin time test, 458
  coagulation disorders and, 498, 499
  in prothrombin time test, 462
Factor X
  in acquired coagulation disorders, 511
  in activated partial thromboplastin time test, 458
  assay for, in coagulation disorders, 506
  in leukemia, 329
  in prothrombin time test, 460, 461
Factor Xa, in prothrombin time test, 460
Factor XI
  in activated partial thromboplastin time test, 458, 459
  coagulation disorders and, 499
  early contact phase in bleeding and, 446
  Fletcher factor and HMW-kininogen deficiency and, 505
Factor XII
  in activated partial thromboplastin time test, 458, 459
  coagulation disorders and, 499
  Fletcher factor and HMW-kininogen deficiency and, 505
  early contact phase in bleeding and, 446
Factor XIII
  in activated partial thromboplastin time, 456
  clotting mechanism and, 455
Family history
  bleeding disorders and, 443
  in hemoglobin disorders, 134
  hereditary spherocytosis and, 98
  in pyruvate kinase deficiency, 109
Fanconi's anemia, 30
Fc disease (see Gamma heavy-chain disease)
Felty's syndrome (see Hypersplenism)

Hexose monophosphate (HMP) shunt (*continued*)
  in glycolysis, 105–107
  hereditary disorders of, 115–125
  hereditary GSH deficiency and, 119
  screening tests for enzymes of, 114

High molecular weight (HMW)-kininogen,
  in activated partial thromboplastin time (APTT) test, 458, 505
  coagulation disorders and, 499

Hippuryl-L-histadyl-L-leucine (HHL), 296

Histalog test, in megaloblastic anemia, 61–62

Histamine, gastric analysis for hydrochloric acid with, 61

Histiocytes, in lymphomas, 372, 373, 388–389, 390, 394

Histoplasma yeast antigen, in lymphadenopathy, 290, 293

Hodgkin's disease, 396–407
  chronic myelomonocytic leukemia diagnosis and, 351
  classification of, 398, 398(table)
  clinical presentation in, 396–397
  diagnostic evaluation in, 397–398
  diffuse lymphomas mistaken for, 382
  eosinophilia differentiated from, 240, 241
  gamma heavy-chain disease and, 435
  hematologic tests in, 402–404
  immunoglobulin E (IgE) in, 240
  laparotomy in, 405–406
  Lennert's lymphoma and, 385
  leukocyte alkaline phosphatase (LAP) scores and, 346
  lymphocytic depletion type, 399–400, 402(figure)
  lymphocytic predominant type, 399, 400(figure), 403–404
  lymphopenia in, 285, 286
  mixed cellularity type, 399, 401(figure), 404
  mononuclear type, 399, 402(figure), 404
  nodular sclerosis category in, 400–401, 403(figure), 404
  non-Hodgkin's lymphomas differentiated from, 396
  radiologic studies in, 404–405
  serum biochemistry in, 406

simultaneous and sequential biopsies in, 401
  skin testing in, 407
  staging in, 404, 405(table)
  tissue biopsy in, 398–401
  types of, 399–401

Howell-Jolly bodies, 13(figure)

Humoral immunity, B cells in, 263

Hydrochloric acid, gastric analysis for, 61–62

Hydrops fetalis, 133

Hyperbilirubinemia
  in hemolysis, 80
  in liver disease with portal hypertension, 306

Hypercalcemia
  in Hodgkin's disease, 406
  in immunoproliferative disorders, 414, 430

Hyperplasia
  reactive follicular, and nodular lymphomas, 380
  reticuloendothelial, and monocytosis, 244

Hypersplenism, 298–310
  definition of, 298
  diagnostic evaluation of, 300
  granulocytopenia and, 247
  hematologic tests in, 300–301
  liver disease with portal hypertension and, 306
  malignant lymphomas and, 390
  mechanisms of splenic enlargement in, 298, 299(table)
  pancytopenia associated with, 32
  radioactive chromium test in, 90, 301–303

Hypertension, portal, in liver disease, 305–310
  blood cell counts in, 306
  bone marrow in, 306
  hematologic tests in, 306
  liver function tests in, 306–307, 308 (table)

Hyperuricemia, in Hodgkin's disease, 406

Hypochromia
  mean corpuscular hemoglobin concentration in, 12
  in thalassemia, 40, 41

568